£24.95
OOP
2/06

APPLIED ANATOMY AND
BIOMECHANICS IN SPORT

APPLIED ANATOMY AND BIOMECHANICS IN SPORT

John Bloomfield
Professor, Department of Human Movement
University of Western Australia

Timothy R. Ackland
Senior Lecturer, Department of Human Movement
University of Western Australia

Bruce C. Elliott
Associate Professor, Department of Human Movement
University of Western Australia

BLACKWELL SCIENTIFIC PUBLICATIONS
MELBOURNE OXFORD LONDON EDINBURGH BOSTON
PARIS BERLIN VIENNA

© 1994 by
Blackwell Scientific Publications
Editorial Offices:
54 University Street, Carlton
  Victoria 3053, Australia
Osney Mead, Oxford OX2 0EL
25 John Street, London WC1N 2BL
23 Ainslie Place, Edinburgh EH3 6AJ
238 Main Street, Cambridge
  Massachusetts 02142, USA

Other Editorial Offices:
Librairie Arnette SA
1, rue de Lille
75007 Paris
France

Blackwell Wissenschafts-Verlag GmbH
Kurfürstendamm 57
10707 Berlin
Germany

Blackwell MZV
Feldgasse 13
A-1238 Wien
Austria

First published 1994

Set by Times Graphics Pte Ltd, Singapore
Printed by Australian Print Group, Maryborough,
Victoria, Australia

DISTRIBUTORS
Australia
  Blackwell Scientific Publications Pty Ltd
  54 University Street
  Carlton, Victoria 3053
  (*Orders*: Tel: 03 347-5552
      Fax: 03 347-5001)

UK and Europe
  Marston Book Services Ltd
  PO Box 87
  Oxford OX2 0DT
  (*Orders:* Tel: 0865 791155
      Fax: 0865 791927
      Telex: 837515)

USA
  Blackwell Scientific Publications, Inc.
  238 Main Street
  Cambridge, MA 02142
  (*Orders:* Tel: 800 759-6102
      617 876-7000)

Canada
  Times Mirror Professional Publishing, Ltd
  130 Flaska Drive
  Markham, Ontario L6G 1B8
  (*Orders:* Tel: 800 268-4178
      416 470-6739)

Cataloguing in Publication Data
Bloomfield, John, 1932–
  Applied anatomy and biomechanics in sport.

  Bibliography.
  Includes index.
  ISBN 0 86793 305 4

  1. Biomechanics. 2. Human anatomy.
  3. Sports - Physiological aspects. 4. Human
  mechanics. I. Ackland, Timothy Robert.
  II. Elliott, Bruce (Bruce C.). III. Title.
612-76

CONTENTS

CONTENTS

SECTION 2   APPLIED ANATOMY

CONTENTS

CONTENTS

CONTENTS

DEDICATION

To Dr Peter Olaf Sigerseth, an
'old style' educator and a great man,
whose influence has encircled the globe.

AUTHORS

PROFESSOR JOHN BLOOMFIELD AM, MSc, PhD, DipPE, FACHPER, FASMF, CBiol, FIBiol, FAIBiol, is a former national champion sportsman, a former high level coach and currently an academic at the University of Western Australia. He has been Chairman of the Australian Institute of Sport, the Australian Sports Science Council and the Australian Sports Medicine Federation, and has written two government reports and numerous papers in the field of sport and sport science. Professor Bloomfield is also the author of one book and co-author of two others.

DR TIMOTHY R. ACKLAND MPE, PhD, is currently a senior lecturer in Human Movement at the University of Western Australia, with teaching and research specialities in Functional Anatomy and Biomechanics. He is currently involved as a practising sport scientist with elite level sailors and has co-authored two books emanating from international level research projects. Dr Ackland has also authored a large number of research papers in his field.

ASSOCIATE PROFESSOR BRUCE C. ELLIOTT MEd, PhD, DipPE, FACHPER, is an academic and a practising sport scientist at the University of Western Australia. He is a former outstanding racquet sports player and a state-level tennis coach and was the major author in an international textbook entitled *The Art and Science of Tennis*. Furthermore, Professor Elliott is a much sought-after international speaker on the application of biomechanics to sport. He is also the author of a large number of research papers in international academic journals.

GUEST AUTHOR

DR GREG WILSON BPE, PhD, is currently a lecturer at Southern Cross University. His academic area is biomechanics and he ranks among the foremost authorities in the world in the development and assessment of strength and explosive power. He is also a former power-lifter, having competed in three world championships, where he gained two medals. This experience has enabled him to combine theory with practice and his success as a sport scientist, advising many young elite athletes in explosive power sports, attests to this.

FOREWORD

Research in sport science and medicine during the past decade has made rapid strides, but much of it can still only be found in the scientific literature. This unique book, which covers the field of sport technique development, has identified this research and combined it with the knowledge of several of the world's leading coaches, in order to present the latest information in this specialized area of coaching.

This book is not a 'rehash' of the many single sport books that have gone before it but rather it encourages a new approach to coaching. The authors have used many sports as examples, which they have placed into several categories in order to illustrate the various sport science theories and their applications.

Before its publication, the final manuscript of *Applied Anatomy and Biomechanics in Sport* was forwarded to several expert reviewers and some of their statements were as follows:

'The book is comprehensive in its areas of focus, very readable and set out in a logical format'

'Each section in the book is "state of the art"'

'[This book] is extremely well illustrated'

'It provides essential background theory while also providing abundant practical information'.

It is my perception also that the book is practical and easy to read and caters for an area of sport coaching which has generally been neglected in the past.

Finally, this timely publication will assist Australian coaches first to identify, then to develop our young athletes, so that their performances will peak as they approach the Sydney Olympic Games to be held in the year 2000. I therefore commend the authors of this book for the outstanding job they have done with its development and strongly recommend it to all practising coaches.

John D. Coates
President
Australian Olympic Committee

PREFACE

The application of sport science to coaching has become the single most important factor behind the rapid advances made in international sport performances during the past decade, yet comprehensive publications in book form have not kept pace with these advances. This publication will partly fill this gap, as it applies sport science to coaching and deals at length with the development of sports technique, an area which has been generally neglected in the past.

Applied Anatomy and Biomechanics in Sport examines coaching from a different perspective and focuses on the *individual* rather than the *en masse* coaching approach of the past. It in no way resembles the majority of the sport books currently in print, but is designed to advise coaches how to appraise the body structure of their athletes, so that their strengths can be fully utilized and their weaknesses improved, using specially designed programmes. In order to do this, the concept of modifying the body and/or the technique of the individual is used throughout and it is expressed in simple language which coaches and teachers at all levels will find easy to understand.

During the past decade the authors of this book have consulted a large number of highly trained and internationally successful coaches from a wide range of sports, in order to glean much of the information which appears in this work. These coaches continually stressed that an athlete can only reach a general level of proficiency with 'group' coaching and that many of the most successful coaches are already aware of the need to tailor a technique to suit each individual if an optimal level of performance is to be attained. They also expressed dissatisfaction with the generalist 'How to do it' books, citing them as no longer relevant for the modern coach.

In the past the majority of books in the coaching field have dealt with only one sport. However, single sports no longer exist in isolation, as they share many common features with other similar activities. In this publication, nine sports groups are systematically dealt with and these include: racquet sports; aquatic sports; gymnastic and power sports; track, field and cycling; mobile field sports; set field sports; court sports; contact field sports; and the martial arts. Within these groups examples are given from 30 national and international sports, so as to promote discussion of their various characteristics and allow 'cross-fertilization' of ideas to occur.

Special features of this book include information from recent research on the development of training methods which will increase explosive power; the utilization of elastic energy in the development of power and speed; and the modification of proportionality and posture to improve performance. Moreover, information available in this publication on proportionality and posture as applied to sport has not previously appeared in other books or recent journals in the coaching or sport science area.

The majority of this text is of an *applied* nature, as it concentrates on the various ways in which both the human body and the individual's technique can be modified to achieve an optimal skill performance, either for the average performer or the elite athlete. The contents at all times take into account the growth, development and sex of the individual, while also making the reader aware of the mechanical overstresses that cause various injuries and impair performance. In order to achieve this, the book has a preventive medical theme throughout.

The final section of this book comprehensively covers the latest assessment techniques currently used by international human movement and sport science specialists to evaluate human physiques and physical capacities. This section will be especially useful for practitioners already in the field who wish to evaluate their athletes objectively, or for students who are currently pursuing their professional training.

J. Bloomfield
T. R. Ackland
B. C. Elliott

ACKNOWLEDGEMENTS

No worthwhile book can be produced today without a great deal of assistance from a number of sources and this work is no exception. The following individuals have contributed in a variety of ways to its development and we wish to thank them for their effort: John Coates, Mark de Jong, Julie Draper, Dave Dunstan, Jim Ferguson, Ken Fitch, Rebecca Hewitt, Bob Hobson, Debbie Kerr, Kerry Langton, Terry Manford, Fiona Miller, Alan Morton, Guillermo Noffal, Paul Slaughter, Ross Smith, Michelle Telfer, Gordon Treble, Joan Williams and Rob Wood. A further group of contributors whose assistance has been invaluable are also mentioned below: Aileen Boyd-Squires of Blackwell Scientific Publications has given positive direction to us at all times; Marnie Hannagan of Blackwell Scientific Publications has capably carried out the task of copy editor; Laurie Woodman of the Australian Coaching Council reviewed the manuscript and in so doing improved its quality; Dianne Newton has done a very thorough job with the typing and organization of the manuscript; Paul Ricketts has demonstrated a high degree of professionalism with the art work; Noelene Bloomfield in her role as a critic has constructively reviewed the manuscript; while Roger Dickinson, who has expertise in many areas of publishing, has been a tower of strength in the development of this work.

J. Bloomfield
T. R. Ackland
B. C. Elliott

INTRODUCTION

CHAPTER 1

THE ROLE OF SCIENCE IN SPORT

While 'raw athletic talent' is the most important factor in the attainment of high levels of sporting performance, coaching based on sound sport science principles is also an essential ingredient if this talent is to be fully developed. Sport science therefore, focuses first on the identification of sporting talent and then on its development, so that an athlete's optimal performance can be achieved. It is generally accepted by coaches and sport scientists that high level performance is dependent upon an identifiable set of basic factors, each one of which carries a relative importance for that activity (Pollock *et al*. 1980; Fig. 1.1). Athletes therefore will only reach their full potential if the following factors are combined:

- The physical characteristics of the athlete that are important in a particular sport must be present (physical capacities)
- Appropriate techniques for the sport need to be developed (biomechanics)
- A level of fitness which is specific to the particular activity must be attained (physiological capacity)
- The psychological factors which enable the performer to compete successfully need to be developed and maintained (psychological make-up)
- A work ethic which includes an appropriate attitude to training must be present
- The opportunity to compete with athletes of a similar or superior level must be available

In order to maximize an athlete's inherent abilities, such factors as a coach's own *past experiences*, either as a competitor or coach, as well as specialized knowledge of *current world trends* in a particular sport are important in the athlete's development, otherwise his or her full potential will not be realized.

Past experience as either a player or a coach provides coaches with a personal knowledge of biological or behavioural factors, such as in the following examples:

- The appropriate grip to be used in a forehand drive in tennis on a clay court
- The need for anaerobic training to compete successfully in squash or American football
- The need for specific psychological skills in shooting sports
- The need to foster group cohesion in interactive team sports
- The progressive sequence of drills that should be used while players are learning a specific skill

These are the aspects of coaching which can be learned through intelligently observing the teaching techniques of others. It is advisable therefore, for young coaches to serve an 'apprenticeship' under a senior coach, so that the younger person is exposed to a wide range of experiences.

Current world trends in performance are also of vital importance and coaches need to be

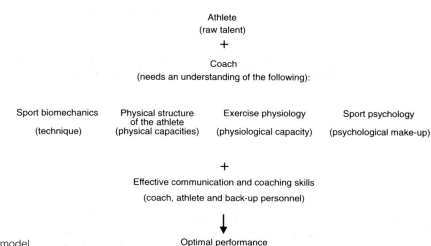

Athlete
(raw talent)

+

Coach
(needs an understanding of the following):

Sport biomechanics   Physical structure   Exercise physiology   Sport psychology
                          of the athlete
(technique)   (physical capacities)   (physiological capacity)   (psychological make-up)

+

Effective communication and coaching skills

(coach, athlete and back-up personnel)

↓

Optimal performance

Fig. 1.1   The performance model.

aware of the techniques of international level performers, so that they can constantly improve the skill levels of their charges. Examples of these trends are:

- The use of the late breathing technique in breast-stroke swimming
- The use of topspin in tennis
- The use of the 'short grip' in squash
- The use of the 'hitch kick' in the long jump
- The use of the 'one knuckle' grip in golf

Coaches must also be aware of the role of athletic *flair* in performance. One of the most puzzling aspects of coaching international level athletes is that it is often difficult to determine whether their natural abilities have made them champions, or whether it is their training which has differentiated them from other talented athletes. The high level coach therefore has to determine which aspects of performance to foster and which to modify, in order for athletes to reach the highest levels of achievement.

The coaches who offer the best guidance to their athletes are those who can integrate the above factors with a thorough understanding of *sport science*, which generally includes the sub-disciplines of sport physiology, sport psychology, social psychology and biomechanics.

UNDERSTANDING PHYSIOLOGICAL PRINCIPLES WHICH RELATE TO PERFORMANCE

In order to physically prepare an athlete for the appropriate level of performance, a sound knowledge of sport physiology is necessary. First, the principles of training and their implementation as they relate to the physiological performance of the athlete must be understood (Table 1.1). Coaches must also be aware of physiological and physical stress and how they manifest themselves in both poor performances and injury. Moreover, they should also possess an understanding of the various stages of an athlete's physical development. If coaches are participating in a state or national development plan, they may not need to outline their own individual training programmes. However, they will still need a thorough understanding of sport physiology in order to apply them.

UNDERSTANDING PSYCHOLOGICAL AND SOCIAL FACTORS WHICH RELATE TO PERFORMANCE

Sport psychology relates in part to the development of mental skills which enable athletes to

Table 1.1 Training schedules for young athletes: summer-based sport (modified from Holm 1987)

	No. and length of training sessions per week			Development of specific biomotor abilities		
Stage of development	No. training sessions per week		Duration of training sessions (min)	Biomotor abilities	Age (years)	
	Winter	Summer			Boys	Girls
Pre-competitive, 6–10 years	2	3–4	30–60	Dexterity/coordination	6–10	6–10
Overall, 11–14 years	3	5–6	60–90	Flexibility (emphasized)	≥13	≥12
Specific, 15–18 years	4	6	60–90	Speed/agility		
				Accelerated run	12–14	10–12
				Slalom run	13	11
				Interval training	15	13
High performance	4	7	60–180 (may include two sessions on 1 day)	Strength		
				Stage I: improving neuro-muscular coordination	10–14	10–12
				Stage II: increasing muscle mass	15–16	13–15
				Stage III: developing maximum strength/endurance	17–18	16–17
				Aerobic capacity		
				Commence training	12–14	11–13
				Endurance maximum	17–18	16–17

perform in their ideal performing state. The acquisition of these skills is generally considered by elite athletes to be an integral part of performance and an important factor in the player's personal growth. A mental skills programme helps to 'short circuit' experience to some extent, by promoting strategies that will teach individuals, from a young age, how to deal effectively with new experiences or how to compete against a difficult opponent.

In the psychological development of an athlete, consideration must be given to a systematic approach to *mental skills development*. Early training for these skills (initiation phase) at a basic level may occur at a young age. Athletes who wish to maximize their performance opportunities need further training both in the sport setting (e.g. on-field, on-court) and away from this environment (e.g. in a quiet room). Weinberg's (1988) publication on the development of mental skills in tennis can be used as a general reference for many other sports.

Athletes are also influenced by social factors both when training and during competition. The family, peer group, media and economic circumstances all influence the athlete's ability to prepare for and then to perform in a competitive environment. Coaches, often with the aid of administrators and/or sports psychologists, must therefore assist their athletes to deal with all these external pressures. If this can be achieved, then it will assist them to alleviate their stress, thus enabling them to train and compete in a reasonably relaxed state.

UNDERSTANDING BIOMECHANICAL PRINCIPLES WHICH RELATE TO PERFORMANCE

This book is oriented towards providing an understanding of how biomechanics and applied anatomy can be used to enhance performance. It basically demonstrates how various sport techniques can be modified to suit the physical characteristics of individuals, and also how the physical capacities of various athletes can be modified to suit biomechanically sound techniques.

The applied discipline of biomechanics is the part of sport science that examines the internal and external forces acting on the body and the effects produced by these forces. In some instances it may also examine sports equipment, surfaces, clothing and protective equipment. An awareness of the mechanics and the anatomy of movement will better equip athletes to acquire correct techniques, while also allowing coaches to detect and correct flaws in their performance. An understanding of movement biomechanics enables the coach to:

- Integrate technique modifications with the athlete's morphology so as to improve performance
- Select the appropriate equipment for the individual's body size and shape so that an optimal performance can be achieved
- Reduce the incidence of overuse and/or impact injuries through an appreciation of the force absorption requirements of a particular skill

Three broad types of biomechanical information can be used by coaches to enhance their understanding of the mechanics of sporting skills and each of these will now be discussed, in order to provide coaches with an understanding of the value of biomechanical data.

Technique Analysis

Technique analysis and its modification are a major concern of the coach. Information on technique which would be useful in coaching can generally be regarded to be of three types:

DESCRIPTIVE INFORMATION

This type of information, for example, enables a coach to appreciate such skills as the following:

- The correct sequence of movement in a kicking action
- The release position with reference to the height of the jump in a basketball jump shot
- The correct orientation of the hand at release when throwing a curveball in baseball

- The trajectory of the racquet needed to impart topspin to the ball in a tennis forehand drive
- The angle of the hand as it enters the water in freestyle swimming
- The ground reaction forces on the members of a rugby scrum, associated with various scrummaging techniques

CAUSAL INFORMATION

This *cause and effect* information enables the coach to correct the cause of an inefficient movement rather than its effect. Examples of this would include the following:

- A coach may observe a butterfly swimmer 'diving' during the stroke. In an attempt to correct this 'dive' (the effect), the coach must check the swimmer's dolphin kick (the cause), in order to see if one of its phases is so strong that it is forcing the body to rise upwards. If this occurs, an equal and opposite reaction will cause the body to plunge downwards, thereby creating unnecessary vertical frontal resistance
- The golfer who has the club face closed at the top of the back-swing (the effect), should not be instructed to gradually 'open' it on the way to the top, because this will artificially manipulate the club into the correct 'slot' position. Rather the golfer should modify the grip (the cause), by rotating the hands 15–20° to the left on the club. This will then place the hands and consequently the club head, into a neutral position at the top of the back-swing, enabling the player to naturally contact the ball squarely on the down-swing
- The coach who tells a basketballer to reduce the excessive forward movement during a jump shot is attempting to modify an effect, and is not addressing the cause of this technical error. It is vital that attention is paid to various aspects of the shot prior to, and at take-off, so that the body moves vertically rather than horizontally during the jump
- Tennis players are often advised to increase the height of the ball toss while serving so as to allow the racquet time to move through its intricate pathway. If the arms do not move in

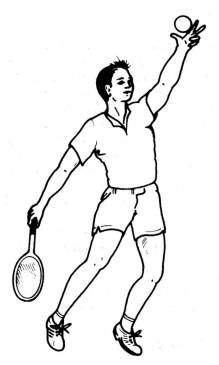

Fig. 1.2 The asynchronous arm action in a tennis serve.

a coordinated manner (i.e. 'arms down and then up together') and if the racquet 'trails' the release of the ball (Fig. 1.2), this increase in ball height (an effect of the asynchronous arm actions) may have a detrimental influence on other aspects of the service action. It would be more appropriate to coach for a coordinated arm movement, thereby removing the need for the increase in ball height

INFORMATION FROM COMPUTER OPTIMIZATION/SIMULATION

In the past it has often been the athlete or coach who has developed new techniques, or modified and improved those currently in existence. In recent times biomechanical data have slowly begun to assist the coach in this area and the following examples illustrate this point:

- Work by Yeadon and Atha (1985) on the twisting techniques of elite springboard divers using three-dimensional computer simulation analysis of cinematographic data, showed that the majority of twist produced by elite divers resulted from asymmetrical arm and hip movements during flight. This important information has changed the way in which twisting dives have since been taught
- Similarly, research in gymnastics using three-dimensional computer analyses has enabled new skills to be taught with safety, as the computer simulation is able to predict whether this new skill is attainable, given the biomechanical variables measured from skills that can already be performed

Stress Reduction

It is important in coaching that training and competition occur in a relatively injury-free environment. Overuse and/or misuse, generally in association with poor technique and an inappropriate physical structure, predispose an athlete to injury. Coaches must therefore be aware of information that will assist them to better understand how the activities they are teaching place stress on the bodies of their athletes. The following examples illustrate this point:

- Coaches of high repetition, moderate force activities such as running, swimming, kicking, fast bowling in cricket, and high velocity throwing, must not only reduce the number of repetitions during training and performance, but also ensure that the physical capacities of their athletes are suitable for the requirements of the activity
- Coaches of moderate repetition, high force activities that require high velocity landings such as in gymnastics, high velocity take-offs such as in jumping, or high velocity body contact such as in the tackle football codes, must not only follow the previous guidelines but must further reduce the number of performance repetitions. Lead-up drills must therefore play a major role in these sports and 'good technique' must be stressed in these drills

Equipment/Clothing Design

The physical characteristics of equipment and clothing, whether used for protection (e.g. a helmet) or as part of the activity (e.g. a bat) have a direct bearing on how movements within given sporting activities are performed.

Coaches, particularly those who deal with children, must ensure that 'correct' movement patterns are not hampered by inappropriate equipment, clothes or shoes. That is, equipment such as baseball helmets must provide head protection, which then permit the young athletes to develop good batting skills; for example, by allowing them to 'step into the ball' without the fear of injury. Likewise the bat, racquet or club selected for performance must be of suitable dimensions and weight so that the athlete can perform the intricate manoeuvres required for that sport.

Equally, coaches must ensure that appropriate footwear is worn to reduce the likelihood of injury both when athletes perform their aerobic and anaerobic training and also during competition. Bindings on ski boots have also improved so that there is now less likelihood of a skier sustaining a serious injury when falling.

Modern clothing can be used to increase comfort (such as padded socks), protect the athlete from injury (such as batting gloves in cricket) or reduce aerodynamic or hydrodynamic drag (e.g. in skiing, cycling or swimming). In the vast majority of cases such clothing has helped to improve an athlete's performance.

CONCLUSION

Coaching is therefore both an art and a science, and an understanding of biomechanics and the anatomy of the athlete is essential in coach development. This book focuses on the way in which the coach can use a knowledge of biomechanics and functional anatomy to improve performance, as well as giving systematic analysis strategies to identify key movement characteristics that may need modification. Chapters which demonstrate how this can best be done are included in the remainder of this book and give specific information on:

- How physical structure relates to performance
- How structural modifications can enhance performance
- How technique may be modified to permit optimal use of physical structures that will remain constant, or relatively constant

REFERENCES

Hohm J. (1987) *Tennis: Play to Win the Czech Way*, pp. 178–222. Sport Books Publications, Toronto.

Pollock M., Jackson A. & Pate R. (1980) Discriminant analysis of physiological differences between good and elite distance runners. *Research Quarterly for Exercise and Sport* **51**, 521–532.

Weinberg R. (1988) *The Mental Advantage*. Leisure Press, Champaign, IL, USA.

Yeadon M. & Atha J. (1985) The production of a sustained aerial twist during a somersault without the use of an asymmetrical arm action. In Winter D., Norman R., Wells R., Hayes K. & Patla A. (eds) *Biomechanics IX-B*, pp. 395–400. Human Kinetics Publishers, Champaign, IL, USA.

SECTION 1

APPLIED BIOMECHANICS

CHAPTER 2

ANALYSIS OF TECHNIQUE IN SPORT

Many people in the field of coach education have emphasized the importance of observation, followed by correction, in successful coaching. High level coaches are first concerned with the evaluation of technique, then with its modification, in order to improve an athlete's performance. Barrett (1983) stressed that a coach's attention must be focused on the identification of 'critical features' if movement is to be successfully analysed. Inexperienced observers are generally not able to identify as many details in a particular movement as are experienced coaches and this is mainly attributed to their difficulty in distinguishing relevant from irrelevant factors (Allison 1987). In sport therefore, a structured analysis and evaluation plan in the observation of technique is frequently used by coaches.

PRE-ANALYSIS METHODS

The coach must ascertain the following factors prior to beginning any analysis of movement. First, which *level* of performer is to be evaluated; and second what are the *aspirations* and the age of the individuals being examined? For example, there is a great difference between the expectations of an under-12 soccer team training 3 h per week, in comparison to an under-12 elite gymnastics squad, who may train 30 h per week in preparation for an international level performance.

While good technique will improve performance and mostly lead to more enjoyment, the continual emphasis on the minor modifications which are needed if an elite level is to be reached, may destroy the enthusiasm of a young athlete who is new to a sport, or who only wishes to participate at a recreational level.

Rather than immediately attempting to correct a flaw in technique, a good coach should first check to see if the real source of the problem is elsewhere. This may require the assessment of the psychological, physical and tactical aspects of the movement, before an assumption is made that the cause of the error is purely technical. The following examples will illustrate these points:

- The coach needs to determine whether the athlete is *psychologically* ready to learn the skill or to perform an already learned skill under pressure. Factors such as stress, which may be from an outside source such as the home or the school, or anxiety caused by fear of failure, can affect technique and need to be addressed before technique modification is attempted

- The coach must also ascertain if *physical* factors are the reason for a technique fault. The reason for a particular error may be low levels of flexibility, strength, or explosive power, or an inappropriate lever system for the activity that is to be performed

- Errors in technique may also be the result of a poor *tactical* situation, rather than the technique itself. A player may have tried to hit or kick the ball too hard for a given court or field position, or may have chosen an inappropriate response to a tactical situation, making the performance of a learned response almost impossible. Or the player may not have had sufficient practice 'under pressure'

SUBJECTIVE ANALYSIS METHODS

Prior to discussing how any skill should be analysed, it is worth reviewing the 'spectator' and 'cause–effect' types of analysis that are commonly part of coaching.

'Spectator' Analysis

It is important for coaches to be constructive in their comments. They may say for example, 'good shot', 'well done', 'bad pass', 'you missed', 'jump higher', and so forth. While feedback at this level does convey some information to the athlete, and if used correctly, can sometimes increase his or her self-concept, it does little to help the individual understand why the performance was good or bad. Examples of more positive feedback are listed below:

- 'Good shot or good hit' may be replaced by 'you kept your head down well during that shot or hit'
- 'Well done' may be replaced by 'you held the tuck for a slightly longer time, which enabled you to complete the somersault'
- 'Bad pass' may be replaced by the comment 'the hands must be kept in line with the arms as you release the ball'

Cause–Effect Analysis

Some coaches have trouble 'seeing the wood for the trees' and spend too much time trying to correct the 'symptom' rather than the cause of the fault. This is often expressed as correcting the *effect* rather than the *cause*. A good example of this can be found in gymnastics, when the gymnast takes a step backwards upon landing after a back somersault has been performed. A coach may then comment, 'next time make your landing stick', whereas the poor landing may well have been the

result of not tucking tightly enough during flight, or opening out too soon. The coach has not identified the cause of the problem and will have the athlete focusing on an inappropriate part of the skill. Telling a gymnast to concentrate on the landing does nothing to improve the performance, if the reason for the poor landing occurs during the flight or take-off phase of the skill. Other examples of this type of coaching error are found in Chapter 1. Unfortunately, a large number of coaches do not discriminate between the *cause* and *effect* and as a result continually mislead their athletes by not giving them the necessary instructions which will correct their faults.

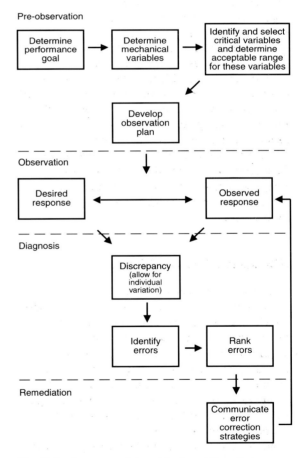

Fig. 2.1 An approach to subjective skill analysis (modified from McPherson 1988).

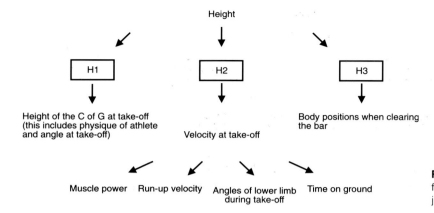

Fig. 2.2 A mechanical model for a distance-based skill: a high jump (modified from Hay 1985).

Skill Analysis

The successful analysis of skill involves planning a routine set of procedures that become easier to structure with practice. In order to analyse a skill, the coach needs to understand the biomechanical principles involved in it and must be completely familiar with its performance (i.e. having a thorough understanding of the purpose and requirements of the skill). With this information in hand the coach can then analyse movement using the framework set out in Fig. 2.1.

The steps a coach would use in implementing such a format would be as follows:

PRE-OBSERVATION PHASE

| Determine performance goal |

What is the coach trying to achieve for the performer: a lower time, greater distance or perhaps a tactical advantage?

| Determine mechanical variables |

Before a technique can be modified, it is essential that a *mechanical model of the performance* is established in the mind of the coach. By developing this model (Figs 2.2, 2.3) one can identify the interrelationships of different factors that influence performance.

| Identify and select critical variables |

Not all the features of these models are of the same importance and therefore critical variables must be identified (e.g. the run-up velocity in the high jump, or the racquet-face angle in the squash drive).

| Determine acceptable range for critical variables |

An acceptable range for the run-up variable may be between 6 and 8 m/s, while a racquet-face angle with reference to the court of ±5° of the vertical may be acceptable. Objective data reported in applied sport science research studies usually provide coaches with such ranges of acceptability.

| Develop observation plan |

The coach must decide such factors as:

- The directions from which the skill should be viewed (i.e. side, front and/or overhead etc.)
- Whether the individual phases of the movement should be viewed separately (i.e. backswing, forward-swing and/or impact etc.)
- Whether an emphasis should be placed on particular segments in the movement (i.e. head, leg and/or trunk etc.)

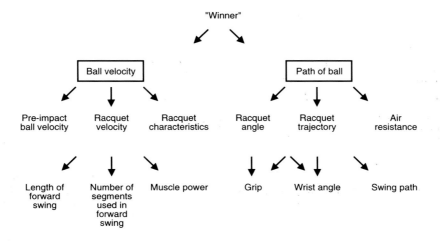

Fig. 2.3 A mechanical model for a tactical-based skill: a down-the-line passing shot in tennis.

OBSERVATION PHASE

In this phase of the skill analysis a coach compares what was observed with the previously established mechanical model. The coach is there-

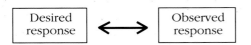

fore identifying those aspects of a skill that need correcting. It is important to consider at this stage whether the error in performance is 'forced' or 'unforced' and whether the effectiveness of the technique is being assessed. That is, the analysis of the skill must not be divorced from the tactical aspects of performance. A diver or skater with a technique flaw must have this error corrected, because it is directly related to the way in which the routine is judged. However, a tennis player with a variation in technique which does not detract from performance and which does not 'break down' under pressure, may be left alone (i.e. the coach must always consider *flair* in assessing performance).

DIAGNOSIS PHASE

> Discrepancy (allow for individual variation)

> Identify errors

> Rank errors

Any errors that are identified must be *ranked* according to their importance, and the time that will be needed for their correction must also be assessed. Therefore, if a major fault is detected, it may be advisable to wait until the off-season before the correction takes place, because this may upset the individual's performance. On the other hand, a minor fault that is not likely to have any deleterious effect on the performance may be easily corrected in the weeks leading up to a major event. It is important not to rank an '*effect*' but to address the '*cause(s)*' of each error.

REMEDIATION

> Communicate error correction strategies

In many respects the ability to communicate with athletes in a manner which they can easily understand is one of the most important characteristics of a successful coach. All the instructions which are given to the performer during error correction must be as simple as possible. First the coach should describe the error, show it on a video or film and/or demonstrate it. The correct technique should then be described and demonstrated so that the athlete can '*picture*' the correct movement. The athlete may then be told how the movement '*feels*' (or in some cases '*sounds*') as this is often the best way to emphasize '*flow*' in the action. Unfortunately, this useful strategy is rarely used by many coaches. Finally, a good coach will check to see that the athletes understand not only how to correct their technique but also why it is necessary.

The coach may then ask questions that determine if the athlete fully understands the changes which are being attempted and the progressions needed to correct this fault in technique. Performance at the completion of practice must then be re-observed to see if the equired changes have occurred.

A coach can then, at least in part, gauge how successful the intervention in technique has been from the athlete's improvement. If a substantial improvement after a reasonable period of practice has not occurred, then the coach may need to re-examine the modification process by asking the following questions:

- Was the error in technique identified correctly and was it clearly a '*cause*' and not the '*effect*' of some other factor?
- Was the correction sequence appropriate?
- Did the athlete understand the modification needed and the reason for the change?

IN SUMMARY

Coaches who wish to improve the technique of their athletes should have a sound working knowledge of both skill analysis and biomechanics, as well as the ability to 'see' the movement in its various phases. The coach also needs a thorough understanding of the requirements of the skill, and the factors which produce the desired result. With this in mind, repeated and specific observations should occur so that the coach can determine how the movement characteristics affect the performance, and individualized instruction should then be given.

Coaches must remember that errors in the technique(s) in any given movement may be the result of other factors. Psychological considerations such as anxiety or poor concentration may influence technique, as may physiological factors such as fatigue. Tactical situations such as poor shot selection may also be the cause of technical errors. Coaches must therefore ensure that they do not develop too narrow a focus when analysing movement.

As athletes improve their technique and are able to perform at a higher level, it may then be necessary for the coach to further consider the tactical implications of a given skill. A squash player, who has learned the techniques needed to hit a ball down-the-wall, must also be able to hit the ball across-court so that an opponent is not able to predict the direction of the shot. This may then mean that additional factors need to be added to the mechanical performance model, so that a player learns how to disguise stroke mechanics and thus tactically gain an advantage over an opponent.

OBJECTIVE ANALYSIS METHODS

At this level of movement analysis, there is often a need for interaction between the coach and a biomechanist, if the maximum amount of information is to be gained. The coach may, however, objectively evaluate skill by recording a permanent copy of a movement or series of movements (e.g. film or video) for a number of trials, so that each can be viewed and analysed. Different types of information may be needed by coaches for different sports and examples of these are illustrated below.

The *swimming coach* may wish to know:

- The muscle groups that need to be specifically trained for an efficient recovery in the butterfly stroke
- The angle of the hand and forearm as they enter the water in the freestyle stroke
- The body position as it enters the water during a racing dive

The *long jump coach* may wish to know:

- The velocity of the body at take-off
- The angle of the front leg at take-off
- The levels of vertical, forward-and-back and side-to-side forces recorded at take-off

The *volleyball coach* may be interested in:

- The height of the centre of gravity at ball impact
- The role of trunk rotation in velocity generation
- The position of the hand at ball impact in the spike

Recording of movement data in a permanent format which will answer questions such as the above, may take a number of different forms, as outlined below.

Image Analysis Techniques

Image analysis techniques, including both cinematography and videography, provide the opportunity to record complex movement sequences on film or videotape so that a detailed analysis can be made.

At the subjective level of analysis, film or video techniques may be used to record movement and allow general comments to be made on various observed characteristics. After watching a video or film of a baseball hit, the coach may subjectively comment on the flexion of the lower limbs

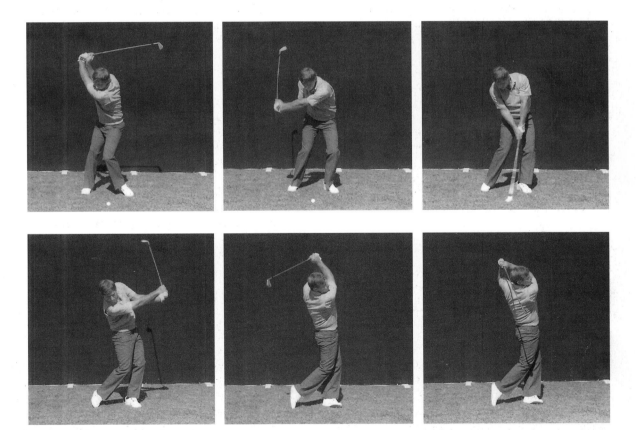

Fig. 2.4 Photographs from a high-speed film of the golf swing.

15

or the position of the bat with reference to the front foot at impact in a baseball drive. At an objective level it is not sufficient to simply record and observe movement, as detailed measurements must be completed and inferences drawn with reference to that movement. Objective data from the above example would be the measurement of the angle of the front and back knee joints and the actual distance of the bat from the front foot at impact. Specific recording equipment and analysis procedures must be used if accurate data are to be collected using image analysis techniques.

In high-speed cinematography a motor driven camera, operating at speeds from 100 to 500 frames per second, can record the motion in such a way that many images of a given activity are collected.

In Fig. 2.4 a number of frames of a golf swing have been printed from 16 mm film shot at 400 frames per second. The majority of these frames have not been included; however, the relative movement sequence is clearly illustrated.

The collection of data from film (digitizing) for analytical purposes is the most time-consuming and tedious aspect of cinematographic research, because the projection of an image by a stop-action projector is needed for frame-by-frame digitizing (Fig. 2.5). In this process, an operator moves an X–Y coordinate system until a pointer lies over the desired anatomical landmark and the coordinates of this point are then stored in a computer. This landmark must therefore be clearly marked

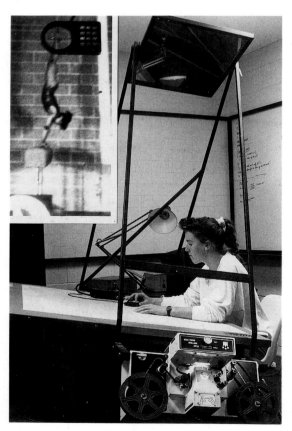

Fig. 2.5 A 16 mm film digitizing facility (from Bloomfield *et al*. 1992).

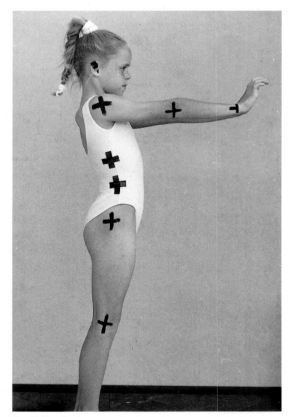

Fig. 2.6 A photograph of a subject ready for digitizing.

16

on the subject being filmed so that an accurate identification of the segment end point or joint centre is possible. Figure 2.6 illustrates the markings which have been placed on a gymnast for a two-dimensional analysis. The angle of the thigh would therefore be calculated from the markers of the hip and knee joints.

It is obvious from Fig. 2.7 that additional information over and above the coordinates of the selected landmarks is required if more than segment angle information is to be calculated. The film or video speed in conjunction with a scaling value and information on the movement of each of the landmarks enable linear or angular velocity and acceleration to be calculated (kinematic data). Kinetic data (force information) can then also be calculated if the physical anthropometry of the athlete (e.g. the mass of each body segment) and the acceleration of each segment are known.

Film data are usually collected from a sagittal (side), transverse (from above), frontal (front) view, or from a combination of camera views that enable three-dimensional information to be collected. Advances in video technology (frame rates >50 or 60 pictures per second) now permit video to compete with film as a convenient, accurate and cost-efficient tool to collect objective data on movement. The packages that best meet the needs of coaches are the Video Image Analysis systems, which enable the user to analyse two-dimensional or three-dimensional patterns of movement, by recording the images from the camera(s) on videotape. This provides not only an image which can be viewed at a later date, but also the opportunity to re-analyse the motion. These data can generally be measured from the video images in the same way as that shown in Fig. 2.7.

Dynamometric Techniques

Dynamometric techniques refer to the measurement of force and the most common dynamometer used in sport biomechanics is the force platform. It enables the measurement of the three perpendicular components of the ground reaction forces (vertical [Fz], forward–backward [Fy] and side-to-side [Fx]) and the point of resultant force application (CPx, CPy) with reference to the centre of the force plate. Illustrations of how these measures are used to assist coaches to understand the forces associated with a number of sporting activities are as follows.

External force data are often used to aid in performance or to approximate levels of internal load placed on the body. In Fig. 2.8 the forces associated with a long jump are recorded. From these data it is evident that this jumper may adopt the following strategies to improve performance:

- The horizontal braking force should be reduced at footstrike, while an attempt is made to increase the propulsive force by training the jumper to position the landing foot closer to the body at board contact
- The magnitude of the side-to-side force must be reduced, as this does not aid jumping performance but causes lateral movement at take-off
- The large vertical impact force of approximately 6.5 body weights at footstrike on the board shows that long jumping is a high impact activity. Coaches of long jumpers must therefore carefully monitor the number of repetitions performed so as to reduce the likelihood of overuse injuries

Fast bowling in cricket has been shown to be a high impact activity, where the bowler experiences a series of 'collisions' or minor impacts with the ground during the run-up, followed by a large impact when landing on the front foot during the delivery stride. A force platform can be used to identify the maximum vertical and forward–back ground reaction forces at front foot impact during the delivery stride (Fig. 2.9). As the front foot impacts with the platform, a peak vertical force of five times the bowler's body weight and a peak forward–back force of twice the body weight are recorded. At release, when the upper limb is near the vertical, it can be seen that these forces have reduced considerably. While research has not directly linked these forces to the development of back injuries in fast bowlers, considerable force

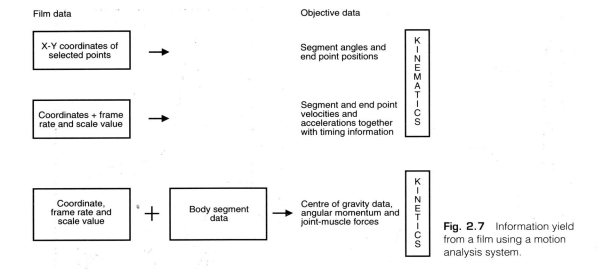

Fig. 2.7 Information yield from a film using a motion analysis system.

must be transmitted through bones, cartilage and muscles to the various joints in the body, especially in the region of the lumbar spine. To avoid overuse injuries, bowlers should reduce impact forces through flexion (bending) of the front knee joint and by inserting 'force absorbing material' in their boots.

In rowing, the forces which are applied by the athlete to the oar during the stroke are of major interest to the coach, and small transducers (force measuring devices) may be attached to the oar and used to determine these forces, which are shown in Fig. 2.10. This figure illustrates how the force applied to the oar varies over the complete stroke. The relationship between the force applied to the oar and the boat speed (Fig. 2.11) provides the coach with valuable information on the mechanical effectiveness of the stroke as well as the boat's 'flow' through the water.

In relatively stationary activities such as archery and the shooting sports, body sway is an important factor, and an analysis of the centre of pressure movement, although not a measure of the motion of the centre of gravity of the body, has been used to monitor sway. Figure 2.12 represents the total area over which the centre of pressure of an archer moved during the aiming period and may be used to represent the sway of the archer.

The overall direction of the sway may also be used to approximate the angle of stance with reference to the target.

The centre of pressure movement may also be used to indicate the type of foot strike pattern common in running. Figure 2.13 demonstrates the typical pattern for centre of pressure changes, from foot-strike to toe-off, for runners with mid-foot and rear-foot landing characteristics. In both situations the runner landed on the lateral (outside) border of the foot and then the centre of pressure moved medially (inwards), prior to the last contact being made with the area under the big toe.

Electromyographic Techniques

Muscle action is initiated by electrical activity and the detection and recording of these signals is a technique known as electromyography (EMG). In its most basic form, EMG provides an indication of the electrical activity in a particular muscle or muscle group. Comparisons of levels of electromyographic activity between muscles however, can only be made with extreme caution.

While coaches may never use this technique with their own athletes, awareness of data from controlled studies will certainly assist in planning training programmes. Figure 2.14 depicts the surface

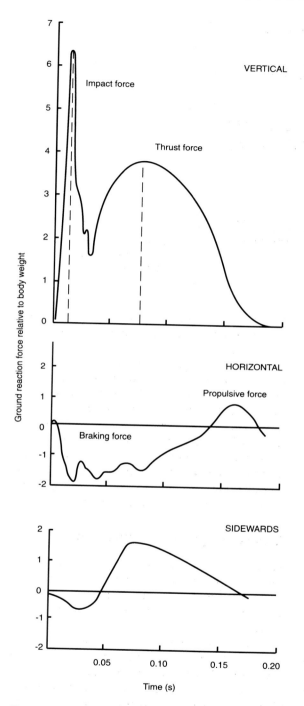

VERTICAL

Impact force

Thrust force

HORIZONTAL

Propulsive force

Braking force

SIDEWARDS

Fig. 2.8 The ground reaction force data for the long jump take-off.

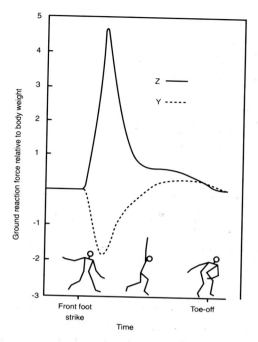

Fig. 2.9 Vertical (Z) and horizontal (Y) ground reaction forces which occur during the bowling stride.

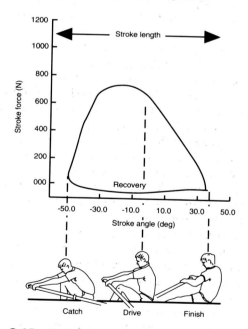

Fig. 2.10 The force profile of a rowing stroke (modified from Smith & Spinks 1989).

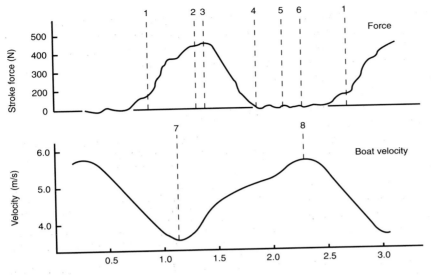

Key:
1. Beginning of catch
2. Oar vertical to boat during drive
3. Peak force
4. End of drive phase
5. Beginning of recovery phase
6. Oar vertical to boat during recovery

7. Lowest velocity
8. Peak velocity

Fig. 2.11 The relationship between force and boat speed during a rowing stroke (modified from Angst *et al.* 1985).

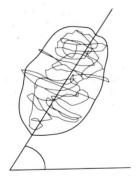

Fig. 2.12 Diagrammatic representation of the area over which the centre of pressure moved with relation to the angle of stance of an archer.

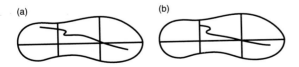

Fig. 2.13 The centre of pressure patterns for runners with (a) rear-foot and (b) mid-foot foot strike patterns.

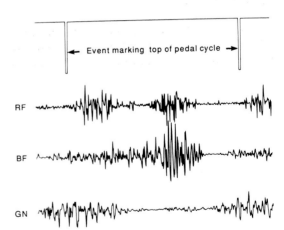

Fig. 2.14 Electromyographic activity in lower extremity musculature during stationary cycling: RF, rectus femoris; BF, biceps femoris; GN, gastrocnemius (from Bloomfield *et al.* 1992).

EMG activity of selected muscles of the lower extremity during stationary cycling. The rectus femoris (RF), a major extensor of the leg at the knee joint, shows two bursts of activity. One begins just after the top of the pedal stroke and ends slightly before the leg is fully extended at the bottom of the stroke cycle. A second burst is seen starting at about the bottom of the stroke and finishing about half-way through the recovery (upward) movement. The leg flexors, represented by the biceps femoris muscle (BF), show slight to moderate activity during the propulsive (downward) stroke and a major burst at the start of the recovery movement. The gastrocnemius muscle (GN) assists with the final aspect of leg flexion prior to the top of the cycle, and is then active in the early part of the propulsive phase either in producing plantar flexion, or in ensuring good force transmission through to the pedal by holding the foot in a static position. Studies of the muscle activity which occurs during swimming, as reported by Piette and Clarys (1979) illustrate how the muscles identified as playing a role in the freestyle stroke must then be the ones which are trained in a muscle strength/endurance programme for freestyle swimming.

CONCLUSION

The ability to both identify faults using subjective and/or objective analysis methods and then communicate learning strategies to the athlete are essential skills for any coach. Those coaches who can assist their athletes to refine their techniques using the methods which have been described in this chapter, will greatly improve their performances.

REFERENCES

Allison P. (1987) What and how pre-service physical education teachers observe during an early field experience. *Research Quarterly for Exercise and Sport* **58**, 242–249.

Angst F., Gerber H. & Stussi E. (1985) Physical and biomechanical foundations of the rowing motion, pp. 10–11. Paper presented at the Olympic Solidarity Seminar, Canberra, Australia.

Barrett K. (1983) A hypothetical model of observing as a teaching skill. *Journal of Teaching Physical Education* **3**, 22–33.

Bloomfield J., Fricker P. & Fitch K. (eds) (1992) *Textbook of Science and Medicine in Sport*, pp. 50, 61. Blackwell Scientific Publications, Melbourne.

Hay J. (1985) *The Biomechanics of Sports Techniques*. 3rd edn, p. 449. Prentice-Hall Inc., Englewood Cliffs, NJ, USA.

McPherson M. (1988) The development, implementation and evaluation of a program designed to promote competency in skill analysis. PhD thesis, University of Alberta, Edmonton, Canada (unpubl.).

Piette G. & Clarys J. (1979) Telemetric electromyography of the front crawl movement. In Terauds J. & Bedingfield E. (eds) *Swimming III*, pp. 153–159. University Park Press, Baltimore.

Smith R. & Spinks W. (1989) Matching technology to coaching needs: On water rowing analysis. In Morrison W. (ed.) *Proceedings of the VIIth International Symposium of the Society of Biomechanics in Sports*, pp. 277–287. Footscray Institute of Technology Press, Melbourne.

CHAPTER 3

THE ROLE OF BIOMECHANICS IN IMPROVING SPORT PERFORMANCE

Coaches who understand the mechanical basis of a skill, who can analyse movement and who are also able to communicate with their athletes, will provide the best opportunity for the optimal development of that skill with the minimum risk of injury. The ways in which biomechanical information may generally benefit the coach and athlete were briefly dealt with in Chapter 1. However, this chapter discusses in detail the role of biomechanics, first in the development of technique and second in creating a performance environment where the potential for injury is reduced. A number of biomechanical considerations which are important in the teaching of high velocity movement will also be discussed.

TECHNIQUE DEVELOPMENT

It is generally accepted by coaches that high level performance is dependent upon a number of factors, one of the most important being the technique needed to demonstrate a given skill. The coach relies to a large extent on an understanding of the existing information in his or her sport to identify the critical features in a movement and these were described in Chapter 2. Descriptive data are generally provided by applied research articles, and these should be used to assist in deciding which technique should be adopted. Without such data, it is extremely difficult for a coach to modify technique in an effort to improve performance.

For example, in the tennis service action, descriptive research has identified the following as being some of the characteristics which are common to high performance players (Elliott *et al.* 1986):

- Approximately 50° of leg flexion during the preparatory movements with a range of ±20°
- An impact position of approximately 150% of standing height with a range of ±10%
- A racquet angle to the court of 92° at impact with a range of ±2°

It is important to remember that descriptive data such as the above form the basis for the structure of the mechanical model of the tennis serve, as well as for the establishment of ranges of acceptability for each important characteristic.

Tennis coaches may, in addition to the data above, be interested in knowing if specific changes to the service motion produce a higher racquet speed. Preliminary research by Sprigings *et al.* (1994) has shown the importance of upper limb rotations in producing racquet speed in the tennis serve. At the time of impact, forearm pronation only contributed 4 m/s, while horizontal flexion of the upper arm contributed 6.5 m/s to racquet speed.

Computer simulation as described in Chapter 2, allows issues such as those mentioned below to be clarified for the tennis coach.

- The influence of an increase in forearm pronation on racquet speed

- The influence of an increase in horizontal flexion of the arm on racquet speed

Computer simulation and optimization are beginning to play an important role in the development of sporting excellence. The general aim of this area of research when applied to athletic performance is to predict changes that would occur as a result of alterations to selected aspects of technique. The coach is then able to obtain answers to a question such as: *What would happen in a given skill if a critical feature was modified?* For example:

- Optimum release characteristics of the new javelin (post-1986) were investigated by Hubbard and Alaways (1987), who reported that release conditions were velocity-dependent. They found that success with the new javelin depended to a large extent on strength and power and that finesse and skill were of less importance
- In gymnastics, a coach may be interested to know the influence of changes to release conditions from the horizontal or uneven bars, on skills that may be performed after release. Nissinen and co-workers (1983) showed how the initial release values, calculated from a double-back somersault with straight-body dismount on the horizontal bar, were sufficient to enable the gymnast to perform a triple back-tucked somersault dismount. This new skill could then be attempted by the gymnast with relative safety

Preparation of elite athletes is changing from a situation where in the past the coaches or athletes themselves often led the innovative changes in technique, usually through a trial and error approach, to where biomechanists can now assist coaches to predict which further modifications may be desirable.

PROBLEM OF OVERUSE INJURIES

Increased participation by children and adolescents in highly organized sport has resulted in an in-creased number of injuries, particularly overuse ones; these are generally due to a loading of the musculoskeletal system where a number of repetitive forces, each lower than the acute injury threshold for any tissue, produces a combined fatigue effect in that tissue over a period of time. An important consideration in the cause of sporting injuries is the load on the body during training or performance. A diagram of the principal factors influencing load in sporting movements is shown in Fig. 3.1. Key contributing factors to overuse injuries include 'poor technique'; an excessive number of attempts at an activity; inappropriate footwear, particularly when performing on 'hard surfaces'; musculoskeletal immaturity; and/or a body build that may predispose an athlete to injury in a particular sport or activity.

The potential of a specific activity or technique to cause an overuse injury is best determined by epidemiological or prospective studies. In epidemiological studies, changes in injury statistics are carefully assessed following a change in technique, equipment, playing surface, or the rules of play. In prospective studies, factors such as techniques and/or the physical capacities of athletes are measured prior to the commencement of the season and any resulting injuries are then related back to these characteristics. As these studies are difficult to administer when working with high performance athletes and are also costly to run, biomechanists generally use the forces acting on the body during a particular performance as an indicator of the potential for an overuse injury. It must be understood however, that external forces (which are usually measured using a force platform, see Chapter 2) of the same magnitude and direction may produce different internal forces, at least in part because of the morphology of the athlete. That is, the athlete with a flat foot arch would generally experience greater forces in the Achilles' tendon than would an athlete with a high foot arch, for equivalent external forces acting on the ball of the foot. The higher arch is thus able to absorb the external forces more effectively than the low arch. Nevertheless, when assessing impacts against a hard concrete or 'plexipave' surface, these

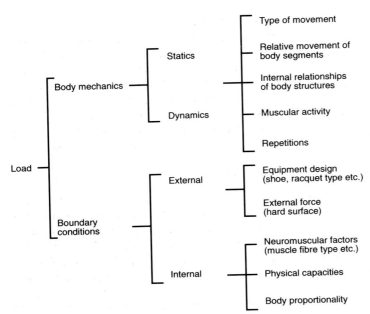

Fig. 3.1 The factors that influence load in sports performance (modified from Nigg *et al.* 1984).

external forces are approximate measures of the forces acting on the body and are at least an indicator of the potential for overuse injury with high performance athletes, who all perform the activity in a similar manner.

The loads experienced in sport are generally of two types. The first is associated with a high number of repetitions of an activity, such as in endurance training or fast bowling where, at each footstrike, forces from the ground (ground reaction forces) and associated turning forces (torques) must be absorbed by footwear and the body, or in swimming, where the high number of upper limb rotations place stress on the shoulder region. The second type is associated with a smaller number of repeated performances requiring high levels of skill/technique and power, such as in gymnastics or in jumping, where much higher forces are usually generated than in the first classification.

High Repetition, Moderate Force Activities

The type of overuse injury to muscle, tendon, bursa or bone associated with high repetition, moderate force activities is generally caused either by fric-

tional forces associated with a high number of repetitions (as in swimming) or by repetitive loading of a high number of exposures of the body to a force. Examples of these repetitive loading activities include fast bowling in cricket; selected movements during aerobic dance classes; running, both as an activity in itself or as part of a training programme for another sport; netball and/or basketball, where a player is required to land on a hard surface after jumping and catching a pass; and pitching or throwing for speed in baseball, where large internal muscle forces are needed to produce very fast movements of body segments.

SWIMMING

The potential for overuse injuries in swimming, particularly in the shoulder region, is obvious, as swimmers may rotate each arm 2500 times while completing 5000 m of freestyle. Tenosynovitis of the long head of the biceps brachii tendon or of the supraspinatus muscle attachment, as well as inflammation of the subacromial bursa ('swimmer's shoulder') can result from repeated upper limb movements, particularly during freestyle and butterfly swimming (Fricker 1992).

FAST BOWLING IN CRICKET

Fast bowling is an impact activity in which the bowler experiences a series of 'collisions' or minor impacts with the grass surface in the run-up. This is followed by two heavy impacts when landing on the rear foot and then on the front foot, on a very hard turf or concrete surface during the delivery stride. Peak vertical ground reaction forces (GRF) of approximately five times the bowler's body weight (BW) have been recorded when the front foot is planted and these impact forces are transmitted through bones, cartilages, tendons and muscles to the joints of the body (Nigg *et al.* 1984). Stress fractures in the spine (primarily to the L4 – L5 region) are the most serious injury a fast bowler can sustain, although injuries to the body musculature and joints, particularly of the lower limb and back, are also commonplace (Foster *et al.* 1989).

SELECTED MOVEMENTS IN AEROBIC DANCE

Rates of injury sustained in aerobic classes, particularly to the lower limb, have been reported to be as high as 76% for instructors and 43% for students (Ritchie *et al.* 1985; Garrick *et al.* 1986). One of the major causes of this spate of impact and/or overuse injuries has been attributed to the need for the body to absorb repeated forces at each foot contact with the floor (Francis & Francis 1986).

Elliott *et al.* (1991) compared, both biomechanically and physiologically, two low impact (walking and high intensity walking at 2.1 m/s) and two high impact (jogging at 2.1 m/s and running at 2.9 m/s) movements used in aerobic dance classes, in an attempt to find activities that provided sufficient physiological intensity, while reducing the level of GRF at foot contact. While all four movement patterns caused stress on the cardio-respiratory system above the minimum guidelines for training as recommended by the American College of Sports Medicine (1991), differences were also apparent in the force data. Walking (1.4 BW) and high intensity walking (1.3 BW) produced lower peak vertical GRF than did jogging (2.2 BW) and running (2.4 BW).

The suitability of each of these movements for use in an aerobic dance class will depend on the prescribed intensity and impact levels of the routine as well as the fitness levels of the participants. The risk of injury, however, from any of these movements seems mainly to arise from excessive repetitions of the activity, insufficient preparation of the participant for the stress of the particular movement pattern, or poor technique when performing these movements, rather than from the forces generated during any single activity.

RUNNING

Running as a means of maintaining general cardiovascular fitness, as a form of aerobic and anaerobic preparation for sport or as part of a sport, has always produced a relatively high proportion of lower back and lower limb injuries. Knee injuries, Achilles tendonitis, tibial pain ('shin splints' or compartmental pressure syndrome) and, to a lesser extent, stress fractures, are all lower limb injuries common to runners or joggers. One could speculate that the injury level may have been even higher with recent increases in the intensity of training and distances covered, if shoe design had not improved so much.

Depending on the direction and point of application, GRF at each footstrike produce different effects on the body. The level of these GRF is velocity-dependent. Maximum vertical and retarding horizontal GRF of 1.2 and 0.2 BW, respectively, for walking, increase to approximately 2.5 and 0.5 BW, respectively, for running and to levels of approximately 3.6 and 0.8 BW, respectively, for sprinting. Unfortunately the internal forces associated with these locomotor activities can easily be a multiple of the external GRF and therefore, depending on the direction of the acting forces and the geometry of the locomotor system, the stress pattern on the body can be greater than the GRF would signify (Nigg 1986).

NETBALL

Netball, a game played primarily on hard surfaces, requires players to continually accelerate–decelerate and to jump and land in an attempt to receive a pass. It is not surprising therefore that injuries occur, particularly in the lower limb.

A study by Hopper (1986), reported that 5.2% of a total of 3108 players (158 injuries) were injured during one season. It was also demonstrated that the ankle (58.2%) and then the knee joints (15.2%) were the most common injury sites, although the injuries to the knee joint were more disabling.

A study by Steele and Lafortune (1989) reported that peak vertical GRF of 5.2 BW (heel landing) and 5.7 BW (forefoot landing) were recorded for high performance players landing on one foot, after catching a ball propelled to a point 20 cm above the head. These players also generated lower braking forces when landing on the forefoot (2.0 BW) compared to landing on the heel (3.3 BW). The time to peak braking force was, however, shorter when landing on the forefoot in comparison to landing on the heel. Therefore, the rate of loading and thus an increased risk of injury associated with this higher rate, may offset any advantage gained from a lower peak braking force recorded when landing on the forefoot in preference to landing on the heel.

BASKETBALL

In basketball, peak vertical GRF of 2.3–7.1 BW have been recorded on landing following a rebound (Valiant & Cavanagh 1985). If basketballers were required to train on plexipave and bitumen surfaces like netballers and not on 'sprung' gymnasium floors, then they too would face similar injury problems. The majority of their injuries are the result of landing in an inappropriate manner and thus many may be classified as either 'impact or overuse injuries'.

HIGH VELOCITY THROWING (e.g. Baseball Pitching)

Studies by Adams (1968) and Torg et al. (1972) on young pitchers have clearly shown that overuse injuries are apparent in baseball pitching, the most common being 'elbow' soreness and separation of the medial epicondylar epiphysis. If a high number of repetitions is combined with poor technique, then an overuse injury is almost inevitable (English et al. 1984).

The underlying mechanism for injury primarily to the elbow region appears to be related to the large forces associated with the forward-swing phase of the upper limb during the pitching action, in conjunction with the position of the forearm with respect to the upper arm during this phase. Very high turning forces are needed to cause the rapid extension of the forearm at the elbow joint, a characteristic of pitching and high velocity throwing (Gainor et al. 1980).

General guidelines for the prevention of overuse injuries in high repetition, moderate force activities are as follows:

- Warm up prior to, and cool down at the completion of practice and competition
- Include specific flexibility and muscle endurance training as part of the general programme
- Emphasize good technique
- Ensure that increases in training load or training location (hill running; change from aerobic to anaerobic conditioning) are introduced gradually
- Vary training to place the load on different areas of the body
- Practise landing skills, while catching a ball (if appropriate to the sport) to develop 'kinaesthetic sense' with relation to where the body is in space prior to and upon landing
- Carefully monitor the number of repetitions (bowling/throwing) both in practice and when competing
- Wear appropriate footwear with respect to the surface used at practice and in the game situation

Moderate Repetition, High Force Activities

In overuse injuries from moderate repetition, high force activities, the high forces associated with each performance limit the number of repetitions which can be performed if injury, particularly to the musculoskeletal system, is to be avoided. With these activities coaches must develop highly specific lead-up drills that enable athletes to practise selected aspects of the final performance without exposing themselves to the potential for injury. Safety precautions, including the use of specialized equipment associated with each of these activities, must be strictly adhered to.

GYMNASTICS

The magnitude of take-off and landing forces in gymnastics clearly show that extremely high forces are associated with gymnastic activities. Peak single limb vertical GRF at take-off for a running forward somersault of 13.6 BW (Miller & Nissinen 1987) and between 8.8 and 14.4 BW on landing after a double-back somersault (Panzer *et al.* 1988) have been recorded. Brüggemann (1987) recorded peak vertical take-off forces of between 3.4 and 5.6 BW for a back somersault following a round-off, which translated into much larger internal forces in the Achilles tendon. While it has been shown that asymmetrical landings produce higher forces than symmetrical ones, there were only minor reductions in GRF in landings with a flexed leg compared to a competition landing where the legs were fully extended (Panzer *et al.* 1988). Therefore if injuries, particularly those which may disturb normal growth, are to be avoided, it is imperative that correct equipment, such as an appropriate floor and good matting, be used for teaching gymnastics.

JUMPING ACTIVITIES

Ramey (1970) in a study of the long jump take-off, recorded peak vertical GRF of almost 7 BW for a jump of only 4.2 m. These GRF increased to levels between 7 and 12 BW in the take-offs for the triple jump (Ramey & Williams 1985). In a high jump of approximately 2.2 m, peak vertical impact forces of between 8.4 and 8.9 BW and peak horizontal retarding impact forces of 5.6 to 6.5 BW (Deporte & van Gheluwe 1989) show the very high forces associated with this activity. It is therefore not surprising that athletes involved in jumping activities or physical education classes emphasizing jumping must be very careful to avoid overuse or even misuse injuries.

JAVELIN THROWING

A mean peak vertical GRF at front foot impact of 9 BW for javelin throwing (Deporte & van Gheluwe 1989) showed that this activity must *not* be excessively repeated if injury to the lower limb or back is to be avoided. The high velocity requirement of the upper limb segments prior to javelin release also means that high internal forces are acting and repeated maximum efforts should be avoided.

General guidelines for reducing injuries in moderate repetition, high force activities are as follows:

- Ensure that a thorough warm-up and cool-down, including both flexibility and moderate power activities, are carried out prior to and after performance
- Stress good technique at all levels of performance. This includes lead-up or practice drills where selected aspects of the total skill are practised
- Carefully monitor the number of repetitions both at practice and during competition
- Physically prepare the athlete for the selected activity
- Vary training, so that emphasis is placed on different skills and activities throughout each session
- Perform in shoes and on surfaces which assist in the reduction of the impact forces at ground contact

Prevention is the key to the alleviation of the majority of overuse injuries, because in many instances they can be avoided or reduced if a sensible approach to training and performance is adopted. When symptoms of overuse injuries such as continual pain are reported, teachers and coaches must evaluate the athlete's total programme. The technique being used must be analysed, the physical preparation evaluated and the intensity of training/play reconsidered. Factors such as the equipment/shoes used and the playing surfaces must also be evaluated. An effective coach/teacher will of course have considered all these aspects of the programme prior to the start of each season.

It may also be prudent to advise a young athlete to undergo a specific medical examination prior to making a total commitment to any sport that requires a vast increase in training. Furthermore, athletes with segment malalignments and inappropriate body dimensions (discussed in Chapter 8) may then follow a programme designed to prepare the body for the forces expected in their sport.

Today, a high degree of perfection in performance is needed for competition at the international level, and therefore long hours of practice are a normal phenomenon of modern training. It is hoped that a greater understanding of the forces which must be absorbed by the body during different activities will enable coaches to allow all athletes to reach their full potential in an environment which is as injury-free as possible.

COACHING FOR HIGH VELOCITY MOVEMENTS

An important characteristic in modern athletic performance is the explosive power which is applied to various skills. It would seem that to be successful, an athlete must throw or hit with greater velocity, kick further or run faster. Coaches are therefore often challenged to improve various aspects of their athletes' skills, so that they are able to:

- Hit or kick a ball with a higher velocity, while still maintaining an acceptable level of control. This often occurs in such sports as tennis, golf, squash, baseball, soccer and rugby
- Generate higher limb velocities, which will in turn enable higher release velocities to be made. This occurs in throwing, or in discus and javelin events
- Rotate segments of the body more quickly to apply more force to an implement. This can either be with a bat, club, oar or pedal, or in a medium such as water, where the body needs to be propelled

This chapter further discusses a number of additional biomechanical considerations which are important in the teaching of high velocity movement and these are as follows:

- The use of elastic energy
- The distance over which velocity can be developed

- The use of coordinated movements
- The role of muscle strength and power
- The role of equipment and clothing design

Use of Elastic Energy

'Prepare early' is a phrase often used by coaches of hitting sports. The logic behind such a statement is that for the ball to be hit at the appropriate time and not 'late' requires early preparation. The question then arises as to whether performance is in fact hindered by this early preparation, as elastic energy stored during the 'stretch cycle' of any movement may not be of benefit during the 'shorten cycle' of the activity.

For example, during the stretching or back-swing phase in some sports the muscles and tendons are placed 'on stretch'. This is demonstrated in the preparation for a volleyball spike (Fig. 3.2), where

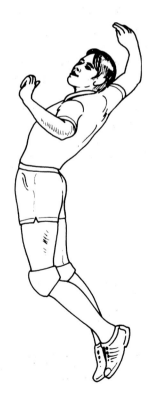

Fig. 3.2 The back-swing or stretching phase of a volleyball spike.

elastic energy is stored in the same way that an elastic band stores energy when it is stretched. Research has shown that by increasing the speed of the stretching phase and resisting the stretching movement by applying greater tension in the muscle(s) being stretched, there is an increase in the storage of elastic energy. On movement reversal, during the shortening phase, the stretched muscles and tendons recoil to their original shape and in so doing a portion of the stored energy is applied, thereby assisting the movement (in this example the forward-swing to the volleyball).

Research has shown that the use of elastic energy accounts for approximately:

- 50% of the total energy requirement of running (Cavagna *et al.* 1964)
- 19% of the weight capable of being lifted in a bench press (Wilson *et al.* 1991a)
- 12% of the total height attained in a vertical jump (Asmussen & Bonde-Petersen 1974)

The key to the recovery of this elastic energy is the timing within the stretch–shorten cycle. The benefit of this stored energy is reduced if a delay occurs between the stretch and shorten phases of the movement. For example, in a recent study using a bench press, Wilson *et al.* (1991a), reported that after a period of approximately 1 s, 55% of the stored energy was lost; after 2 s, 80% of the stored energy was lost; and after a delay of 4 s, all the stored energy was lost (Fig. 3.3). An athlete

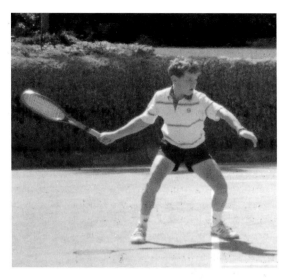

Fig. 3.4 A poor mechanical position at the completion of the back-swing.

who does not pause between the stretch–shorten cycle can therefore lift almost 20% more than would be possible if a 4 s pause occurred between the two phases of the bench press.

The recovery of this stored energy occurs relatively quickly and is therefore of major benefit early in the forward-swing phase of a hit or in a movement to a ball. Chapman and Caldwell (1985) reported that all the elastic energy had been released 0.25 s into the shortening phase of a forearm rotation movement, while Wilson *et al.* (1991b) reported that the majority of stored energy in the bench press had been released 0.2 s into the effort phase. Understanding this is of major benefit to young children, who may often need the assistance of this energy source to overcome inertia (swing weight) of an implement during the early section of the forward-swing (Fig. 3.4). Adults and adolescents also benefit from this energy source during the early part of a forward movement in most hitting sports, as the position reached with the racquet, bat or stick at the completion of the back-swing is often a poor mechanical one from which to apply force; therefore this elastic energy is used in combination with muscle force to initiate a forward movement.

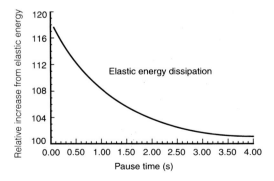

Fig. 3.3 The loss of elastic energy with increased pause time (modified from Wilson *et al.* 1991a).

Furthermore, research has shown that the flexibility of a joint is also related to the elasticity of the muscles and tendons around that joint (Wilson *et al.* 1991c). Specific flexibility training has been shown to not only increase the range of movement, but also to be linked to an increase in performance. Wilson *et al.* (1991d) proposed that this increase in elasticity enabled an increase in the utilization of elastic energy to occur. A more detailed discussion of this finding can be found in Chapter 10, which deals with flexibility in sport.

PRACTICAL IMPLICATIONS RELATING TO ELASTIC ENERGY RELEASE

Coaches must teach players to adopt the following components in their techniques in order to utilize elastic energy:

- The muscles and tendons should be *slightly* overstretched at the completion of the back-swing. They will then vigorously recoil at the commencement of the hitting phase. Care must be taken however not to overstretch to the point where the smooth 'flow' in the technique is affected
- The back-swing and forward-swing phases in hitting or kicking skills should flow from one phase of the movement to the other with *minimal* delay
- Efficient movement skills should be developed when running to the ball. Players must time the leg flexion (bend)–extension (straighten) action when initiating movement, in order to coordinate with the movement of an opponent or the flight of the ball or shuttle, so that these two counter movements flow together, enabling the player to move quickly to intercept the opponent, ball or shuttle
- Plyometrics should be carried out in the majority of training programmes (see Chapter 9 for detailed information on plyometric training), as it will enable athletes to overload their musculature in positions and at velocities more similar to the competitive situation, in comparison to conventional strength training. This type

of training may also enhance an athlete's ability to use elastic energy (Bosco *et al.* 1982), as these researchers suggested that plyometric training may alter the elasticity of the tendons and muscles, making them capable of storing greater quantities of elastic energy in given stretch–shorten cycle movements. Equipment such as the Plyometric Power System permits many strength training activities to be performed in a plyometric fashion. By incorporating the proven benefits of traditional strength training with plyometric techniques, this machine, described in Chapter 9, affords the opportunity to powerfully perform resistance exercises at high velocities

- Flexibility training needs to be carried out as it permits an increase in performance through a better use of elastic energy

The rapid velocity at which plyometric training is performed promotes the storage of elastic energy by stretching the muscle and tendon with great force. Moreover, in such training the delay time between the stretch–shorten cycle is *minimized* thereby ensuring a maximal recovery of stored energy. Thus a further benefit of plyometric training, when compared to conventional strength or power training, is that it appears to involve the implementation of those movement strategies which maximize the contribution of elastic energy to stretch–shorten cycle movements.

However, the performance of high impact movements involving stretching, when performed in plyometric training, may result in some muscle soreness in the days following training. Hence the use of plyometrics in a training routine requires several days of recovery time between exercise sessions of this type. This may not be the case if the Plyometric Power System is used for this type of exercise. With this system, a set of dampeners serve to reduce the initial eccentric loading of the movement and therefore lessen the muscle and tissue damage that is often associated with plyometric exercise. Other appropriate periodization procedures should also be implemented in plyometric training to avoid over-training and injury.

Distance over which Velocity can be Developed

One of the main reasons for having a back-swing or a series of preparatory movements in many activities is to increase the distance over which velocity can be developed during the forward-swing. The potential to generate velocity over this increased distance will only occur if the time needed to perform the activity does not increase proportionately. It is important to remember that there is always the potential for increasing velocity, even in the absence of greater displacement, simply by decreasing the time interval from the completion of the back-swing to release or impact.

In a straight back-swing (often taught to beginners) the implement (i.e. racquet, bat, stick or club) is taken back in a relatively straight line, before pausing in the back-swing position, prior to then swinging forward to the ball. This type of back-swing, which is easy to learn, is very good for developing ball control and it may even use some of the elastic energy stored when the muscles are stretched; however, the distance the implement or limb moves forward to the ball is often not sufficient to allow the development of a high velocity for impact.

The *looped* or *curved* back-swing has been developed in many sports in order to increase the velocity at impact. Some examples of this are as follows:

- A ground stroke in tennis (Fig. 3.5a)
- A golf back-swing
- A baseball pitch back-swing or 'wind-up'
- The rotation of the lower limb in preparation for a kick (Fig. 3.5b) in the various football codes

If a player does not pause between the back-swing and the forward-swing phases of the movement, such as when using a looped back-swing, the elastic energy stored during it will be optimally used to assist velocity generation in the forward-swing. If a pause is required between the back-swing or forward-swing phases of a movement, such as a tennis forehand, then the racquet should stop at position B and not C (Fig. 3.6) to increase

the distance over which velocity can be generated for impact. If the racquet had been stopped at position C, this would be similar to using a straight back-swing from A to C.

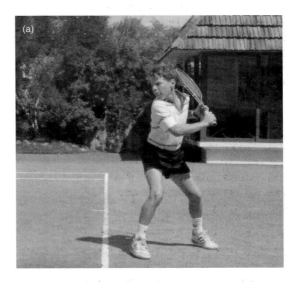

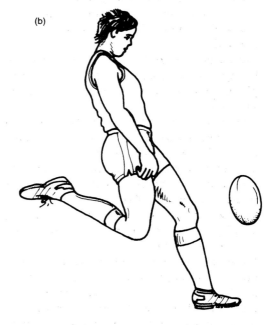

Fig. 3.5 (a) A looped back-swing in tennis; (b) a curved back-swing in a punt kick.

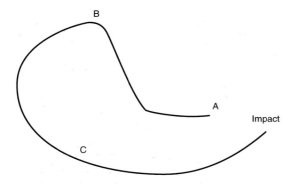

Fig. 3.6 A diagrammatic representation of a looped forehand back-swing and forward-swing in tennis.

PRACTICAL IMPLICATIONS FOR INCREASED MOVEMENT

Coaches should teach their athletes to adopt the following general *technique principles* in order to improve their performance:

- There should be no pause or only a *very brief* pause or 'change-over' between the back-swing and forward-swing phases during power hits such as in the tennis serve or the volleyball spike. By almost eliminating the pause, the stored elastic energy will be used in the forward-swing
- Athletes should be taught to use a looped or curved back-swing to increase the 'power' potential of the forward-swing. Many coaches also believe that a curved approach in the soccer kick, or kicking for goal in rugby, enables the player to make better contact (a higher effective mass) with the ball
- Athletes should strive to improve flexibility at a particular joint, such as at the shoulder joint in backstroke swimming, to enable performers to rotate the upper limb through a greater range of movement and therefore increase their potential for better performance. Chapter 10 provides a number of flexibility programmes which may be used by athletes in many different sports which will enable this increased movement to occur

Use of Coordinated Movements

In sports where a high velocity, and yet control of an implement is required, a number of body segments must be coordinated in such a way that this high velocity is achieved at impact or release. The progressive movement of segments participating in high velocity striking or throwing skills are generally sequenced in a *proximal-to-distal* fashion. That is, the sequence of the segments involved in a movement if maximal hand velocity is to be achieved would be the lower limbs and trunk, followed by upper arm, forearm and then the hand. One of the most popular principles underlining the description of this sequencing in sport movements is the *summation of velocity principle* (Bunn 1972), which suggests that the velocity of the distal end of a linked system is built up by summing the individual velocities of all the segments participating in the sequence. However, the principle does not provide a mechanical explanation of how this is achieved. This coordination occurs so that the movement of one segment begins as the velocity of the previous moving segment has reached its maximum, in a 'staircase effect' (Fig. 3.7a). The sequential rotation of the body segments shown in Fig. 3.7a is usually measured in hitting sports by the velocity of the segment end-points (the wrist joint is the end of the forearm segment and so on). In Fig. 3.7b the velocities of these end-points are shown for a forehand drive in tennis. The arrows represent the commencement of movement for each of the segments used in the stroke. Note how the velocities of all the segments add together to assist in developing racquet velocity for impact.

Putnam (1993) presented the view that joint angular velocity data provide the best description of proximal-to-distal sequencing. Furthermore, these data enable coaches to visualize a movement, as motion is generally characterized as a series of segment rotations about a number of joints. Other researchers such as van Gheluwe and Hebbelinck (1985) and Joris *et al.* (1985) have proposed an optimal coordination principle, where to achieve maximum speed at the distal end of an open-linked system, the rate of rotation of all segments should reach a maximum value simultaneously. While this

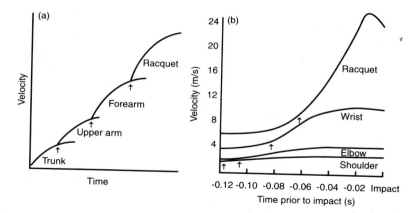

Fig. 3.7 Summation of segment velocities in the tennis forehand (a, theoretical; b, tennis data).

sequence has been observed in some striking activities such as the old-style unit forehand in tennis (Deporte *et al.* 1990), most striking and throwing actions where high velocity is an important factor in the movement now follow the summation of velocity principle (Putnam 1993).

PRACTICAL IMPLICATIONS FOR COORDINATED MOVEMENTS

In sport, the summation of a number of body segments in a coordinated manner plays a part in velocity generation in the following ways:

- The first example relates to situations where forward movement of the body is added to the rotation of a body segment or number of segments. In fast bowling in cricket, the velocity of the body developed during the run-up is added to the velocity developed by trunk and upper limb rotations, to produce the release velocity of the ball. In kicking skills, the velocity developed in the forward movement of the body is added to that developed from trunk and lower limb rotations, to produce a high foot velocity at impact

- Another example is where a body segment (a forward step) increases the distance over which velocity can be developed. That is, in baseball or hockey the player 'steps into' the ball to enable a higher velocity to be developed. It is often preferable as a coach to visualize this as adding another segment to the movement, so as to increase the potential to develop a high

velocity and also to increase the distance over which velocity can be developed

- Players often attempt to generate higher velocities by adding more segments to the movement. In a basketball jump shot, beginners may first be taught to use forearm extension to generate ball velocity at the peak of the jump. They may later add hand flexion to this action, so as to develop a higher release velocity and thus enable the player to shoot further from the basket

Movement patterns that require the coordinated action of total body movements are usually the sign of a mature action. The following examples illustrate this point.

- *The forward-swing phase of the squash forehand drive consists of:*
  — a forward step and trunk rotation
  — continuous trunk rotation as the upper arm moves forward
  — extension and pronation of the forearm at the elbow and upper arm inward rotation
  — minor hand flexion at the wrist to complete the forward-swing to impact
- *The forward-swing phase of the overhand throw for distance consists of:*
  — a forward step and trunk rotation
  — horizontal flexion and inward rotation of the upper arm
  — extension of the forearm at the elbow
  — hand flexion at the wrist to complete the forward-swing to release

The removal of any of these movements from the respective actions illustrated above will have the effect of reducing the potential velocity. If accuracy, however, is a major factor in the skill being performed, such as in a jump shot in basketball or chip shot in golf, a player reduces the number of segments used in the performance and often coordinates the movement so that the segments move in unison.

- In the basketball jump shot, ball velocity is generated primarily by two segments (forearm extension and hand flexion). The accuracy of shooting is decreased if a player uses the forward and upward movement of the body to generate ball velocity, rather than shooting from the peak of a vertical jump, where the shooting-shoulder velocity is close to zero (Elliott 1992)
- In a chip shot in golf, the hands are not 'cocked' at the wrist joint on the back-swing and as a result the hands and forearms are kept firm at ball impact. The accuracy of the chip will be decreased if the wrists are cocked and then uncocked during the shot

Role of Muscle Strength and Power

The relationship between selected physical capacities such as muscle strength and/or explosive power and performance is relatively easy to assess in sports such as weightlifting, or in activities such as shot putting and discus throwing. However, such a relationship is very difficult to quantify in the majority of sporting movements where it is not so obvious. For example, one must consider how much muscle strength and/or power is needed to carry out the following skills:

- Pitching with a high velocity in baseball
- Punting a ball a long distance in rugby
- Hitting a long and accurate drive in golf, baseball or cricket

No significant relationship has been found between muscle strength and serving velocity in tennis (Ellenbecker 1989) or between muscle strength

and kicking velocity in soccer (McClean & Jamieson 1991). However, a significant relationship was found with increased tennis racquet acceleration, following a specific strength and power training programme (Kleinöder 1990). Therefore it would seem that more research must be undertaken which investigates the relationships between increases in muscle strength and/or power and the capacity to rotate segments of the body more rapidly.

The absence of consistent research data that provide a definitive amount of strength and power required for most sporting activities should not prevent coaches ensuring that their young athletes, who aspire to high levels of performance, include strength and explosive power training as part of their total programme. Players must develop sufficient muscle strength (the ability to perform one maximal effort) and muscle endurance (the ability to repeat the above action many times) to perform effectively in a long match or over a large number of efforts. An increase in muscle strength means that a smaller percentage of total strength is needed for each movement, and this assists the athlete to repeat the performance with 'good technique' over the entire match or competition. Muscle power is needed, as in a practical sense it may be considered as the velocity at which a muscle force can be applied and therefore relates to the speed at which a segment can be rotated. There appears to be a definite need for many of the exercises which are performed in a muscle power programme to be carried out at a rate and in a posture similar to that of the relevant sport. The principle of specificity is an important one if the best results are to be obtained. Chapter 9 provides coaches with a number of programmes which demonstrate how specific strength, strength–endurance and explosive power training may be included as part of the total development of an athlete.

PRACTICAL IMPLICATIONS FOR MUSCLE STRENGTH AND POWER DEVELOPMENT

The coaching emphasis during pre-adolescence in almost all sports should be on skill training with only a small amount of strength and power training being done. The greatest gains in muscle strength and power are achieved in mid-adolescence, that is, at around age 14 in boys and 12–13 years in girls. However, because the adolescent growth spurt is not as marked in girls as in boys and more oestrogen is being secreted at this time in girls, its value is not as great as for boys. Not all athletes may need a strength and power training programme; however, those who lack 'power' or 'penetration' during performance, as well as those who aspire to elite performance should include this form of training as part of their total programme.

Role of Equipment and Clothing Design

While it is beyond the scope of this chapter to fully discuss the implications of equipment and clothing design on all sporting movements, some mention of the relationship between these and performance should be made.

In a sport such as tennis, a great deal of technological effort has been directed towards racquet development in an endeavour to increase 'power' and 'control', while reducing the unpleasant vibrations produced by off-centre impacts. 'Today the new breed of thicker, stiffer and more powerful racquets have gained immediate favour with the masses, and in the last year and half have taken over the market' (Sparrow 1989). Many players who had difficulty rotating the racquet quickly are using these new racquets to increase their ability to develop ball speed.

It is often stated that children are not 'miniature adults' and that the individual physical characteristics of a young athlete should be taken into account when selecting sporting equipment. In tennis the size of the racquet must be related to the player's physical characteristics if optimal skill development is sought (Elliott 1981). When using a shorter length racquet, the individual may have to sacrifice range of movement in favour of control and the ability to master the fundamental tennis skills.

In running shoe selection, it is imperative that the design of the shoe selected matches the running characteristics of the athlete. A runner with high levels of pronation must select a shoe which helps to stabilize the foot during the running cycle in preference to one that merely offers high levels of cushioning.

In cycling it is necessary that the physical characteristics of the rider are matched to the size of the bike. This obviously requires specific physical characteristics, such as lower limb length to be matched to seat-pedal height, if an efficient movement pattern is to be achieved.

Golf is a good example of a sport where improvement to equipment has altered performance. The most important change has come with perimeter-weighted club heads, which increase the size of the area of percussion (sweet spot), giving the player more accurate shots than the traditional bladed club. Another change has been in the quality and composition of modern shafts, many of which are now made of boron or graphite. For the average player, these high quality materials give slightly more length to the shot than the old steel shafts. Therefore players with different physical capacities should choose their equipment to suit them. For example, a powerful golfer should use a stiff-shafted club in order to cut down on blade rotation, which will give a less accurate shot. The golfer who is less powerful and who cannot generate enough club-head velocity should use a 'softer' or more 'whippy' shaft in order to get as much distance as possible. It should be understood however that a golfer runs the risk of less accurate shots by using a more flexible shaft.

In many sporting activities (e.g. cycling, speed skating, skiing) high velocities are achieved and therefore aerodynamic drag must be reduced if optimal performance is to be achieved. The type and fit of clothing worn by athletes in the above sports has been shown to play an important role in reducing this drag. Work by Kyle and Caiozzo (1986) in wind tunnels further showed the importance of appropriate clothing in running events. They reported that proper clothing lowered the drag on a competitor and provided an advantage over opponents with loose-fitting and wrinkled clothing. Athletes who are therefore involved in high velocity sports must seriously consider wearing appropriate clothing made of materials such as lycra or spandex to help reduce the influence of aerodynamic drag on their performance.

CONCLUSION

The role of biomechanics in improving sport performance should not be underestimated. Not only is an understanding of biomechanical principles essential for technique development and its modification, but it is also important in assisting athletes to avoid injuries caused by the overuse of various joints and muscles. Coaches also need to be aware of the importance of coaching for high velocity movements and the ways in which elastic energy can be utilized in various sporting movements. Such elements as clothing and equipment design are also important factors which must be considered if athletes are to reach their full potential.

REFERENCES

Adams, J. (1968) Bone injuries in very young athletes. *Clinical Orthopaedics and Related Research* **58**, 129–140.

American College of Sports Medicine (1991) *Guidelines for Exercise Testing and Prescription*, 4th edn, pp. 93–120. Lea & Febiger, Philadelphia.

Asmussen E. & Bonde-Petersen F. (1974) Storage of elastic energy in skeletal muscle in man. *Acta Physiologica Scandinavica* **91**, 385–392.

Bosco C., Komi P., Pulli M., Pittera C. & Montonev H. (1982) Considerations of the training of the elastic potential of the human skeletal muscle. *Volleyball Technical Journal* **6**, 75–80.

Brüggemann P. (1987) Biomechanics in gymnastics. In van Gheluwe B. & Atha J. (eds) *Current Research in Sports Biomechanics*, pp. 142–176. Karger, Sydney.

Bunn J. (1972) *Scientific Principles of Coaching*, pp. 142–143. Prentice-Hall Inc., Englewood Cliffs, NJ, USA.

Cavagna G., Saibene F. & Margaria R. (1964) Mechanical work in running. *Journal of Applied Physiology* **19**, 249–256.

Chapman A. & Caldwell G. (1985) The use of muscle stretch in inertial loading. In Winter D., Norman R., Wells R., Hayes K. & Patla A. (eds) *Biomechanics IX-A*, pp. 44–49. Human Kinetics Publishers, Champaign, IL, USA.

Deporte E. & van Gheluwe B. (1989) Ground reaction forces in elite high jumping. In Gregor R., Zernicke R. & Whiting W. (eds) *Congress Proceedings XII International Congress of Biomechanics*, p. 202. UCLA Press, Los Angeles.

Deporte E., van Gheluwe B. & Hebbelinck M. (1990) A three-dimensional cinematographical analysis and racket at impact in tennis. In Berme N. & Capozzo A. (eds) *Biomechanics of Human Movement Applications in Rehabilitation Sports and Ergonomics*, pp. 460–467. Bertic Corp., Worthington, USA.

Ellenbecker T. (1989) A total arm strength isokinetic profile of highly skilled tennis players and its relation to a functional performance measurement. In Gregor R., Zernicke R. & Whiting W. (eds) *Congress Proceedings XII International Congress of Biomechanics*, p. 141. UCLA Press, Los Angeles, USA.

Elliott B. (1981) Tennis racquet selection: A factor in early skill development. *Australian Journal of Sport Sciences* **1**, 23–25.

Elliott B., Marsh T. & Blanksby B. (1986) A three-dimensional cinematographic analysis of the tennis serve. *International Journal of Sports Biomechanics* **2**, 260–271.

Elliott B., Morton A. & Johnston R. (1991) Biomechanical and physiological responses to modes of locomotion used in aerobic dance. *Australian Journal of Science and Medicine in Sport* **23**, 89–95.

Elliott B. (1992) A kinematic comparison of the male and female two-point and three-point jump shots in basketball. *Australian Journal of Science and Medicine in Sport* **24**, 111–118.

English W., Young D., Moss R. & Raven P. (1984) Chronic muscle overuse syndrome in baseball. *The Physician and Sports Medicine* **12**, 111–115.

Foster D., John D., Elliott B., Ackland T. & Fitch K. (1989) Back injuries to fast bowlers in cricket: A prospective study. *British Journal of Sports Medicine* **23**, 150–154.

Francis P. & Francis L. (1986) Low-impact aerobics: Part 2. *Dance Exercise Today* September, 31–32.

Fricker P. (1992) Injuries to the shoulder. In Bloomfield J., Fricker P., & Fitch K., (eds) *Textbook of Science and Medicine in Sport* p. 365. Blackwell Scientific Publications, Melbourne.

Gainor B., Piotrowski G., Puhl J., Allen W. & Hagen R. (1980) The throw: Biomechanics and acute injury. *The American Journal of Sports Medicine* **8**, 114–118.

Garrick J., Gillien D. & Whiteside P. (1986) Epidemiology of aerobic dance injuries. *American Journal of Sports Medicine* **14**, 67–72.

Hopper D. (1986) A survey of netball injuries and conditions related to these injuries. *The Australian Journal of Physiotherapy* **32**, 231–239.

Hubbard M. & Alaways L. (1987) Optimum release conditions for the new rules javelin. *International Journal of Sport Biomechanics* **3**, 207–221.

Joris H., Edwards van Muven A., van Ingen Schenau G. & Kemper H. (1985) Force, velocity and energy flow during the overarm throw in female handball players. *Journal of Biomechanics* **18**, 409–414.

Kleinöder H. (1990) The effect of tennis specific power-training towards an increase of service speed and speed of leg movements. PhD thesis, Deutsche Sporthochschule, Köln. (unpubl.)

Kyle C. & Caiozzo V. (1986) The effect of athletic clothing aerodynamics upon running speed. *Medicine and Science in Sports and Exercise* **18**, 509–515.

McClean B. & Jamieson I. (1991) The relationship between strength and kicking velocity in elite soccer players. Abstract, 1991 Annual Scientific Conference in Sports Medicine, Canberra, Australia.

Miller D. & Nissinen M. (1987) Critical examination of ground reaction force in the running forward somersault. *International Journal of Sports Biomechanics* **3**, 189–207.

Nigg B., Denoth J., Kerr B., Leuthi S., Smith D. & Stacoff A. (1984) Load, sports shoes and playing surfaces. In Frederick E. (ed.), *Sport Shoes and Playing Surfaces*, pp. 1–23. Human Kinetics Publishers, Champaign, IL, USA.

Nigg B. (1986) Biomechanical aspects of running. In Nigg B. (ed.) *Biomechanics of Running Shoes*, pp. 1–26. Human Kinetics Publishers, Champaign, IL, USA.

Nissinen M., Preiss R. & Brüggemann P. (1983) Simulation of human airborne movements on the horizontal bar. In Winter D., Norman R., Wells R., Hayes K. & Patla A. (eds) *Biomechanics IX-B*, pp. 373–376. Human Kinetics Publishers, Champaign IL, USA.

Panzer V., Wood G., Bates B. & Mason B. (1988). Lower extremity loads in landings of elite gymnasts. In de Groot G., Hollander P., Huijing P. & van Ingen Schenau G. (eds) *Biomechanics XI-B*, pp. 727–735. Free University Press, Amsterdam.

Putnam C. (1993) Sequential motions of the body segments in striking and throwing skills: Descriptions and explanations. *Journal of Biomechanics* **26** (Suppl. 1), 125–135.

Ramey M. (1970) Force relationships of the running long jump. *Medicine and Science in Sport* **2**, 146–151.

Ramey M. & Williams, K. (1985) Ground reaction forces in the triple jump. *International Journal of Sports Biomechanics* **1**, 233–239.

Ritchie J., Kelso S. & Belluci P. (1985) Aerobic dance injuries: A retrospective study of instructors and participants. *The Physician and Sports Medicine* **13**, 130–140.

Sparrow D. (1989) Racket almanac. *World Tennis* November, 47–49.

Sprigings E., Marshall R., Elliott B. & Jennings W. (1994) The effectiveness of upper limb rotations in producing racket-head speed in the tennis serve. *Journal of Biomechanics* **27**, 245–254.

Steele J. & Lafortune M. (1989) A kinetic analysis of footfall patterns at landing in netball; a follow-up study. In Morrison W. (ed.) *Proceedings of VII International Symposium of Biomechanics in Sports*, pp. 101–112. Footscray Institute of Technology Press, Melbourne.

Torg J., Pollack H. & Sweterlitsch P. (1972) The effects of competitive pitching on the shoulders and elbows of pre-adolescent baseball players. *Pediatrics* **49**, 267–270.

Valiant G. & Cavanagh P. (1985) A study of landing from a jump: Implications for the design of a basketball shoe. In Winter D., Norman R., Wells R., Hayes K. & Patla A. (eds), *Biomechanics IX-B*, pp. 117–122. Human Kinetics Publishers, Champaign, IL, USA.

van Gheluwe B. & Hebbelinck M. (1985) The kinematics of the service movement in tennis: A three-dimensional cinematographical approach. In Winter D., Norman R., Wells R., Hayes K. & Patla A. (eds) *Biomechanics IX-B*, pp. 521–526. Human Kinetics Publishers, Champaign, IL, USA.

Wilson G., Elliott B. & Wood G. (1991a) The effect of imposing a delay between the eccentric and concentric phases of a stretch–shorten cycle movement. *Medicine and Science in Sports and Exercise* **23**, 364–370.

Wilson G., Wood G. & Elliott B. (1991b) Optimal stiffness of series elastic component in a stretch–shorten cycle activity. *Journal of Applied Physiology* **70**, 825–833.

Wilson G., Wood G. & Elliott B. (1991c) The relationship between stiffness of the musculature and static flexibility: An alternative explanation for the occurrence of muscular injury. *International Journal of Sports Medicine* **12**, 403–407.

Wilson G., Elliott B. & Wood G. (1991d) Performance benefits through flexibility training. *Sports Coach* **14**, 7–9.

SECTION 2

APPLIED ANATOMY

CHAPTER 4

MODIFICATION OF PHYSIQUE AND/OR TECHNIQUE TO IMPROVE PERFORMANCE

Section 1 of this book has discussed the role that the discipline of biomechanics plays in improving sport performance and its orientation has traditionally been much more mechanical than anatomical. However when analysing physical performance it is impossible to separate these components, because the working human body consists of a large number of integrated systems which work in unison. Section 2 however, is more oriented towards the application of anatomy to performance, but it must be kept in mind that because the human body consists of a series of links connected by joints which act as levers, various mechanical principles dictate what it can and cannot do.

The following chapters therefore deal primarily with the various physical capacities of the human body, first by assessing their role in sport and then by suggesting ways in which these capacities, or the individual's technique, can be modified in order to improve performance.

BODY MODIFICATION–TECHNIQUE MODIFICATION CONCEPT

During the past 20 years there has been a rapid development in sport performance standards. There are many reasons for this, including such factors as better living conditions, a much larger number of people playing sport and more participants from those racial types whose physiques are highly suitable for certain sports or events within

them. However, the contribution of sport science and medicine is probably the major reason for these improvements, because the knowledge base in this field is now extensive. Further, coaching standards have risen dramatically during this time and much of the information which successful coaches now have to pass on to their athletes has its basis in sport science and medicine.

One area of sport science which has not yet had as much attention as the others, is the modification of an individual's physique and/or technique to improve performance (Bloomfield 1979). In the past, coaches have tended to teach standard techniques, especially those that have been used by world or Olympic champions, whether they suited their own athletes or not. Bloomfield and Blanksby (1973) in discussing this point stated that 'it is sometimes disturbing to be able to identify the coach of a certain group of swimmers by the similarity of their stroke technique(s) regardless of the obvious differences in their body type'. They further suggested that performances would be improved considerably if coaches were able to objectively assess the physical strengths and weaknesses of their swimmers, as this would enable them to develop a stroke which better suited their specific physical capacities.

Observations Relating to the Concept

One of the authors became aware of the differences in performance levels between individuals while teaching beginning swimmers in the late 1950s. It must be stressed that the following observations and subsequent actions were not part of a formal research study, merely a series of critical evaluations in response to the circumstances. After the first 10 lessons it was very obvious that many of the subjects performed quite differently in the final technique test, despite the fact that they had all received almost identical instruction throughout the lessons. It was clear that during the lesson series the majority of the swimmers understood the verbal and physical instructions they had been given, but that the poorer performers had not been able to apply these particularly well. Their lack of skill appeared to be a combination of their internal information processing ability and their body build, that is, such physical capacities as body composition, strength, flexibility and lever lengths. When several of the poorer performers in the group progressed to junior squad training, the above capacities were assessed using field tests, and intervention programmes were instigated to improve these physical deficiencies. At a later time some technique modification was also carried out, especially with the longer levered swimmers. Both programmes appeared to work reasonably well for those children who participated, as their techniques steadily improved (Bloomfield 1979).

A series of similar observations and actions were performed several years later using third year physical education students, who took part in a beginning golf instruction course. After 10 h of tuition, their swings were rated from a high speed (slow motion) film and great disparities were obvious between them. They had all been given identical information and appeared to understand it when questioned, which again pointed to the fact that it was a combination of internal information processing and their body build which brought about the differences. With further individual instruction, when an effort was made to 'fit the swing' to suit their individual physical capacities, the poorer performers improved their basic swing.

While neither of the above examples was anything more than systematic observation, they both point to something which intelligent coaches have known for some time. This is that performance will often improve if the relationship between an individual's physique and technique are considered when modifying skill. The greatest exponent of this concept was Dr James Counsilman from the University of Indiana, whose record as a scientific swimming coach over a 30 year period was unsurpassed. Counsilman was able to make an appraisal of a swimmer's body, then 'tailor' both the body and the technique to achieve an optimal performance.

Appraising Body Morphology

Coaches with a knowledge of sport science are usually more aware of the various physical characteristics of their athletes and are often able to appraise them more quickly than those who are untrained. They are able to assess strength and power well by simply observing the individual's size, shape, proportionality, posture and musculature. Likewise, flexibility levels can be assessed by examining technique, while speed and agility can be appraised reasonably well by observing game performance. This subjective appraisal is of great value and experienced coaches may need only this information in order to 'bring out the best' in their athletes. However, coaches without this knowledge may need a sport scientist to assist them with their initial appraisal. This is often possible in locations where members of university departments are available to assist coaches with such problems, or in institutes of sport or intensive training centres where there are sport scientists on staff.

At the international level, it is useful for the coach to collect appropriate data for each athlete on the following physical capacities: shape; body composition; proportionality; posture; strength and power; flexibility; speed; and agility. Chapter 14 of this text covers the various tests and measurements which are needed to do this thoroughly, using the most recent international testing protocols. On the other hand, the sections on

Talent Identification and Development in Chapter 13 demonstrate how to apply it.

Examples of Optimal Physique Characteristics for Various Sports

Some elite athletes at the international level have almost the perfect physique for their sport, combined with all the other characteristics which go to make up the optimal performance. These specific physical characteristics, especially in the technique-oriented sports, are often the very reason that the athlete selected that particular sport in the first place. In the past 30 years, since other races, especially African Americans and Asians, have been competing against European athletes, we have seen almost complete dominance of some events, for example in the male 100 m sprint in track, which is now dominated by African Americans. Several other events have a preponderance of one race of people performing better than the others and in technique-oriented sports this can, in many cases, be explained by differences in racial physical characteristics. It is important, however, not to overemphasize these characteristics, but merely to point out that even within racial groups, there is also a great divergence of physiques. The following examples illustrate the types of physical advantages some athletes have over others:

- *Gymnasts* who possess long bodies and short upper and lower limbs have a mechanical advantage in strength and power over their opponents, as well as a rotatory advantage with their short extremities
- *Sprint runners* who have postures which accentuate the anterior pelvic tilt (APT) and the protruding or 'high' buttocks, accompanied by a well developed musculature in the buttocks and thighs, are usually very fast athletes (Fig. 8.9). This body shape enables them to powerfully extend their thighs at an optimal driving angle which is essential for top sprinters
- Competitive *weightlifters* who have long bodies and short extremities have a mechanical advantage over other lifters; if they also

possess optimal *muscle insertion points* they will be considerably stronger than their competitors. It is well known that if the insertion point of the tendon is further away from the joint, it will give the individual a mechanical advantage in his performance

- If *contact sports* players have partially rounded shoulders and a reasonably flexible spine, rather than a rigid upright posture where the spine has little flexibility, then they have a natural advantage because they are able to 'tuck in' or 'cover up' when running into rucks, mauls, packs, while tackling or in closed field running
- Racquet sports players in *tennis, badminton, squash* and *racquetball* who have slightly inverted feet or 'pigeon toes' have a speed advantage over short distances, in comparison to other players with a conventional foot posture
- *Agility athletes* with the overhanging thigh (Fig. 8.10) have an advantage over those athletes with straight legs or genu recurvartum (hyperextension of the knee joint) because the knee joint is slightly flexed in this posture. This places them in an advantageous mechanical position for rapid agile movements
- *Butterfly swimmers* who are partially hypermobile in the shoulder joints will have a definite advantage over their competitors, because this physical capacity enables them to recover their arms during the stroke with great ease. As a result, their 'rise and fall' in the water will not be so extreme, thus cutting down considerably on frontal resistance
- *High jumpers* who are tall, with long lower limbs in comparison to their trunk and high crural indices (short thighs in comparison to their lower legs) have definite mechanical advantages over their competitors who do not possess these extreme proportionality characteristics

Body Modification

Athletes who do not have the physique advantages of the competitors quoted in the previous section can, however, carry out intervention programmes so as to modify their morphology to improve their performance. These programmes can enable athletes to greatly strengthen their weak points. Those human physical capacities which can be modified to a greater or lesser extent are as follows:

- *Strength, body bulk, power* and *flexibility* are the most easily modified capacities and very good results can be obtained in many sports, if these can be improved. Chapters 9 and 10 cover the above capacities in detail
- *Body type, body composition, speed* and *agility* are more difficult than the above group to change; however, there have been intensive intervention programmes developed during the past decade which will considerably improve these capacities. Chapters 5, 6, 11 and part of 12 explain ways in which they can be modified
- *Posture* and *dynamic balance* are not easy to modify and a long term intervention programme over several years is needed to accomplish this. Chapter 8 and part of 12 cover the above capacities in detail
- *Proportionality* or *body lever lengths* are capacities which can only be marginally changed during childhood and early adolescence, because bone lengths are finite once the adult has reached full maturity. It is important to mention at this point however that they can be modified within the context of the athlete's *technique*, with intelligent coaching. Chapter 7 covers proportionality in detail

Before giving examples of body modification, it is important to state that the capacities mentioned above are in some cases closely related. For example, body type and body composition have many factors in common, while strength, power, speed and agility are closely related. Flexibility and posture are partially related, while proportionality has some relationship to body type, strength, power, speed, balance and agility.

EXAMPLES OF MODIFICATIONS THAT CAN BE MADE TO ATHLETES

The following examples are cited to illustrate the fact that various physical characteristics can be modified with *intensive* intervention programmes in order for athletes to improve their performance:

- A *butterfly swimmer* who has all the other physical capacities to swim at the top level, may lack the shoulder flexibility that is needed for an effortless and effective technique. By embarking on a long-term intensive static and/or a proprioceptive neuromuscular facilitation (PNF) stretching programme, particularly for the shoulder joint, flexibility, and consequently technique, can be greatly improved. Chapter 10 outlines such a programme
- *Contact and mobile field athletes* who lack natural speed and agility can greatly improve these capacities by embarking on a special speed and agility training programme, which if continued over several seasons, will certainly improve this aspect of their performance. Chapters 11 and 12 cover such programmes
- It is desirable for a *male gymnast* to have long arms in order to perform well on the pommel horse. Unfortunately however, long arms present strength problems when a gymnast is performing on the rings. In order to perform optimally in this event, it is necessary to develop very high levels of strength in the upper trunk and arms. Chapter 9 outlines such a programme
- *Basketballers, volleyballers, netball players* and *field games jumpers* all need to develop their jumping ability in order to be effective in their sports. Modern power training methods can improve their performances, especially if combined with flexibility training, by increasing the amount of energy recovered for the concentric movement from the stretch–shorten cycle, where elastic energy is stored in the musculotendinous unit, then released during various ballistic skills. Chapters 9 and 10 cover such programmes

- A *contact sports* player taking part in one of the football codes may have the great majority of the capacities that are needed to perform well, but may lack the body bulk necessary for that sport. A body building programme will considerably improve this physical characteristic, with a resultant improvement in overall performance. Chapter 9 outlines a programme that will enable this to occur
- *Cricket fast bowlers* may wish to increase the speed of their delivery. To do this and protect themselves from injury, they should improve their strength and power as well as their flexibility levels, especially in the trunk and shoulder joints. The combination of these programmes will give them the body bulk, power and elastic energy needed to increase the velocity of their ball delivery. Chapters 9 and 10 cover such a programme
- A *female gymnast* may find that as she progresses through adolescence, her body fat level rises, thus affecting her power to weight ratio. She will, at this point, need professional advice from a nutritionist to enable her to reduce her fat mass to an acceptable level

Technique Modification

Many athletes will be able to achieve their goals by simply undergoing a body modification programme. There are situations, however, where individuals are not able to modify their physical capacities enough to give them an optimal performance and if this is the case, other approaches need to be adopted.

Technique modification should then be considered, but before discussing this, it is important to point out one of the problems that may occur if the coach is not aware of the *mechanical principles*, which are determined by the *laws of motion* (Wiren 1976). These principles must be observed at all times for an optimal result to be obtained. However, because humans demonstrate many anatomical differences, the way in which these principles can be applied varies considerably, and certain physical characteristics will be

advantageous for one sport, whereas they may be a handicap in others. Therefore, the coach must develop a set of *preferences* (Wiren 1976) which can be applied in a particular sport and these must be chosen to suit an individual, or particular circumstance. These preferences are the ways in which athletes will perform the skill within the framework of the mechanical principles mentioned above. There are many such preferences available to the athlete in every sport and their selection often relates to the physique of the player, the environmental conditions (wind, heat, cold, humidity etc.), the playing surface, the opposition and a myriad of other variables which need to be taken into account in every sport. In order to illustrate these *technique preferences* two examples are given below:

- *Tennis* players who perform on different surfaces, or against a particular player, need to adapt their shot to suit each circumstance and one option is to change their grip on the racquet in order to do this. For example, if they wish to predominantly use top spin, then they will probably opt for a Western grip. However, if they are more concerned with hitting the ball 'flat' and very powerfully, they may choose an Eastern or more neutral grip. If an undercut shot is needed, then a Continental grip is probably the best option
- Right-handed *golfers* who wish to 'move the ball' from right to left during flight (a draw) because of a 'dog-leg' or windy conditions, can adopt a closed position at address. This means that the left foot will be further forward than the right one and the feet will be aligned with the body up to 15° to the right of the target. If they wish to hit a straight ball, the feet and the body should be square to the target line; if a left to right shot (a fade) is needed, then they should set up with the left foot further behind the right foot and with the body facing about 15° to the left of the target

These preferences can only be determined when coaches have a good knowledge of the physique of their athletes as well as of their movement and psychological capacities. This approach is the very essence of scientific coaching, where the coach decides what suits the individual best, according to his or her physical strengths and weaknesses, rather than teaching a general technique which is mechanically efficient but may not suit that athlete particularly well.

The following examples illustrate technique modification which is undertaken when the body's physical capacities can be modified no further, or not at all, as is the case with proportionality:

- If a *butterfly swimmer's* flexibility level has not improved to the point where the style is economical and mechanically effective, despite an intensive stretching programme for the shoulder joints, then the coach should teach that competitor the side-breathing technique
- In *combative sports*, individuals with long lower limbs compared to their trunk lengths should flex them at the knees a little more than shorter legged athletes, in order to lower their centre of gravity, thus increasing their dynamic stability
- The *swimmer* who has not been able to develop enough power to adopt an optimal pulling lever during the stroke, must shorten the upper limb by flexing the forearm at the elbow in order to develop an efficient lever system (Fig. 7.14)
- The *contact sports* player who has square shoulders and an immobile spine needs to consciously practise a round-shouldered posture as well as do flexibility exercises for the spine, in order to be more physically effective and less prone to injury
- The *breast-stroke swimmer* with a poor kicking posture (i.e. slightly inverted feet or a conventional foot posture) should concentrate more on the synchronization of the body and the arm pull, in order to overcome this postural deficiency in the stroke
- The *female tennis* player who is not particularly strong should consider flexing the forearm more in order to shorten the hitting lever, or use a double-handed technique so as to produce more powerful ground strokes (Fig. 7.13)

- *Contact sports* players with long legs tend to stride out during on-field running, and this lowers their level of dynamic balance. In order to increase it, they should bend their legs a little more and consciously take short, very fast steps, especially when near or contacting opponents. By adopting such a technique, they keep their base of support under their body, thereby improving their dynamic balance

CONCLUSION

The aim of this chapter has been to assist coaches to apply the body modification–technique modification concept. This is done by either modifying the body to suit a mechanically sound technique and/or altering the technique to suit the individual. The combination of both, however, is frequently the best solution to the problem. Throughout the history of sport we have seen various 'technique fads' sweep through the sporting world. New jumping, hitting, throwing, running and swimming techniques have evolved at a rapid rate, especially during the past 20 years. These techniques have obviously suited the athletes for whom they have been developed and other individuals with similar physiques have adopted them successfully. However, those competitors with different physical capacities have often copied these techniques blindly and have been disappointed with their poor performances.

It is the responsibility of coaches to equip themselves with enough scientific knowledge to enable them to tailor a technique to suit each individual athlete. The remainder of this book is therefore dedicated to this end.

REFERENCES

Bloomfield J. (1979) Modifying human physical capacities and technique to improve performance. *Sports Coach* **3**, 14–19.

Bloomfield J. & Blanksby B. (1973) Anatomical features (involved) in developing the ideal swimming stroke. *International Swimmer* **8**, July, 8–9.

Wiren G. (1976) Introduction to laws, principles and preferences. *PGA Magazine*, April, 1–4.

CHAPTER 5

BODY TYPING IN SPORT

The scientific measurement of human physique has only occurred in the past 60 years; however, human biologists and medical doctors have been interested in the field for many centuries. Throughout history there have been several attempts to group or classify the human form into appropriate categories, but it was Hippocrates the Greek physician who formally classified two fundamental body types in the 5th century BC. The first he called *phthisic habitus*, which was characterized by a long thin body dominated by a vertical dimension; and the second *apoplectic habitus*, whose main physical characteristic was a short thick body which was strong in the horizontal dimension. The first group he suggested was prone to respiratory disorders, especially tuberculosis, while the second tended to develop cardiovascular disease. He made almost no distinction between muscle and fat in the second type; however, this may have been because in ancient Greece, with little automation, people expended significant amounts of energy in their daily lives and were therefore not as obese as many individuals in the 20th century. Rostan, a Frenchman, was the first person to develop the three category classification in the early part of the 19th century and his descriptions of the *type digestif, type musculaire* and *type cérébral* were very close to the modern somatotype classifications.

However, none of those individuals who classified and then described the various body types in the past did any objective measuring. This was first carried out by Dr William H. Sheldon, a med-

ical doctor from the USA, who in 1939 devised a method to classify body types, using anthropometric measurements from 4000 male subjects. His method, which indicated the presence of three basic body types, became the standard for all the systems which were to develop in the latter part of the 20th century.

BASIC SOMATOTYPES

The somatotype or body type names of *endomorph, mesomorph* and *ectomorph* were derived by Sheldon *et al.* (1940) from the embryonic tissue layers of the body, with the *endoderm* representing the digestive layer, the *mesoderm* the muscle and skeletal layer and the *ectoderm* the sensory layer. Sheldon *et al.* (1940) described these three basic body types (Fig. 5.1), which are the extremes of their group, in the following way:

- *Endomorph* — the obese individual whose most conspicuous feature is body fat
- *Mesomorph* — the muscular athletic type who has a predominance of bone, muscle and connective tissue
- *Ectomorph* — the tall lean individual whose body surface area predominates over the body mass

Second Order Variables

In addition to the three basic components outlined above, there are several other characteristics

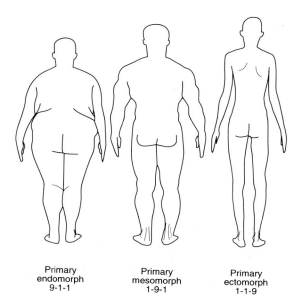

Primary
endomorph
9-1-1

Primary
mesomorph
1-9-1

Primary
ectomorph
1-1-9

Fig. 5.1 The three basic body types.

that play a part in body typing to a greater or lesser extent. These are as follows:

- *Dysplasia* — the physical disharmony between different regions of the same physique. When, for example, a body is of one somatotype in the region of the head, neck and trunk and of another in the buttocks and legs, the individual is described as dysplasic
- *Gynandromorphy* — the bisexuality of physique. This occurs when members of one sex exhibit several secondary characteristics of the opposite sex
- *Hirsutism* — the hairiness of the body and the abundance and location of body hair. This characteristic is basically related to hormonal secretions, with males normally having much more body hair than females

DEVELOPMENT OF THE SOMATOTYPE RATING SYSTEM

The Sheldon System

Sheldon *et al.* (1940) classified the basic body types mentioned above from 4000 subjects, then later

increased the sample to 46 000. This sample was derived from 18 to 65 year old males who had anthropometric measures taken on the head, face and neck, the thoracic trunk, the arms, shoulders and hands, the abdomen, trunk and pelvis, as well as the buttocks, legs and feet. Their general appearance was also assessed and photographs were taken anteriorly, laterally and posteriorly. From these data he ultimately isolated 88 body types within the three basic somatotypes (Sheldon 1954).

As each individual had, to a greater or lesser extent, all the physical characteristics mentioned above, they were rated on the predominance of endomorphy, mesomorphy and ectomorphy on a 7 point scale. A rating of 7 displayed primary dominance, while 1 had little dominance. Each physique was expressed in 3 numbers which denoted the amounts of endomorphy, mesomorphy and ectomorphy, in that order. Therefore, an individual with a rating of **7–1–1** had a very high endomorphic component, whereas a **1–7–1** was very high in mesomorphy. The primary ectomorph's rating was **1–1–7**. Most humans demonstrate a combination of two body types, with one usually greater than the other and the third one only playing a minor role. There is, however, a balanced central type (Fig. 14.14) with the components being present in equal amounts. Finally, in order to rate the body types, Sheldon (1954) developed an 'atlas' where photographs of 1175 men were displayed. A method was set out in which photographs of the subject were compared with those in the atlas.

The Parnell System

Parnell (1958) a medical doctor from Oxford who was interested in the relationship between physique and behaviour, developed a more objective method than that of Sheldon for both males and females. He used anthropometric measurements and constructed a Deviation Chart, or M4 rating chart, on which to place these measures, thus eliminating the need for a photograph. Parnell also raised the question of the *phenotype*, because body typing up until that time was said to represent only the *genotype* or the genetic body type. Because the phenotype represents the living body at any given moment in time, human biologists have more recently accepted it as a more valid representation of the somatotype. It is well known by coaches that various body types can be altered over time by intervention programmes, which can change the somatotype by the use of dietary or strength training regimens, so this is a more realistic criterion for the field of sport science.

The Heath–Carter System

The most recent development in body typing is that of Heath and Carter (1967) who refined both the Sheldon and Parnell systems to a point where an objective assessment can now be made of the body type. These investigators extended the scale from 1 to 9, which turned out to be an important addition to the system, because it had become obvious to specialists working in the fields of medicine and sport science that various subpopulations around the world, such as the Nilotic peoples of northeastern Africa, had some individuals who were more than 7 in ectomorphy (Fig. 5.2a). Furthermore, several cases of grossly obese individuals have been isolated in various parts of the world who rated well over 7 in endomorphy (Fig. 5.2b). Similarly, highly mesomorphic athletes have developed, especially those competing in gymnastics, weight- and power-lifting as well, as in the sport of body building, who score well over 7 in mesomorphy (Fig. 5.2c). In addition, in this system there is also the provision for an open-ended scale where *very extreme* body types can be rated above 9, especially in the endomorphic component.

Heath and Carter (1967) further developed their measuring system and devised a rating chart or somatotype rating form on which to record the measures (Fig. 14.13). These ratings were then placed on a somatochart (Fig. 14.14) and as well as having a 3 figure rating, subjects were described with relation to their position on the somatochart (Fig. 5.3).

BODY TYPE AND HEALTH

Various investigators have reported that there is a strong relationship between body type and physical health and this is briefly outlined below:

- *The endomorph* is the shortest lived of the three types and is not well adapted to prolonged physical work, tending to avoid it if possible. Endomorphs do well in intellectual pursuits, are sociable with a pleasant disposition, and can stay relatively healthy if their obesity is

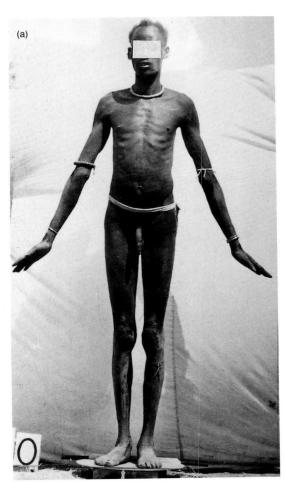

Fig. 5.2 (a) An example of an extreme ectomorph whose rating was classified above 7 using the Health–Carter system (courtesy of D. Roberts, reprinted with permission of Cambridge University Press).

48

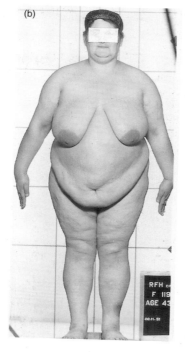 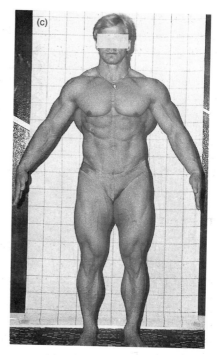

Fig. 5.2 Examples of extreme body types whose ratings were classified above 7 using the Heath–Carter system. (b) Endomorph (courtesy of B. Heath Roll). (c) Mesomorph (courtesy of J. Borms, reprinted with permission of Cambridge University Press).

controlled with a low kilojoule diet and regular exercise. If their obesity levels rise, they then become prone to cardiovascular and associated diseases. Aquatic and non-weight bearing sports, weightlifting and combative sports are usually suitable for many endomorphs

- *The mesomorph* is generally an energetic and healthy individual who is capable of more physical work than the other body types. Mesomorphs can become obese if they cease physical activity and do not control their kilojoule intake. If this occurs, they become susceptible to the degenerative diseases, mainly cardiovascular disease. Members of this group are aggressive and athletically skilled with little aversion to contact sport. They do well in sports that require strength, power, speed and agility.

- *The ectomorph* is usually active with better than average longevity. Ectomorphs need to be aware, however, that they are prone to respiratory disease and in some cases nervous disorders, but they are generally healthy types. Extreme ectomorphs sometimes need health

counselling with regard to their diet, relaxation habits and their physical activity. Because they have light bones, less musculature and weak joint capsules they are more easily injured in contact sports, but do well in many sports where endurance and agility are needed

CHANGES IN BODY TYPE DURING GROWTH

The question as to whether one can accurately predict the final adult somatotype from ratings made during childhood and adolescence has not been fully answered, mainly because too few longitudinal studies have as yet been completed. However, both Carter and Heath (1990) and Malina and Bouchard (1991) have suggested that there are general trends which the somatotype usually follows, but that there are some individuals who do not conform to these.

In general, young boys move from endo-mesomorphy toward balanced mesomorphy, then tend to decrease in mesomorphy, moving slightly towards ectomorphy in mid-adolescence. After this

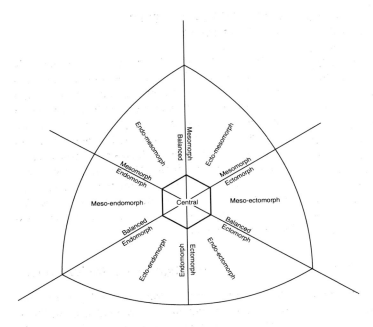

Fig. 5.3 A diagrammatic representation of the location of the somatotype categories.

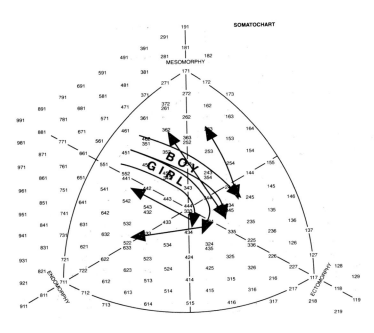

Fig. 5.4 The general pathway which is followed by the majority of somatotypes from infancy to adulthood (courtesy of Carter & Heath 1990, reprinted with permission of Cambridge University Press).

point they generally move back towards mesomorphy as their muscle mass increases. Girls, on the other hand, move from endo-mesomorphy towards central somatotypes, thereby decreasing their mesomorphy in adolescence. They then move towards endo-mesomorphy and balanced endomorphy–mesomorphy in late adolescence (Fig. 5.4). Carter and Heath (1990) suggest that individuals may differ considerably from these trends and that genetic factors play an important part in the above process. They further state that nutrition and exercise also play important roles.

A thorough knowledge of these trends can be important in talent identification for selected sports, because the informed coach will be better able to predict what the ultimate body type will generally be like. Experienced coaches and teachers in the areas of gymnastics and dance have been able to make quite accurate predictions, especially with females, while many coaches of males in sports which require body bulk, explosive power, agility and speed in their athletes have also made reasonably accurate forecasts.

BODY TYPE AND SPORT PERFORMANCE

It must be remembered that the somatotype is only a general physical capacity and as such it is only one indicator of an athlete's suitability to perform at a high level. It must be combined with other capacities such as body composition, proportionality, strength and power, flexibility, posture, speed and agility, when one evaluates the physical characteristics of an athlete. However, in the wider performance context the athlete's level of skill, cardiovascular fitness and psychological profile must also be carefully considered, as was discussed in Chapter 1.

Body Type and High Level Performance

Body shape plays an important role in the self-selection of individuals for competitive sport. There is also a considerable amount of information in the sport science literature on the suitability of various body types, not only for particular sports,

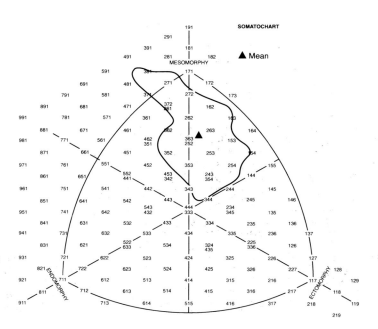

Fig. 5.5 Divers who competed in the World Championships in 1991 illustrate how athletes cluster around the mean (adapted from Carter & Marfell-Jones 1994).

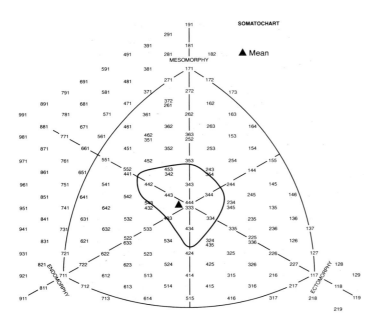

Fig. 5.6 The region of the somatochart which is occupied by high level female volleyball players (adapted from Carter & Heath 1990).

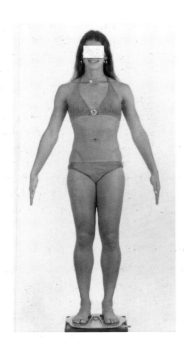

Fig. 5.7 The body type of a typical high level female volleyball player (courtesy of Carter & Heath 1990, reprinted with permission of Cambridge University Press).

but also for specific events or positions within many sports. As a large number of factors are involved in the physical make-up of a champion sportsman or sportswoman, there is not necessarily one perfect body shape for a particular sport or event within that sport. Much of the literature gives mean somatotype ratings of high level athletes in a large number of sports. However, it should be kept in mind that there will be a range of shapes which will cluster around the mean body type in each group. Figure 5.5 illustrates this point, as it demonstrates the spread of divers who competed in the World Championships in 1991. Figure 5.6 represents the region of the somatochart occupied by high level female volleyball players and Fig. 5.7 shows one of them.

DIFFERENCES BETWEEN THE SEXES

The majority of data collected over the past 40 years on high level athletes has been on males; however, this deficiency is now being steadily redressed. Unfortunately, there are no accurate formulae by which male data can be transposed and used to predict the ideal body type for females for particular sports. However, existing data would indicate that high level female athletes are more

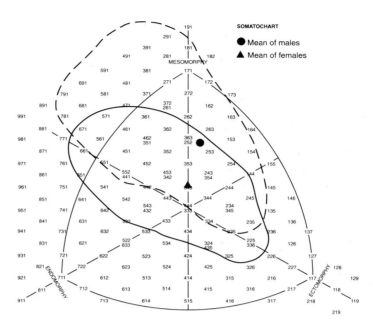

Fig. 5.8 Somatotype distributions of male and female Olympic athletes. (– – –) Males; (—) females. (Adapted from Carter & Heath 1990.)

endomorphic and less mesomorphic than their male counterparts, but have a similar ectomorphy rating (Fig. 5.8). The rough guide which has been used in the past by sport scientists in sports where a reasonable amount of data have been gathered is as follows:

- In sprint running, the female is usually about 1 component more in endomorphy and 1–1.5 less in mesomorphy, with ectomorphy at a similar level. In middle distance running, the female is generally about 0.5 more in endomorphy and 1 less in mesomorphy, with ectomorphy again similar
- There is the same range of differences between male and female swimmers. However, when greater body bulk and/or explosive power are needed in sports such as field games or judo, then females are up to 2 components higher in endomorphy and 2 lower in mesomorphy than males. Ectomorphy is generally similar, but may vary by 0.5 in some cases

Carter and Heath (1990) suggested that more intensive training does not significantly modify the abovementioned differences and that 'this may help to account for the continued differences in the performance of trained male and female athletes'.

DIFFERENCES BETWEEN ATHLETES AND NON-ATHLETES

High level male and female athletes generally place themselves into the top to middle left side of the somatochart, when compared to individuals from the normal population, who are more randomly spread around the somatochart. Figure 5.9 demonstrates these differences, with the male athletes tending to be much more mesomorphic than the normal male population, with a mean somatotype of approximately **2.0–5.0–2.5**, while female athletes have higher levels of meso-endomorphy, mesomorphy–endomorphy and endomesomorphy than non-athletes (Fig. 5.10). The mean somatotype for the female athletes was approximately **3.0–4.0–3.0**.

ATHLETE BODY TYPE CHANGES OVER TIME

Carter and Heath (1990) stated that somatotypes of athletes whose photographs have been assessed over the past 60 years have undergone various changes. In this period male swimmers have become less endomorphic and field games athletes have developed more mesomorphy, while high jumpers and 400 m runners are now less mesomorphic and more ectomorphic. Track sprinters however have had very little change. Furthermore,

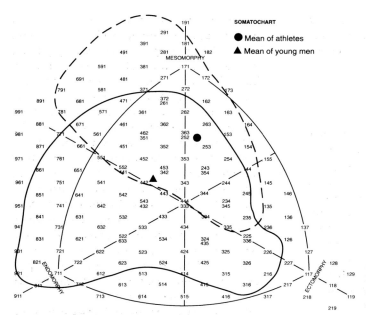

Fig. 5.9 Somatotype distributions of male Olympic athletes and young United States males. (– – –) Athletes; (—) young males. (Adapted from Carter & Heath 1990.)

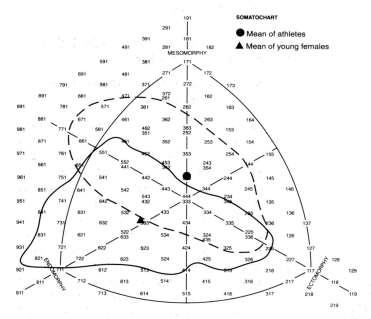

Fig. 5.10 Somatotype distributions of female Olympic athletes and young United States females. (– – –) Athletes; (—) young females. (Adapted from Carter & Heath 1990.)

a shift was noted by Štěpnička (1986) towards higher mesomorphy in cross-country skiing, judo and basketball, where power is an important element in the sport.

These changes are probably the result of several factors which are outlined below:

- The *first* would be self-selection for the sport, where more individuals with suitable body types are now selecting themselves for various sports or events. They are also coming from a considerably larger population interested in sport participation than was the case before the 1970s. Further, various races and ethnic groups, who have some very special physical features which suit particular sports, are now competing regularly in international sport
- The *second* factor relates to the very intensive endurance training which has been carried out during the past 10–15 years. Depending on the sport, many endurance athletes now spend from 4–5 h training each day and expend a great deal of energy while doing so. This reduces their endomorphy, while at the same time increasing their ectomorphy in some sports, such as distance running, or their mesomorphy in such sports as swimming (Fig. 5.11), rowing and canoeing, where very intensive anaerobic/aerobic training is carried out
- The *third* reason is that sport scientists have been able to tailor athletes' nutritional needs to suit them personally. In some cases they need 'force-feeding' to gain bulk or more endomorphy and in other sports they need to reduce adipose tissue in order to 'make the weight' and to compete at an optimal performance weight with a very low fat mass (FM), thus increasing their ectomorphy
- The *fourth* factor is the universal use of intensive strength and explosive power training through which competitors now increase their lean body mass (LBM), as well as their mesomorphy rating

DESIRABLE BODY TYPES FOR HIGH LEVEL PERFORMANCE

Racquet Sports (Tennis, Badminton, Squash, Racquetball)

Competitors in racquet sports have variable body types. The mean somatotype for male *tennis* players is **2.0–4.5–3.0**, while females rate **3.5–3.5–3.0**. Carter and Heath (1990) have surveyed the literature on high level female tennis players and stated that 'the somatoplots of tennis players cover a fairly wide circular area, with most means (of the various groups) just to the left of the centre of the somatochart'. Male *badminton* players have very similar body types to male tennis players; however, *squash* players of both sexes were higher in mesomorphy than tennis players. Finally, it should be noted that male US *racquetball* professionals are lower in mesomorphy and higher in endomorphy than international level performers in other racquet sports (Table 5.1).

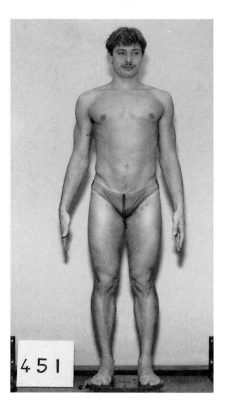

Fig. 5.11 The mesomorphy of a swimmer increases with very intensive anaerobic/aerobic training.

Table 5.1 Somatotypes of high level sportsmen and sportswomen

Sport	Males	Females
Racquet sports		
Tennis	2.0–4.5–3.0	3.5–3.5–3.0
Badminton	2.5–4.5–3.0	— — —
Squash	2.5–5.0–3.0	3.5–4.0–3.0
Racquetball	3.0–3.5–3.0	— — —
Aquatic sports		
Swimming	2.0–5.0–3.0	3.0–4.0–3.0
Waterpolo	2.5–5.5–2.5	3.5–4.0–3.0
Rowing	2.5–5.5–2.5	3.0–4.0–3.0
Canoeing	2.0–5.5–2.5	3.0–4.5–2.5
Gymnastic and power sports		
Gymnastics	1.5–6.0–2.0	2.0–4.0–3.0*
Skating	1.5–5.0–3.0	2.5–4.0–3.0
Diving	2.0–5.5–2.5	3.0–4.0–3.0
Weightlifting (<60 kg)	1.5–7.0–1.0	— — —
(60–79.9 kg)	2.0–7.0–1.0	— — —
(80–99.9 kg)	2.5–8.0–0.5	— — —
(>100 kg)	5.0–9.0–0.5	— — —
Track, field and cycling		
Sprint running and hurdles	1.5–5.0–3.0†	2.5–4.0–3.0
400 m, 400 m hurdles	1.5–4.5–3.5	2.0–3.5–3.5
800 m, 1500 m	1.5–4.5–3.5	2.0–3.5–3.5
5000 m, 10 000 m	1.5–4.0–3.5	— — —
Marathon	1.5–4.5–3.5	— — —
Shot, discus, hammer	3.0–7.0–1.0	5.5–5.5–1.5
High, long, triple jump	1.5–4.0–3.5	2.5–3.0–4.0
Cycling: Track	2.0–5.5–2.5	— — —
Road	1.5–4.5–3.0	— — —
Mobile field sports		
Field hockey	2.5–4.5–2.5	— — —
Soccer	2.5–5.0–2.5	4.0–4.5–2.0
Lacrosse	3.0–5.5–2.5	4.0–4.5–2.5
Contact field sports		
Rugby	3.0–6.0–2.0	— — —
Australian football	2.0–5.5–2.5	— — —
American football: Linemen	5.0–7.5–1.0	— — —
Backs	3.0–5.5–1.5	— — —
Set field sports		
Baseball (males only), softball (females only)	2.5–5.5–2.0	3.5–4.5–2.0
Cricket	— — —	5.0–4.5–2.0
Golf	4.0–5.0–2.0	4.0–4.0–2.5
Court sports		
Basketball	2.0–4.5–3.5	4.0–4.0–3.0
Netball	— — —	3.0–4.0–3.5
Volleyball	2.5–4.5–3.5	3.5–4.0–3.0
Martial arts		
Judo	2.0–6.5–1.5	4.0–4.0–2.0
Wrestling (<60 kg)	1.5–5.5–2.5	— — —
(60–79.9 kg)	2.0–6.5–1.5	— — —
(80–99.9 kg)	2.5–7.0–1.0	— — —
(>100 kg)	4.0–7.5–1.0	— — —
Boxing (<60 kg)	1.5–5.0–3.0	— — —
(60–79.9 kg)	2.0–5.5–2.5	— — —
(80–89.9 kg)	2.5–6.0–2.0	— — —

* More mature gymnasts 3.0–4.0–3.0. † Most specialist 100 m sprinters score at least 5.5 on mesomorphy.

Aquatic Sports

SWIMMING

From a very large sample of *swimmers* taken at the 1991 World Swimming Championships, the male somatotype (n = 231) was **2.0–5.0–3.0**, which placed them in the ecto-mesomorphic region of the somatochart. This group was characterized by a low level of fatness, moderate to high musculoskeletal robustness and moderate linearity (Carter & Marfell-Jones 1994). The female swimmers (n = 170) were rated at **3.0–4.0–3.0** and demonstrated a higher musculoskeletal rating than the other components of linearity or fatness (Carter & Marfell-Jones 1994). Most studies on high level swimmers during the past 20 years have revealed very similar body types, particularly those individuals competing in freestyle, butterfly and breast-stroke events. Backstrokers however have tended to be a little more ectomorphic than swimmers competing in the other strokes (Carter & Heath 1990; Table 5.1).

WATERPOLO

Two hundred and ninety-nine elite *waterpolo* players were tested at the 1991 World Swimming Championships (Carter & Marfell-Jones 1994). The male players' (n = 190) mean somatotype rating was **2.5–5.5–2.5**, which classified them as balanced mesomorphs. Previous data from De Garay *et al.* (1974) and Hebbelinck *et al.* (1975) of Olympic waterpolo players placed them in the endo-mesomorphic (**3.0–5.5–2.5**) sector of the somatochart. The more intense training required of players since 1974 is the most likely reason why the endomorphy rating has been reduced by 0.5 to 2.5. Female players at the above championships (n = 109), recorded a mean somatotype rating of **3.5–4.0–3.0**, which placed them on the border between the central and endo-mesomorphic somatotype categories, with mesomorphy being the dominant feature of their body type (Table 5.1).

ROWING

Heavyweight *rowers* at the international level have a somatotype rating of **2.5–5.5–2.5**, which gives them a high mesomorphic and low endomorphic rating. This is quite understandable because of the requirement for both strength and power to pull the boat through the water, while they also need a high level of cardiovascular endurance because the event continues for 5–6 min. Female rowers at the elite level have central or balanced mesomorphic somatotypes, with a mean rating of **3.0–4.0–3.0**, which is almost identical to that of swimmers (Hebbelinck *et al.* 1980; Carter *et al.* 1982). However, when one examines their heights and weights they are generally greater than those of swimmers (Table 5.1).

CANOEING

When the data from Olympic male (Carter 1984) and high level Eastern European *canoeists* are combined (Štěpnička 1974; Meszáros & Mohácsi 1982) these athletes have a mean somatotype rating of **2.0–5.5–2.5**. This is an identical somatotype to that reported previously for international oarsmen, which is understandable because of the similar demands of canoeing and rowing. Female canoeists on the other hand, have a mean rating of **3.0–4.5–2.5** (Carter 1984) on data taken from competitors in the 1968 and 1976 Olympic Games. It is interesting to note that although male rowers and canoeists have almost identical body types, female canoeists are more mesomorphic and less ectomorphic than female rowers (Table 5.1).

Gymnastic and Power Sports

GYMNASTICS

The majority of high level male *gymnasts* are either balanced mesomorphs or ecto-mesomorphs with a mean rating of **1.5–6.0–2.0**. They are mature in comparison to female competitors and are very powerful athletes, with heavy musculature and little fat. However, modern female gymnasts at the highest level are mostly pre- or mid-adolescent, which makes them younger than most other international athletes, except perhaps for some swimmers. These athletes are ecto-mesomorphic or central types, with a mean rating of approximately **2.0–4.0–3.0**; however, older competitors usually rate 1 component higher in endomorphy. Carter and Heath (1990) suggested that body type was a very important factor from an early age in gymnastics; therefore it is important in talent identification for coaches to select their future gymnasts carefully (Table 5.1).

SKATING

Male *skaters* who compete in figure skating and ice dancing have high levels of mesomorphy, are reasonably high in ectomorphy and are low in endomorphy, with a rating of **1.5–5.0–3.0**. When they are compared with other gymnastic types, notably gymnasts and divers, they are lower in mesomorphy but higher in ectomorphy. Conversely, female skaters have a mean rating of **2.5–4.0–3.0**, which gives them an almost identical body type to their counterparts in gymnastics and diving (Ross *et al.* 1977; Table 5.1).

DIVING

It is commonly believed that *divers* have almost identical body types to gymnasts, but this is not correct when comparisons are made at the highest level. A sample of 82 divers assessed at the 1991 World Championships (Carter & Marfell-Jones 1994) revealed the following body types. The mean somatotype of male divers ($n = 43$) was **2.0–5.5–2.5**, which classified them as balanced mesomorphs; when they were compared with gymnasts they had slightly more endomorphy, less mesomorphy and more ectomorphy. Female divers ($n = 39$) from the same championships (Carter & Marfell-Jones 1994) were found to be central somatotypes with mean ratings of **3.0–4.0–3.0**. They were very similar to the gymnasts in mesomorphy and ectomorphy but rated 1 component higher in endomorphy (Table 5.1).

WEIGHTLIFTING

Carter (1984), in his paper on the combined data from three Olympic Games, found that the higher the weight class, the higher were the endomorphy and mesomorphy ratings, but the lower the ectomorphy component (Table 5.1). All *weightlifters* require heavy muscle mass which gives them very high ratings in mesomorphy (Fig. 7.4). They

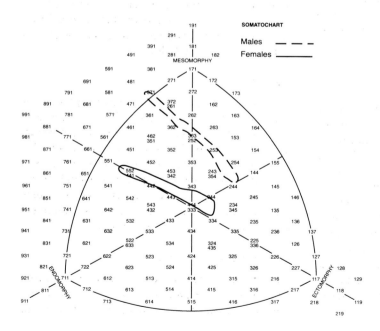

Fig. 5.12 Somatotype distributions of male and female Olympic track and field athletes (adapted from Carter & Heath 1990).

are in fact the most mesomorphic of all the high level athletes, with lifters over 80 kg being the least ectomorphic (Table 5.1). The combined mean of this group was **2.5–7.5–1.0**.

Track, Field and Cycling

TRACK AND FIELD

Athletes from three Olympic Games (*n* = 452) were studied by Carter (1984), who plotted the somatotypes of male athletes in 11 *track and field* events (Fig. 5.12). He found that the somatoplots were almost on a straight line, running from extreme endo-mesomorphy for the throwers, to ectomorphy–mesomorphy for the distance runners. The only group which did not fit this pattern were marathon runners, who were slightly more mesomorphic and less ectomorphic than 5000 and 10 000 m runners. Table 5.1 gives the specific mean body types of the above sample.

Carter (1984) found relatively similar results for female Olympic athletes to those for males and stated that the means of the female athletes are approximately parallel to those of the males but lower down on the somatochart (Carter & Heath 1990). Table 5.1 also gives the specific mean body types of the female sample.

CYCLING

In the past it was common for *cyclists* to compete both on the track and on the road. However, the last two decades have seen specialization occur with two distinct body types emerging. Male track cyclists are a powerful group with a somatotype of **2.0–5.5–2.5**, while road racers have lower mesomorphy and endomorphy ratings, yet are higher in ectomorphy. The body type rating of **1.5–4.5–3.0** (White *et al.* 1982) is quite understandable for an endurance athlete, who at times needs a reasonable amount of power in this event. This will often occur either during hill climbs or short sprints, where a tactical advantage is required (Table 5.1).

Mobile Field Sports (Field Hockey, Soccer, Lacrosse)

Male competitors in mobile field sports are low in both endomorphy and ectomorphy, with reasonably high levels of mesomorphy, enabling them to perform with speed and agility. Female competitors in this group are high in mesomorphy with reasonably high levels of endomorphy, but are low in ectomorphy. Table 5.1 illustrates the individual body types for players in this category.

Contact Field Sports

Individuals competing in contact field sports tend to be basically mesomorphic with some degree of endomorphy, depending on their position on the field. This type of athlete must sustain 'hard knocks' for prolonged periods of time, and thus they are generally low in ectomorphy. Contact sports players need to be fast and powerful and if they are not basically mesomorphic, they need special skills with high levels of agility, speed and dynamic balance. If they possess these qualities there is more chance that they will avoid serious injuries, which have been increasing in incidence and severity as players become bigger and faster. Table 5.1 gives the various body types for players in the following football codes.

RUGBY

The mean somatotype of *rugby* players is **3.0–6.0–2.0**; however, they divide themselves into forwards who tend to be endo-mesomorphic, and backs who tend to be balanced mesomorphs. In both groups in recent years there has been a slight increase in mesomorphy with a similar drop in endomorphy. Anecdotal evidence attributes these minor shifts to more strenuous endurance and more intensive strength training.

AUSTRALIAN FOOTBALL

Australian football is a very mobile game with a large field to be covered by only 18 players, and therefore these athletes need a high level of cardiovascular endurance. Although there is heavy contact from time to time, this is not as sustained as in rugby or American football. The mean somatotype for Australian football is **2.0–5.5–2.5** (Withers *et al.* 1986), which reflects the dynamic nature of the game. However, it should be understood that some specialist players, such as ball gatherers, who need high levels of speed, are short and mesomorphic, whereas others, such as ball markers, who need jumping and catching skills, are tall and more ecto-mesomorphic. Therefore, the spread of body types in Australian football is quite diverse.

AMERICAN FOOTBALL (PROFESSIONAL)

This is a highly specialized and controlled contact sport where player tasks are clearly defined. Linemen, whose task it is to impede or stop the progress of the opposing team members, have high levels of endo-mesomorphy and have an approximate mean somatotype rating of **5.0–7.5–1.0**, from data reported by Carter and Heath (1990). Backfield players on the other hand, who are responsible for the majority of the ball-carrying, passing and defensive tackling, need to be fast and agile. Recent computed data from Carter and Heath (1990) give an approximate body type rating of **3.0–5.5–1.5** for the latter group.

Set Field Sports (Baseball, Cricket, Golf)

Set field sports are generally played in set field positions and therefore do not have the cardiovascular requirements of the more mobile field sports. *Baseball, cricket* and *golf* have very special skill requirements and running speed is also important in the first two. This situation gives rise to a wide spread of body types in these sports in comparison to many others. However, the past 20 years have seen a slight rise in their mesomorphy component, as these athletes have become more concerned about the development of explosive power, which is basically developed by strength and power training. See Table 5.1 for the mean somatotypes in this sport category.

Court Sports

BASKETBALL

The majority of the data on elite male *basketballers* has been gathered on Olympic and amateur players in Europe and North America. As shown in Table 5.1, the mean somatotype of these athletes was **2.0–4.5–3.5** when data reported by Carter and Heath (1990) were computed. The spread of the above players classified them as ecto-mesomorphs, ectomorph–mesomorphs and meso-ectomorphs, which seems perfectly logical when one takes into consideration the different playing positions on the court. Unfortunately almost no data are available on US National Basketball Association professionals, who appear to be larger and slightly more ectomorphic than the above sample. When they examined female basketball players, Carter and Heath (1990) stated that 'there was a large somatotype variation in basketball, partly due to the different functions of the playing positions'. In adult samples the mean female somatotypes were to the left of the somatochart, rating a **4.0–4.0–3.0** body type (Table 5.1).

NETBALL

This is a similar game to basketball, played mainly by females, and limited to the British Commonwealth or countries that at some time were associated with it. Withers *et al.* (1987) found the mean somatotype of players in South Australia to be **3.0–4.0–3.5**, with a spread on the somatochart that accounted for the various player positions. When players in this sport are compared to female basketballers, they have lower levels of endomorphy and higher levels of ectomorphy. However, no logical explanation has yet been given as to why this should be so and whether it is advantageous or not (Table 5.1).

VOLLEYBALL

The distribution of male *volleyball* players covers the range from endo-mesomorphy to meso-ectomorphy, with the majority of the somatotypes being ecto-mesomorphic (Carter & Heath 1990).

The mean rating for high level players is **2.5–4.5–3.5**, which is similar to that for international basketballers. Female volleyball players are reasonably varied in their body types, with an approximate mean somatotype of **3.5–4.0–3.0**, which places them in the central region of the somatochart (Carter & Heath 1990; Table 5.1).

Martial Arts

Those athletes who compete in the various martial arts are highly mesomorphic in somatotype mainly because strength, power, speed and agility are very basic to all of them. However, they do vary in both their endomorphy and ectomorphy ratings according to the weight divisions in which they compete. Table 5.1 gives the various body types for athletes in this category.

JUDO

Male *judoists* at the elite level are predominantly endo-mesomorphs, with the remainder being mainly in the balanced mesomorph region of the somatochart. Their mean somatotype is approximately **2.0–6.5–1.5**; however, if classified by weight, those athletes in the heavyweight classes often rate higher in both mesomorphy and endomorphy, with an ectomorphy rating lower than lighter judoists. On the other hand, females who compete in judo at a high level distribute themselves mainly in the mesomorph–endomorph and central regions, with a mean somatotype of **4.0–4.0–2.0** (Carter & Heath 1990).

WRESTLING

As with other *combative sports*, endomorphy and mesomorphy increase and ectomorphy decreases in the higher weight classes in wrestling (Table 5.1). The lighter wrestlers tend to be balanced mesomorphs and the heavier ones endomesomorphs (Fig. 7.10). Their mean somatotype is **2.5–6.5–1.5**, but they range from **1.5–5.5–2.5** in the under 60 kg class, to **4.0–7.5–1.0** in the heavyweight class (Carter 1984).

BOXING

Boxers demonstrate the same characteristics as wrestlers and judoists with relation to increases in endomorphy and mesomorphy and a decrease in ectomorphy as their weight class increases (Table 5.1). The mean somatotype of this group is approximately **2.0–5.5–2.5**, with a range from **1.5–5.0–3.0** with lighter competitors, to **2.5–6.0–2.0** for heavier boxers (Carter & Heath 1990).

EXCEPTIONS TO THE STANDARD BODY SHAPE AND SIZE

It is not common to find athletes at the state or national level and occasionally at the international level, whose physiques do not appear to be suited to the sport or a specialized event within a sport (Auckland & Bloomfield 1992). One must decide when not to interfere with an individual's body build, and Peter Snell from New Zealand provided a good example of this Phenomenon (Fig. 5.13) Snell was an outstanding middle distance runner, winning gold medals at Tokyo in 1964 for the 800 and 1500 m events, despite the fact that his muscular physique appeared more suited to the 200 m distance. However, with a maximal oxygen uptake ($\dot{V}_{O_2 max}$) of 5.502 L·min^{-1} (73.3 mL·min^{-1}·kg^{-1}), Snell possessed the circulatory capacity to successfully compete in the middle distance events (Pyke & Watson 1978), even though he was carrying much more body mass than his competitors.

More recently, the marathon performances of Robert De Castella (Fig. 5.14) from Australia have interested sport scientists. Between 1981 and 1986 De Castella won six international marathons, including the World Championship in 1983, despite being approximately 5 cm taller than other elite runners and 10–12 kg greater in body mass (R. D. Telford pers. comm. 1990). However, with a $\dot{V}_{O_2 max}$ of 83 mL·min^{-1}·kg^{-1}, he possessed the endurance capacity needed for the marathon event.

When one carefully examines participants in every sport, it is possible to find these 'exceptions to the rule' because of the many factors which make up a championship performance and it is obvious that some champions will succeed des-

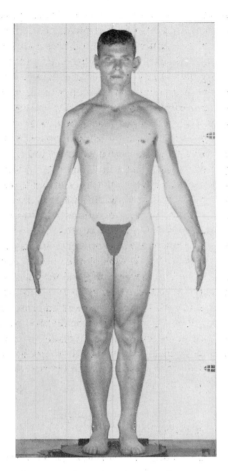

Fig. 5.13 An exception to the standard body type of a world champion 1500 m runner (courtesy of Tanner 1964).

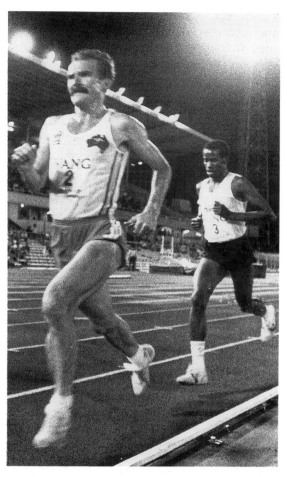

Fig. 5.14 A notable exception to the normal size and body shape of a world champion marathon runner (reproduced by permission of *The Age*, Melbourne).

pite what appears to be an unsuitable body type. With this in mind therefore, coaches should not place too much pressure on their athletes with intervention programmes which are stressful, because somatotype is only one of the general physical capacities. On the other hand, if all the other variables which are needed for a top performance are present, then an almost perfect body type will give competitors an advantage over their opponents.

SPORT SELECTION AND SOMATOTYPE

The term 'self-selection for various sports and events' has been used for a long period of time because physically talented children find they are better at some sports than others. Intelligent coaches also recognize that various physical capacities are important in certain sports and are 'on the lookout' for children who possess them. One of these capacities is body type, because it is well known that an individual with a highly suitable body shape will probably do well in a particular sport. Of the three basic somatotype components, mesomorphy is the most important because strength, explosive power, speed and agility are highly related to this characteristic.

Somatotyping has now reached the stage where there are enough data on junior and senior athletes to enable coaches or sport scientists to predict with some degree of accuracy the most appropriate sport or event for their athletes. One must always be aware however that predictions of this type are not foolproof and if too much emphasis is placed on this variable the athlete and coach may be disappointed. The following statement by Carter and Heath (1990) sums it up well:

> The guidance of coaches, aware of the varying patterns of somatotypic development, is crucial in helping young athletes to discover their aptitudes for particular sports. With the somatotypes of successful athletes for models, the objective is to predict the most likely adult somatotypes, and to estimate the influence of appropriate nutrition and training in modifying the somatotype for optimal performance in the chosen sport.

SOMATOTYPE MODIFICATION

Guidance with diet and exercise can help to modify body type within the limits of the individual's genotype. Athletes should know their somatotype and where they are placed on the somatochart in relation to other high level performers in their sport. If they are within 1 rating of the mean of the group on any of the components, very little modification is needed; however, if they are outside it, an attempt must be made to move them closer to that mean.

In order to modify the body type of the individual, a personal intervention programme should be developed in order to make appropriate changes in one or more of the components. This can be achieved in the following ways:

- *Endomorphy* — athletes may wish to either increase or decrease this component in order to move closer to the mean of their group. Large amounts of complex carbohydrates and some additional protein are needed to increase fat mass (FM). If the athlete wishes to reduce this rating then a low kilojoule diet should be followed in conjunction with endurance training
- *Mesomorphy* — in the majority of cases athletes will wish to increase their mesomorphy rating. This is done by using a low repetition–high resistance strength and power training programme, as outlined in Chapter 9. If competitors wish to reduce their mesomorphy rating, they will find this very difficult to achieve, because testosterone secretions determine the rating in this category to a great extent. However, if no strength and power training are carried out and a low kilojoule diet is accompanied by light endurance training, it may be possible to achieve a slightly lower rating
- *Ectomorphy* — this component can be slightly reduced using a high kilojoule diet and strength and power training. Or conversely, it can also be increased by reducing the kilojoule intake and placing the athlete on an intensive endurance training programme

Junior Athletes

Any efficient talent development programme will cater for young athletes who are at the margins of the various somatotypes that make up a champion sportsperson. (See Chapter 13 for further details.) The same procedure should be followed as the one outlined above, if the competitors wish to change one or more of their somatotype components. However, there is one additional factor which should be taken into account and that is growth during the adolescent period, which was discussed earlier in this chapter. Females should be aware that during adolescence, there is a slight drop in mesomorphy, followed by an increase in endomorphy. Males, on the other hand, will first decrease their mesomorphy rating, then slightly increase their level of ectomorphy. A reversal then occurs which moves the male somatotype back towards the mesomorphic area (Fig. 5.4).

Body type is therefore a variable that must be taken into account in any high quality junior training programme, because its modification can have a significant effect on some athletes. Several examples are available in the literature where at least two, and in some cases three, basic somatotype components have been changed, particularly in males where mesomorphy was an important factor in their success.

CONCLUSION

Body type, although a general physical capacity, can be important to athletes when almost all the other variables that go to make up a high level performance are equal. There are several procedures which can be used to modify the individual's body type, but the most widely used are strength and power training and nutrition. It is also important for the coach to take maturation into account, because it is during this period that hormones can have a significant influence on body type.

REFERENCES

Ackland T. & Bloomfield J. (1992) Functional anatomy. In Bloomfield J., Fricker P. & Fitch K. (eds) *Textbook of Science and Medicine in Sport* p. 4. Blackwell Scientific Publications, Melbourne.

Carter J., Aubry S. & Sleet D. (1982) Somatotypes of Montreal Olympic athletes. In Carter J. (ed.) *Physical Structure of Olympic Athletes Part I*, pp. 53–80. Karger, Basel.

Carter J. (1984) Somatotypes of Olympic athletes from 1948 to 1976. In Carter J. (ed.) *Physical Structure of Olympic Athletes Part II*, pp. 80–109. Karger, Basel.

Carter J. & Heath B. (1990) *Somatotyping — Development and Applications*, pp. 83, 176, 201, 208, 211–218, 220–229, 232–238, 244–258, 261–284, 287. Cambridge University Press, Cambridge.

Carter J. & Marfell-Jones M. (1994) Somatotypes. In Carter J. & Ackland T. (eds) *Kinanthropometry in Aquatic Sports*. Human Kinetics Publishers, Champaign, IL, USA.

De Garay A., Levine L. & Carter J. (1974) *Genetic and Anthropological Studies of Olympic Athletes*, p. 39. Academic Press, New York.

Heath B. & Carter J. (1967) A modified somatotype method. *American Journal of Physical Anthropology* **27**, 57–74.

Hebbelinck M., Carter J. & De Garay A. (1975) Body build and somatotype of Olympic swimmers, divers and water polo players. In Lewillie L. & Clarys J. (eds) *Swimming II*, pp. 285–305. University Park Press, Baltimore.

Hebbelinck M., Ross W., Carter J. & Borms, J. (1980) Anthropometric characteristics of female Olympic rowers. *Canadian Journal of Applied Sport Sciences* **5**, 255–262.

Malina R. & Bouchard C. (1991) *Growth, Maturation and Physical Activity*, pp. 83–85. Human Kinetics Books, Champaign, IL, USA.

Mészáros J. & Mohácsi J. (1982) The somatotype of Hungarian male and female class I paddlers and rowers. *Anthropologiai Közlemények* **26**, 175–179.

Parnell R. (1958) *Behaviour and Physique*, pp. 4–35. Edward Arnold, London.

Pyke F. & Watson G. (1978) *Focus on Running*, pp. 47–48. Pelham Books, London.

Ross W., Brown S., Yu, J. & Faulkner R. (1977) Somatotypes of Canadian figure skaters. *Journal of Sports Medicine and Physical Fitness* **17**, 195–205.

Sheldon W., Stevens S. & Tucker W. (1940) *The Varieties of Human Physique*, pp. 37–46. Harper and Brothers, New York.

Sheldon W. (1954) *Atlas of Men*, pp. 11–22. Harper and Brothers, New York.

Štěpnička J. (1974) Typology of sportsmen. *Acta Universitatis Carolinae Gymnica* **1**, 67–90.

Štěpnička J. (1986) Somatotype in relation to physical performance, sports and body posture. In Reilly T., Watkins J. & Borms J. (eds) *Kinanthropometry III*, pp. 39–52. Spon, London.

Tanner J. (1964) *The Physique of the Olympic Athlete*, pp. 112–113. George Allen and Unwin, London.

White J., Quinn G., Al-Dawalibi M. & Mulhall J. (1982) Seasonal changes in cyclists' performance. Part 1, the British Olympic road race squad. *British Journal of Sports Medicine* **16**, 4–12.

Withers R., Craig N. & Norton K. (1986) Somatotypes of South Australian male athletes. *Human Biology* **58**, 337–356.

Withers R., Wittingham N., Norton K. & Dutton M. (1987) Somatotypes of South Australian female games players. *Human Biology* **59**, 575–589.

CHAPTER 6

BODY COMPOSITION IN SPORT

In seeking to understand the interrelationships between the magnitude of various tissue compartments within the body and their influence on human performance, researchers have been hampered with problems of mixed terminology, poor or non-standardized measurement protocols, and the difficulty of distinguishing the environmental influence of training from the effect of genetic inheritance.

These limitations will be addressed in this chapter and in Section 3, where the factors affecting body composition and the techniques for assessing this capacity are discussed. Further, the relationship between body composition and performance will be examined for a number of sports, and various means of modifying the component tissues will be discussed.

In the literature on human body composition there exists an abundance of interrelated terminology and methods of partitioning the body into fundamental components. Many authors favour an anatomical separation of the body into compartments such as adipose tissue, bone, muscle, organs and extracellular fluid, while others suggest dividing the body into fluid–mineral divisions such as extracellular fluid, intracellular fluid and solids. In order to simplify the above, a two-compartment model has been adopted by researchers for ease of parameter estimation. These compartments have been termed the lean body mass (LBM) and fat mass (FM).

For the purpose of this chapter, an anatomical partitioning of the body will be used in dis-

cussions of body composition. With respect to body composition assessment, reference to FM will be taken to include all components of adipose tissue (lipid plus cellular matrix) and LBM will be employed to describe all other tissues not included in FM.

FACTORS AFFECTING BODY COMPOSITION

A number of factors affect the size, mass and structure of each of the anatomical compartments of the human body. These may be broadly classified as:

- *Genetic* — the influence of heredity
- *Hormonal* — the variable influences of secretions from the endocrine glands
- *Environmental* — the additional influences such as exercise, training, nutrition and emotional stress

In the following section the effects of growth, age, gender and exercise will be examined for the various tissue compartments.

Adipose Tissue

Adipose tissue fulfils many roles within the human body, as it is a site for the storage of lipids and a means for providing insulation, thermogenesis and energy. A strong genetic effect has been reported by Brook *et al.* (1975) who suggested that the tendency towards fatness among the population may be an inheritable trait. This genetic influence however, may be overridden by strong environmental forces such as diet and intensive exercise (Brook 1978).

CHANGES IN ADIPOSE TISSUE DURING GROWTH

Typical growth in adipose tissue (Fig. 6.1) includes a period of rapid increase in the first year and a half of life, in which the tissue reaches a maximum level of approximately 20% of total body mass. This percentage decreases during childhood in response to the body's increased energy requirements for growth and movement, then reaches a plateau just prior to adolescence. It should be understood that the absolute amount of adipose tissue actually increases during this period (Marshall 1978); however, when viewed in rela-

tion to the change in total body mass, a decrease in relative composition results.

During pubertal growth the gain in adipose tissue drops markedly for both males and females in response to an increase in energy requirements. The absolute level of adipose tissue may even decline for males between the ages of 15 and 17 years (Marshall 1978). This growth phenomenon has the effect of sharply lowering the proportion of adipose tissue in relation to total mass (Fig. 6.1).

Following the adolescent growth spurt in size, the typical development of the adipose tissue compartment differs for males and females. While absolute tissue gains are reported for both sexes, the increasing deposition of fat among females is much more marked than for males. As a result, the percentage of adipose tissue with respect to total mass increases sharply for females, whereas among

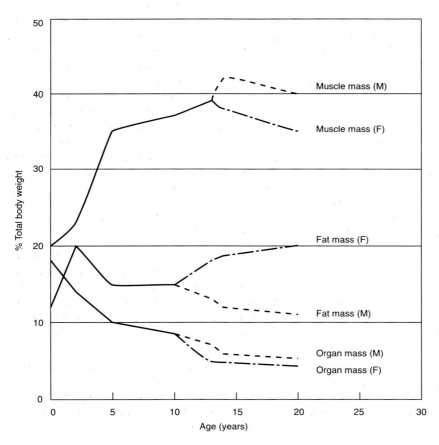

Fig. 6.1 Body composition changes during growth (adapted from data reported by Holliday 1978). M = males; F = females.

males the influence of a rapidly developing musculoskeletal system predominates, so that no net change in the proportion of adipose tissue occurs.

After the attainment of adult status when the energy demands for growth have diminished, the influence of environmental factors such as nutrition and exercise play a most important role. Generally, among adult women skinfold thicknesses steadily increase up to age 60 and then decline again (Wessel *et al.* 1963). For the adult male, the proportion of body fat remains fairly constant; however, a redistribution of fat has been observed (Norris *et al.* 1963) whereby relative gains were noted for the trunk region.

EFFECT OF NUTRITION ON ADIPOSE TISSUE

The influence of nutrition on the amount of adipose tissue is clearly documented, especially for over- and under-nourished populations. There exists a greater variation in body fat among the population at all stages of growth than for other tissue compartments. Short-term changes in nutrition appear to be accommodated by modification of the size of the adipose tissue cell, as the store of lipids reacts to the balance between energy intake and usage. However, long-term stresses of over- and under-nutrition would appear to alter the number as well as the size of adipose tissue cells. Salans *et al.* (1973) reported that there were two distinct periods in life during which excessive feeding may lead to hypercellularity of the adipose tissue. These periods were in the first year of life and again between 9 and 13 years of age.

EFFECT OF EXERCISE ON ADIPOSE TISSUE

Exercise plays an influential role in modifying the amount of adipose tissue an individual has because of the increasing requirement for energy it creates; however, it is clear that the amount and intensity of activity is of critical importance to the resulting effect. Moody *et al.* (1972) reported no change in body composition among girls with a mean age of 16.5 years, despite a 15 week programme of walking and jogging. Conversely, Wells *et al.* (1963) showed a significant reduction in fat

for a group of 34 adolescent girls, who were subjected to daily physical training for a 5 month period. Further discussion of the roles of nutrition and exercise in the modification of body composition is contained later in this chapter.

Muscle Tissue

CHANGES IN MUSCLE TISSUE DURING GROWTH

The composite data reported in Holliday (1978) showed that muscle mass increased from 20% of total body mass in the newborn, up to 35% at 5 years of age (Fig. 6.1). The major increase in muscle mass occurs particularly from 1.5 to 5 years and corresponds to a shift in energy requirements from growth to greater activity levels.

A second growth spurt in muscle mass occurs during the adolescent growth period and is consistent with this time of increased activity and food consumption. Muscle mass reaches a level of greater than 40% of total body mass in adult males, while for females the maximum level of about 39% is achieved during adolescence. However, this value declines at full maturity for females to about 37%, due to the rapid increase in adipose tissue growth at this time. Malina (1978) argued that these adult values are somewhat deflated since they are derived from elderly cadaver dissections. He suggested that the true proportion of muscle mass to total body mass would be more in the order of 45% for the adult male.

EFFECT OF ENVIRONMENTAL FACTORS ON MUSCLE TISSUE

This template for growth may be further affected by environmental factors such as physical activity and nutrition. Increased physical activity results in hypertrophy of muscle, but the intensity of the work is the critical factor. This hypertrophy is accompanied by increases in the number of myofibrils (Fig. 9.4), that is, the cross-sectional area of the muscle fibre, as well as by an increase in strength. Good nutrition and in particular, the availability of protein in the diet, are important factors for muscle hypertrophy. These relationships will be dealt with in more detail in Chapter 9.

Bone Tissue

CHANGES IN BONE TISSUE DURING GROWTH

The longitudinal growth of the human skeleton has usually occurred by early adulthood. That is, the process of ossification of long and short bones is completed and no more increase in bone length will occur after the epiphyseal growth plates have closed. Bone will, however, continue to adapt to the environmental stresses placed upon it by changing in width, mineral density and internal architecture.

EFFECT OF EXERCISE ON BONE TISSUE

Exercise is known to cause an increase in bone density, while inactivity leads to its decline. Buskirk *et al.* (1956) observed, for example, that the bones of the dominant forearm and hand of tennis players were more robust than those in the non-dominant limb and similar phenomena have been seen with athletes in other unilateral sports (Fig. 8.8). This suggests that bone growth had responded positively to the increase in imposed forces. Nilsson and Westlin (1971) reported that young adult athletes possessed greater bone densities compared to non-athletes. Furthermore, the greatest bone density values were generally found for those athletes in whom the lower limbs were typically subjected to heavy loads.

Several reports emanating from some Eastern European countries prior to 1990, suggested that pre-adolescent and adolescent weightlifters were being subjected to intensive training with heavy loads so that an increase in the bone density of their legs would occur. Not only would this improve their base of support for lifting, but it would also compact the epiphyseal growth plates, thus keeping the legs a little shorter than they might otherwise have been.

Research by Abramson (1948) and Donaldson *et al.* (1970) showed that inactivity due to prolonged bed rest or enforced immobilization due to limb casting causes an increased urinary excretion of calcium leading to a decalcification of bone. This process may be reversed on the resumption of normal activity; however, the attainment of pretreatment levels of bone mineral content requires more than 12 months of reconditioning (Kottke 1966).

BODY COMPOSITION ASSESSMENT

Fat is deposited at a variety of sites in the body. Some of it appears to play an essential role in human function, while the majority is seen as an excess beyond normal requirements. This excess fat may be deposited internally in storage sites such as the greater omentum, within the pericardial sac or as epiploic appendages on the intestine. Superficially, fat is deposited in a subcutaneous layer of varying thickness throughout the body.

In the assessment of body composition, scientists and clinicians are normally interested in estimates of the fat compartment relative to the amount of lean body tissue; however, more recently, estimates of skeletal and muscle compartments have become possible. Regardless of the method used, the total mass of all fat deposition sites must be accounted for. The only truly direct method available to date is that of cadaver dissection. Although limited in sample, the cadaver dissection studies (Clarys *et al.* 1984) provide valuable criteria against which other indirect methods can be validated. It is only through appropriate validation studies using results of this direct method, that one may assess the accuracy and applicability of proposed *in vivo* techniques. Unfortunately, very few techniques have been evaluated in this manner and therefore the validity of the others remains questionable.

The indirect methodologies may be classified into one of five groups: weight for height indices; densitometry; skinfolds; tissue fractionation models; and other techniques. A full discussion of the problems associated with the assessment techniques and the application of raw data, together with specific test protocols, is presented in Section 3.

BODY COMPOSITION AND SPORT PERFORMANCE

Since the 1960s a glut of information has become available on the body compositional requirements for various sports and events, or positions within those sports. This interest in body composition has flourished as coaches and athletes observed that success not only demands a particular physique but also a certain ratio of LBM to FM. However, extreme caution is required before there is wholesale application of this information, because of the great variation in data collection and treatment methods. A lack of standardization of techniques and sampling sites in the past, together with the use of a variety of data treatment strategies, has meant that pooling of some of the results for profiling and comparative purposes cannot be done with any real accuracy.

In the following section an attempt will be made to relate the current knowledge in the field to athletic performance in a number of different sports. Where available, only data for the sum of skinfolds or body density from hydrostatic weighing will be presented for the various sport categories. Other sources which report values for per cent body fat or estimates of body density from anthropometry are disregarded, for reasons which will be outlined in Section 3. Although this severely limits the volume of available reference data, at least the reader can be confident that the values have been collected and treated in a manner which limits the adoption of spurious assumptions. Unless otherwise indicated, data are presented for national or international class athletes.

Racquet Sports

Limited body composition data exist for racquet sports. Vodak *et al.* (1980) reported the sum of six skinfolds for male and female recreational *tennis* players (Table 6.1); however, these results are relatively high and would certainly not reflect the body composition characteristics of professional players. A mean sum of seven skinfolds was reported by Pipes (1979) to be 71.8 mm for professional *racquetball* players, which also appears somewhat higher than values expected for this sport.

Aquatic Sports

Data from the Kinanthropometric Aquatic Sports Project (KASP); (Carter & Ackland 1994) were used

to provide results for the *swimmers* and *waterpolo* players in Table 6.1.

Among the swimmers, little difference was shown in body size between sprint distance and middle distance performers, but the latter had smaller skinfold thicknesses. This leaner composition for the 800 and 1500 m competitors probably reflected the need for economy of motion among the middle distance swimmers, compared to the dominance of muscular power development for the sprinters. Competitors in the 25 km open water event (long distance) were significantly smaller than the sprinters, but possessed a much greater amount of fat. In this event the extra fat would assist the swimmer's buoyancy, as well as providing thermal insulation which would protect the swimmer from hypothermia.

Waterpolo players, both male and female, possess higher levels of body fat than most swimmers, however they are generally larger in stature and body mass, and as a result this extra fat is also accompanied by greater amounts of lean tissue. In relative terms, waterpolo players possess a greater proportion of body fat than swimmers and this may provide them with added buoyancy and extra protection against body contact during the game.

Body fat values for *rowers* are influenced by the type of event, with lightweight crew members having lower scores than the heavyweights (Hagerman *et al.* 1979). All rowers possess high levels of lean body tissue due to the power output demands of the sport, while little difference in body composition exists between sweep oar and sculling competitors (Telford *et al.* 1988).

Competitors in *canoeing* and *kayaking* possess low levels of body fat as demonstrated in Table 6.1, while the results of Telford *et al.* (1988) show marathon paddlers to be leaner than their slalom and sprint counterparts.

Gymnastic and Power Sports

Data from the Montreal Olympic Games Anthropological Project (MOGAP) and KASP studies (Carter 1982; Carter & Ackland 1994) are shown in Table 6.2 for *gymnasts* and *divers*. Both groups

Table 6.1 Body composition characteristics in racquet and aquatic sports

Group	Males					Females				
	n	Age (years)	Mass (kg)	SUMSF (mm)	D (g/mL)	n	Age (years)	Mass (kg)	SUMSF (mm)	D (g/mL)
RACQUET SPORTS Tennis Recreational (Vodak *et al.* 1980)	25	42.0	77.1	86.0*	—	25	39.0	55.7	87.8	—
Racquetball Professional (Pipes 1979)	10	25.0	80.3	71.8†	1.080					
AQUATIC SPORTS Swimming SD‡	187	—	78.7	47.0*	—	133	20.0	63.1	70.8	—
MD	10	—	74.3	41.8	—	6	19.3	63.5	62.3	—
LD (Carter & Ackland 1994)	13	21.8	78.1	60.3	—	10	22.8	62.2	104.6	—
Waterpolo All positions (Carter & Ackland 1994)	190	25.2	86.1	62.5*	—	109	23.7	64.8	89.8	—
Rowing All groups (Carter 1982)	65	24.2	90.0	49.5*	—	51	23.8	67.4	75.2	—
Sweep oar	39	—	87.3	54.7§	—	30	—	71.4	93.5**	
Sculling (Telford *et al.* 1988)	16	—	86.8	53.7	—	8	—	73.8	88.5	—
Canoeing All events (Carter 1982)	12	25.1	79.1	37.1*	—	8	20.6	63.0	75.3	—
Kayaking White water (Sidney & Shephard 1973)	10	23.0	68.6	22.7††	—	2	18.0	57.3	28.0	—
Marathon	10	—	74.6	40.1§	—	4	—	67.8	76.8**	—
Slalom	14	—	68.7	45.3	—	5	—	58.0	83.1	—
Sprint (Telford *et al.* 1988)	21	—	78.6	47.4	—					

* SUMSF = sum of triceps, subscapular, supraspinale, abdominal, thigh and calf skinfolds.
† SUMSF = sum of triceps, subscapular, supraspinale, abdominal, thigh, calf and axilla skinfolds.
‡ SD (short distance) = 50, 100 and 200 m competitors in FR (freestyle), BK (backstroke), BR (breast-stroke) and FL (butterfly); MD (middle distance) = 1500 m FR for males and 800 m FR for females; LD (long distance) = 25 km open water swim.
§ SUMSF = sum of triceps, biceps, subscapular, supraspinale, abdominal, thigh, calf and axilla skinfolds.
** SUMSF = sum of triceps, biceps, subscapular, supraspinale, abdominal, thigh and calf skinfolds.
†† SUMSF = sum of triceps, subscapular and supraspinale skinfolds.
D = density.

Table 6.2 Body composition characteristics in gymnastic and track and field sports

Group		Males					Females			
	n	Age (years)	Mass (kg)	SUMSF (mm)	D (g/mL)	n	Age (years)	Mass (kg)	SUMSF (mm)	D (g/mL)
GYMNASTIC SPORTS										
Gymnastics										
All events (Carter & Ackland 1994)	11	25.4	63.5	32.9*	—	15	17.0	50.9	49.4	—
Diving										
All events (Carter 1982)	43	22.2	66.7	45.9*	—	39	20.9	53.7	65.6	—
TRACK AND FIELD										
All athletes (Carter 1982)	40	23.8	73.4	37.4*	—	34	21.8	57.2	56.8	—
Track events										
Distance runners (Costill et al. 1970)	114	26.1	64.2	31.4†						
Distance runners						12	19.9	53.0	42.0‡	—
Sprinters (Malina et al. 1971)						24	20.1	57.1	44.0	
Sprinters	22	—	73.9	41.6§	—	5	—	64.5	66.5**	—
Middle distance	8	—	69.9	37.7	—	7	—	57.9	62.8	—
Long distance	13	—	64.9	39.0	—					
Walkers (Telford et al. 1988)	3	—	69.5	33.7	—	4	—	59.6	68.5	—
Field events										
Pentathletes (Krahenbuhl et al. 1979)						9	21.5	65.4	90.8†	
Throwers (Brown & Wilmore 1974)						7	—	78.6	102.8††	—
Jumpers						11	20.3	59.0	49.0††	—
Discus and javelin						10	21.1	71.1	64.0	—
Shot putters (Malina et al. 1971)						9	21.5	77.0	86.0	—
Jumpers	8	—	75.1	56.8§	—	6	—	62.7	56.8**	—
Throwers (Telford et al. 1988)	12	—	103.5	107.2	—	8	—	85.2	135.0	—

* SUMSF = sum of triceps, subscapular, supraspinale, abdominal, thigh and calf skinfolds.
† SUMSF = sum of triceps, subscapular, abdominal, thigh and calf skinfolds.
‡ SUMSF = sum of triceps, biceps, subscapular and supraspinale skinfolds.
§ SUMSF = sum of triceps, biceps, subscapular, supraspinale, abdominal, thigh, calf and axilla skinfolds.
** SUMSF = sum of triceps, biceps, subscapular, supraspinale, abdominal, thigh and calf skinfolds.
†† SUMSF = sum of triceps, subscapular, supraspinale, abdominal and thigh skinfolds.
D = density.

have low levels of body fat compared to other sports, with the gymnasts possessing particularly low skinfold scores due to the weight-supportive nature of their sport. Female divers are generally older than gymnasts and this would probably account for most of the difference in the sum of their skinfolds. No differences were found between competitors in the three diving events (1 and 3 m springboard, or 10 m platform) at the 1991 World Championships (Carter & Ackland 1994).

While no suitable body composition data could be found for *weightlifting*, it is possible to make an observation based on the somatotype data in Table 5.1. As the weight class of male lifters increases from 60.0 to 99.9 kg, the average endomorphy rating rises from 1.5 to 2.5. This indicates a gradual increase in proportional fat mass. However, for the lifters who weigh >100.0 kg, the endomorphy rating jumps to 5.0. No longer does the lifter need to make a weight limit and so the proportion of body fat is greater than for other lifters since he does not need to restrict his kilojoule intake. It should be noted that this additional mass gives the lifter a greater base of support, which is essential if *very heavy* weights are to be lifted.

Track, Field and Cycling

Combined values for track and field athletes who participated in the MOGAP study (Carter 1982) are shown in Table 6.2. However, this treatment of the data masks the differences shown for track events of varying length by Costill *et al.* (1970), Malina *et al.* (1971) and Telford *et al.* (1988). *Sprinters* possess the greatest sum of skinfold scores of all track athletes, reflecting the importance of muscular power generation as opposed to economy of motion in these events. This is in contrast to the lower fat levels possessed by the *middle* and *long distance runners*, who rely on movement economy for success in their events.

Among the *field event* performers (Table 6.2), the *jumpers* have the lowest levels of body fat (Malina *et al.* 1971; Telford *et al.* 1988). The throwers typically have higher levels of fat, since this does not hinder their performance (Brown &

Wilmore 1974; Telford *et al.* 1988). Within this group however, the javelin and discus throwers are generally leaner than the shot putters (Malina *et al.* 1971).

Telford *et al.* (1988) also provided body fatness information for Australian *cyclists* (Table 6.3). No significant differences were shown between male road cyclists and male track cyclists for the sum of eight skinfolds (46.4 and 48.1 mm, respectively). Female cyclists however, recorded a mean sum of seven skinfolds of 74.9 mm.

Mobile Field Sports

Limited data exist for the mobile field sports at the international level. In Table 6.3 the mean sum of six skinfolds from male *field hockey* participants in the MOGAP study (Carter 1982) was reported as 55.1 mm. This value appears to have significantly decreased over the past half decade, as Telford *et al.* (1988) reported the mean sum of eight skinfolds for Australian players to be 49.1 mm. Even women players averaged only 71.1 mm for the sum of seven skinfolds in this study. Such a vast difference in scores probably reflects the more intensive training which is now part of the professional approach adopted in the preparation of recent Australian hockey teams.

Davis *et al.* (1992) reported body composition information for English professional *soccer* players with respect to playing position. The goalkeepers had a greater sum of four skinfolds compared to other positional players, reflecting their relatively stationary role compared to the mobile nature of the other players. Centre backs were heavier than other positional players, yet their average sum of skinfolds was of similar magnitude, suggesting that they possessed more lean body mass.

Contact Field Sports

Three codes of football are represented in contact field sports and differences in body composition are clearly evident among the positional players in some codes. In *Australian football*, the difference in fatness between set position players and

Table 6.3 Body composition characteristics in cycling and mobile field sports

Group	Males					Females				
	n	Age (years)	Mass (kg)	SUMSF (mm)	D (g/mL)	n	Age (years)	Mass (kg)	SUMSF (mm)	D (g/mL)
CYCLING										
Road	15	—	73.7	46.4*	—					
Track	12	—	75.8	48.1	—	9	—	57.9	74.9[†]	—
(Telford et al. 1988)										
MOBILE FIELD SPORTS										
Field hockey										
All positions	33	25.3	70.4	55.1[‡]	—					
(Carter 1982)										
All positions	17	—	75.9	49.1*	—	16	—	61.8	71.1[†]	
(Telford et al. 1988)										
Soccer										
Goalkeepers	13	26.7	86.1	28.3[§]	—					
Full backs	22	23.5	75.4	23.7	—					
Centre backs	24	24.0	83.3	23.6	—					
Midfielders	35	24.7	73.2	23.4	—					
Forwards	41	23.1	76.4	22.4	—					
Outfielders	122	23.8	77.1	23.2	—					
(Davis et al. 1992)										

* SUMSF = sum of triceps, biceps, subscapular, supraspinale, abdominal, thigh, calf and axilla skinfolds.
[†] SUMSF = sum of triceps, biceps, subscapular, supraspinale, abdominal, thigh and calf skinfolds.
[‡] SUMSF = sum of triceps, subscapular, supraspinale, abdominal, thigh and calf skinfolds.
[§] SUMSF = sum of triceps, biceps, subscapular and iliac crest skinfolds.
 D = density.

mobile players (Ackland et al. 1984) was not significant (Table 6.4), whereas the backs in *rugby* were leaner and lighter than the forwards (Maud & Shultz 1984). These scores accurately reflected the evasive running versus the rucking and mauling roles of these players, respectively.

In *American football*, where the role of players is more strictly defined than in the other two codes, body composition differences between backfield players and linemen are more extreme. Wilmore et al. (1976) reported values of 70–94 mm for the sum of seven skinfolds for backs (Table 6.4), compared to values in excess of 120 mm for linemen. Similar differences were also reported by Wickkiser and Kelly (1975) for college-level players. Extra body fat may be advantageous for linemen as it increases their inertia, thus enhancing their ability to block the progression of their opponent.

Set Field Sports

Coleman (1981) described the body composition of US major league *baseball* players with respect to their fielding position. While few differences were noted in body mass between positions, pitchers possessed the highest level of body fat, with infielders having the next highest sum of three skinfolds. Baseball is not a sport which relies on aerobic fitness or economy of movement for successful participation and this is reflected in the mean scores shown in Table 6.5.

Court Sports

Data exist for two sports at the national and international level in court sports. Professional male *basketball* players were studied by Parr et al.

Table 6.4 Body composition characteristics in contact field sports

		Males					Females			
Group	n	Age (years)	Mass (kg)	SUMSF (mm)	D (g/mL)	n	Age (years)	Mass (kg)	SUMSF (mm)	D (g/mL)
AUSTRALIAN FOOTBALL										
Set position	93	20.7	81.3	35.5*	—					
Followers	96	21.2	78.7	36.0	—					
Ruckmen	12	23.1	92.7	37.5	—					
Field umpires	18	29.2	74.5	48.6	—					
Boundary umpires	18	25.9	71.9	33.5	—					
(Ackland et al. 1984)										
RUGBY										
All players	20	28.1	—	—	—					
Forwards	10	—	94.4	33.6†	—					
Backs	10	—	78.2	27.5	—					
(Maud & Shultz 1984)										
AMERICAN FOOTBALL										
Professional										
All positions	29	26.8	96.1	—	1.0900					
(Adams et al. 1982)										
Defensive backs	26	24.5	84.8	70.5‡	1.770					
Offensive backs and receivers	40	24.7	90.7	83.2	1.0774					
Linebacks	28	24.2	102.2	93.7	1.0668					
Offensive linemen and tight ends	38	24.7	112.6	133.9	1.0631					
Defensive linemen	32	25.7	117.1	119.1	1.0572					
Quarterbacks and kickers	16	24.1	90.1	117.5	1.0659					
(Wilmore et al. 1976)										
College										
Defensive backs	15	—	77.3	—	1.0736					
Offensive backs and receivers	15	—	79.8	—	1.0714					
Linebacks	7	—	82.7	—	1.0687					
Offensive linemen and tight ends	13	—	99.2	—	1.0549					
Defensive linemen	15	—	97.8	—	1.0561					
(Wickkiser & Kelly 1975)										

* SUMSF = sum of triceps, subscapular, supraspinale and abdominal skinfolds.

† SUMSF = sum of triceps, abdominal and chest skinfolds.

‡ SUMSF = sum of triceps, subscapular, supraspinale, abdominal, thigh, axilla and chest skinfolds.

D = density.

(1978), who reported low values for the sum of six skinfolds (Table 6.5). These scores are particularly significant when the size of the player is taken into account. However, the difference shown in Table 6.5 between centres when they were compared to forwards and guards, may be due to the small sample and should not be interpreted as a selection characteristic.

Among national level basketballers, Piechaczek (1990) and Telford et al. (1988) showed that female players possessed higher levels of body fat than their male counterparts.

Puhl et al. (1982) reported body density values for national level *volleyball* players. The male competitors were similar in body density to professional basketballers, but the women volleyball

Table 6.5 Body composition characteristics in set field sports, court sports and the martial arts

Group	n	Males Age (years)	Mass (kg)	SUMSF (mm)	D (g/mL)	n	Females Age (years)	Mass (kg)	SUMSF (mm)	D (g/mL)
SET FIELD SPORTS										
Baseball										
Pitchers	56	26.7	89.8	49.9*	—					
Infield	50	27.4	83.2	39.9	—					
Outfield	30	28.3	85.6	34.0	—					
(Coleman 1981)										
COURT SPORTS										
Basketball										
Professional										
Centres	1	27.7	109.2	37.5†	1.0829					
Forwards	7	25.3	96.9	61.5	1.0784					
Guards	5	25.2	83.6	60.2	1.0747					
(Parr *et al.* 1978)										
College										
All positions						14	19.1	62.6	—	1.0506
(Sinning 1973)										
National team										
All positions	29	—	90.5	29.4‡	—	26	—	70.2	37.1	—
(Piechaczek 1990)										
National team										
All positions	12	—	99.2	67.1§	—	36	—	68.7	83.7**	—
(Telford *et al.* 1988)										
Volleyball										
National level	8	26.1	85.5	—	1.0724	14	21.6	70.5	—	1.0577
(Puhl *et al.* 1982)										
College level						10	20.5	61.0	—	1.0543
(Kovaleski *et al.* 1980)										
MARTIAL ARTS										
Judo										
All competitors	13	23.4	76.5	44.1†	—					
(Carter 1982)										
Wrestling										
All competitors	15	22.5	82.2	51.1†	—					
(Carter 1982)										

* SUMSF = sum of triceps, abdominal and chest skinfolds.
† SUMSF = sum of triceps, subscapular, supraspinale, abdominal, thigh and calf skinfolds.
‡ Reported sites ambiguous. Assume SUMSF = sum of triceps, subscapular and abdominal skinfolds.
§ SUMSF = sum of triceps, biceps, subscapular, supraspinale, abdominal, thigh and calf skinfolds.
** SUMSF = sum of triceps, biceps, subscapular, supraspinale, abdominal, thigh, calf and axilla skinfolds.
    D = density.

players were leaner than female college basket-ballers (Sinning 1973).

Martial Arts

Olympic competitors in the sports of *judo* and *wrestling* were measured in the MOGAP study (Carter 1982). Unfortunately, due to limited sample sizes, the results for these competitors were pooled (Table 6.5). Therefore, it was not possible from these data to observe the differences which exist in body composition for the athletes who must meet a weight criterion, compared to the open competitors. However, data that have been collected on the somatotypes of Olympic martial arts athletes (Table 5.1) show an identical trend to those of weightlifters. That is, endomorphy increases very gradually for those competitors in the weight classes, but when there is no weight limit it increases rapidly.

MODIFYING BODY COMPOSITION

Body composition can be altered by diet, strenuous exercise or a combination of both, which will affect the relative proportions of bone, muscle and fat in the individual. Many athletes are highly conscious of their current body composition status and often undertake dietary regimens to modify this capacity. Whether the aim is to increase or decrease total body mass, LBM or FM, increased knowledge of the degree of modification which can be safely made will ultimately assist the coach to improve the performance of athletes. In addition, the many strategies that may be adopted to achieve this modification need to be assessed in terms of their safety, the effects they have on performance and their effectiveness in achieving the desired goal.

The data presented in the previous section should serve as a guide to the body compositional requirements for each sport. However, many individuals will compete successfully in certain sports despite possessing a body composition which varies from the average. The athlete or coach should not attempt to categorically match these values, especially if the modification regimen affects other facets of the athlete's make-up and becomes detrimental to his or her performance.

Reducing Fat

A reduction in levels of body fat may be achieved by modifying both dietary intake and energy expenditure. Athletes should plan and implement this strategy over a period of several months, rather than succumbing to the temptation to try a 'crash diet'. By reducing the energy intake and increasing aerobic activity levels, the body can draw upon its fat reserves to meet the increased demand for energy. Brukner and Khan (1993) suggest that a realistic goal for safe weight loss is 0.5–1.0 kg per week.

HIGH PROTEIN–LOW CARBOHYDRATE DIETS

According to Brukner and Khan (1993), the body responds to these diets by breaking down glycogen stores and by losing water. Although a reduction in weight will occur, much of the loss will be from the lean body tissues, which may in turn have a detrimental influence on performance.

HIGH CARBOHYDRATE AND FIBRE–LOW FAT AND SUGAR DIETS

This type of diet is generally prescribed for athletes who wish to reduce fat levels, provided adequate amounts of protein and minerals are retained. Athletes are encouraged by Kerr (1993) to avoid fried foods, pastries, take-away foods, oils, cream and snack foods. Instead, carbohydrates in the form of bread, pasta and rice should be maintained at a level which meets the body's requirements for glycogen replacement.

FASTING

Abstaining from food is a strategy often used by athletes as a quick solution to the problem of excess fat. Weight is generally lost, but the loss will occur for lean as well as adipose tissue. In addition, the associated loss of water and severe lack of energy will significantly impair performance.

Gaining Weight

For many athletes an increase in LBM is desirable to improve their performance and, contrary to the opinion of some proponents, this may be achieved without the need for drug therapy. Telford *et al.* (1988) identified three key steps for success in this process and these are as follows:

- Create the correct stimulus. Schmidtbleicher (1986) recommended that training with medium weights and employing a medium to high number of repetitions is best for stimulating muscle hypertrophy. (See Chapter 9 for further discussion on this topic)
- Supply sufficient energy in the form of complex carbohydrates, protein and other nutrients. This process will probably include the need to consume more food than usual
- Provide adequate rest and time for recovery and repair of lean tissue

On a cautionary note, there are a number of commercially available substances such as protein powders and amino acid supplements, as well as banned substances including human growth hormone and anabolic steroids, that have varying effects upon this process. According to Brukner and Khan (1993) no evidence exists to support the claims that ingestion of high quantities of protein or amino acids leads to greater gains in muscular strength. Excess protein, for example, will merely be converted to triglycerides and stored as fat in the adipose tissue.

Making Weight

For many athletes, the trauma of making a weight category dominates their preparation for an event, but this process is rarely managed well. Often athletes undergo last minute dehydration in order to lower total body mass to the required level and this may compromise their performance to some degree. An overview of aids for achieving short-term weight loss is provided by Brukner and Khan (1993), where the effectiveness of appetite suppressants, diuretics, amino acids, saunas and so forth are discussed.

According to Telford *et al.* (1988), weightlifters are least affected by the practice of dehydrating prior to the event, whereas the endurance-oriented class athletes such as rowers, wrestlers, boxers and judoists are most affected. Further, the risk of compromising performance by the adoption of this practice is greatest when the weigh-in is close to the time of the event.

A better management strategy is to reduce body fat levels well before the event and maximize LBM within the weight limit. This process requires constant body composition assessment to monitor each tissue compartment and will allow the athlete to enter the event in peak physical and mental condition. Effective methods for monitoring body composition are outlined and discussed in Section 3.

CONCLUSION

Like other physical capacities such as muscular strength and power, the body composition status of an athlete may be easily modified in order to enhance performance. The relative amounts of fat, muscle and skeletal tissue affect the athlete's ability to perform effectively in weight-supported versus weight-supportive events and in power versus endurance events. Modification of this capacity can be strictly administered and accurately monitored through changes in diet and exercise regimens.

REFERENCES

Abramson A. (1948) Atrophy of disuse. *Archives of Physical Medicine* **29**, 562–570.

Ackland T., Dawson B. & Roberts C. (1984) Pre-season fitness profiles of Australian football players and umpires. *Sports Coach* **8**, 43–48.

Adams J., Mottola M., Bagnall K. & McFadden K. (1982) Total body fat content in a group of professional football players. *Canadian Journal of Applied Sport Science* **7**, 36–40.

Brook C. (1978) Cellular growth: Adipose tissue. In Falkner F., & Tanner J. (eds) *Human Growth Vol. 2*, pp. 21–33. Baillière Tindall, London.

Brook C., Huntley R. & Slack J. (1975) The influence of heredity and environment in determination of skinfold thickness in children. *British Medical Journal* **2**, 719.

Brown C. & Wilmore J. (1974) The effects of maximal resistance training on the strength and body composition of women athletes. *Medicine and Science in Sports* **6**, 174–177.

Brukner P. & Khan K. (1993) *Clinical Sports Medicine*, pp. 493–498. McGraw-Hill, Sydney.

Buskirk E., Andersen K. & Brozek J. (1956) Unilateral activity and bone and muscle development in the forearm. *The Research Quarterly for Exercise and Sport* **27**, 127–131.

Carter J. (1982) *Physical Structure of Olympic Athletes: Part 1, The Montreal Olympic Games Anthropological Project*. Medicine and Sport, Vol. 16, pp. 25–52. Jokl E. (ed.), Karger, Basel.

Carter J. & Ackland T. (1994) *Kinanthropometry in Aquatic Sports*. Human Kinetics Publishers, Champaign, IL, USA.

Clarys J., Martin A. & Drinkwater D. (1984) Gross tissue weights in the human body by cadaver dissection. *Human Biology* **56**, 459–473.

Coleman A. (1981) Skinfold estimates of body fat in major league baseball players. *The Physician and Sportsmedicine* **9**, 77–82.

Costill D., Bowers R. & Kammer W. (1970) Skinfold estimates of body fat among marathon runners. *Medicine and Science in Sports* **2**, 93–95.

Davis J., Brewer J. & Atkin D. (1992) Pre-season physiological characteristics of English first and second division soccer players. *Journal of Sports Sciences* **10**, 541–547.

Donaldson C., Hulley S., Vogel J., Hattner R., Bayers J. & McMillan D. (1970) Effect of prolonged bed rest on bone mineral. *Metabolism* **19**, 1071–1084.

Hagerman F., Hagerman G. & Mickelson T. (1979) Physiological profiles of elite rowers. *The Physician and Sports Medicine* **7**, 74–83.

Holliday M. (1978) Body composition and energy needs during growth. In Falkner F. & Tanner J. (eds) *Human Growth*, Vol. 2, pp. 21–33. Baillière Tindall, London.

Kerr D. (1993) Body weight: Achieving the balance for female athletes. *Sport Health* **11**, 42–44.

Kottke F. (1966) The effects of limitation of activity upon the human body. *Journal of the American Medical Association* **196**, 825–830.

Kovaleski J., Parr R., Hornak J. & Roitman J. (1980) Athletic profile of women college volleyball players. *The Physician and Sportsmedicine* **8**, 112–118.

Krahenbuhl G., Wells C., Brown C. & Ward P. (1979) Characteristics of national and world class female pent-athletes. *Medicine and Science in Sports* **11**, 20–23.

Malina R. (1978) Growth of muscle tissue and muscle mass. In Falkner F. & Tanner J. (eds) *Human Growth*, Vol. 2, pp. 21–33. Baillière Tindall, London.

Malina R., Harper A., Avent H. & Campbell D. (1971) Physique of female track and field athletes. *Medicine and Science in Sports* **3**, 32–38.

Marshall W. (1978) Puberty. In Falkner F. & Tanner J. (eds) *Human Growth*, Vol. 2, pp. 141–178. Baillière Tindall, London.

Maud P. & Shultz B. (1984) The U.S. national rugby team: A physiological and anthropometric assessment. *The Physician and Sportsmedicine* **12**, 86–99.

Moody D., Wilmore J., Girandola R. & Royce J. (1972) The effects of a jogging programme on the body composition of normal and obese high school girls. *Medicine and Science in Sports* **4**, 210–213.

Nilsson B. & Westlin N. (1971) Bone density in athletes. *Clinical Orthopedics* **77**, 179–182.

Norris A., Lundy T. & Shock N. (1963) Trends in selected indices of body composition in men between the ages 30 and 80 years. *Annals of the New York Academy of Science* **110**, 623.

Parr R., Hoover A., Wilmore J., Bachman D. & Kerlan R. (1978) Professional basketball players: Athletic profiles. *The Physician and Sportsmedicine* **6**, 77–84.

Piechaczek H. (1990) Body structure of male and female basketball players. *Biology of Sport* **7**, 273–285.

Pipes T. (1979) The racquetball pro: A physiological profile. *The Physician and Sportsmedicine* **7**, 91–94.

Puhl J., Case S., Fleck S. & Van Handel P. (1982) Physical and physiological characteristics of elite volleyball players. *The Research Quarterly for Exercise and Sport* **53**, 257–262.

Salans L., Cushman S. & Weissman R. (1973) Adipose cell size and number in nonobese and obese patients. *Journal of Clinical Investigation* **52**, 929.

Schmidtbleicher D. (1986) Strength and strength training. *Section 2, The First Elite Coaches' Seminar*. Australian Coaching Council, Canberra, Australia.

Sidney K. & Shephard R. (1973) Physiological characteristics and performance of the white-water paddler. *European Journal of Applied Physiology* **32**, 55–70.

Sinning W. (1973) Body composition, cardiovascular function and rule changes in women's basketball. *The Research Quarterly for Exercise and Sport* **44**, 313–321.

Telford R., Egerton W., Hahn A. & Pang P. (1988) Skinfold measures and weight controls in elite athletes. *Excel* **5**, 21–26.

Vodak P., Savin W., Haskell W. & Wood P. (1980) Physiological profile of middle-aged male and female tennis players. *Medicine and Science in Sports* **12**, 159–163.

Wells J., Parizkova J., Bohanan J. & Jokl E. (1963) Growth, body composition and physical efficiency. *Journal of the Association for Physical and Mental Rehabilitation* **17**, 37–40, 56–57.

Wessel J., Ufer A., Van Huss W. & Cederquist D. (1963) Age trends of various components of body composition and functional characteristics in women aged 20–69 years. *Annals of the New York Academy of Science* **110**, 608.

Wickkiser J. & Kelly J. (1975) The body composition of a college football team. *Medicine and Science in Sports* **7**, 199–202.

Wilmore J., Parr R., Haskell W., Costill D., Milburn L. & Kerlan R. (1976) Football pros' strengths — and CV weaknesses — charted. *The Physician and Sports medicine* **4**, 45–54.

CHAPTER 7

BODY PROPORTIONS AND THEIR EFFECT ON SPORT PERFORMANCE

Human proportionality has been observed for thousands of years, but it was not until the 5th century BC that a Greek named Polykleitos sculpted Doryphoros, the 'Spearbearer' (Fig. 7.1), which was representative of the ideal body form with the proportions of a champion athlete. This figure was then used as a proportional model by sculptors for several centuries. During the Renaissance, Alberti, da Vinci and Vesalius all studied human proportionality and in some cases used linear measures of human proportions for their sculptures and drawings.

It was not until 1887, when Sargent made various observations with relation to the physical build of athletes, that anyone had documented the effect of body proportions on sport performance. During the early 20th century Amar (1920), Kohlrausch (1929), Arnold (1931) and Boardman (1933) measured a large number of athletes and made some very perceptive observations about their suitability for various sports and events. However, it was Cureton in 1951 who did the first definitive work in which a precise knowledge of anatomy was applied to sport, when he reported on his study of 58 Olympic place-getters and world champions in the sports of swimming, track and field, and gymnastics.

SIGNIFICANCE OF PROPORTIONALITY MODIFICATION IN SPORT

Even the casual observer will have noted that human body proportions vary greatly from person to person. These variations play an important part in the self-selection process for various sports and events, and it is obvious that there is little that can be done to alter some anatomical body proportions. With this limitation in mind, it is up to coaches to modify their athletes' technique when their proportions are not suitable for various sports skills, either by shortening or lengthening the various levers of the body in order to obtain an optimal performance. This is the essence of high quality coaching, where coaches cater for each individual and are able to formulate the most efficient technique for their athletes. How to achieve this will be fully discussed later in this chapter.

EFFECT OF GROWTH ON PROPORTIONALITY

During the growth period, every individual undergoes various proportionality changes to a greater or lesser extent, and it is important for coaches to realize this, because there will be times when allowances will need to be made for such changes.

The following information will enable the coach to understand the growth process better from a proportionality perspective:

- Figure 7.2 illustrates the changes which occur during the growth of various parts of the body in both males and females. The head is well

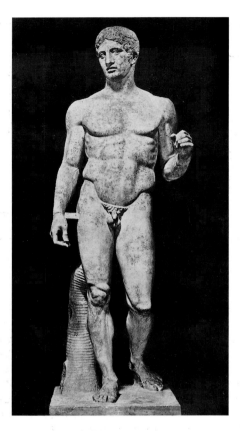

Fig. 7.1 A sculpture of the 'Spearbearer' by Polykleitos.

advanced at birth while the trunk is reasonably developed, with the arms and legs lagging well behind the head and trunk
- From birth, girls are usually more advanced than boys in relation to height. Their height spurt commences at approximately 10.5 years of age and reaches its peak height velocity (PHV) at approximately 12 years of age, with boys following girls by roughly 2 years (Tanner 1989). Bone maturity in boys compared to girls is also approximately 2 years behind
- Malina and Bouchard (1991) stated that 'maximum growth is obtained first by the tibia and then the femur, followed by the fibula and then the bones of the upper extremity. Maximum growth of stature occurs, on the average, more

or less at the same time as maximum growth of the humerus and radius'. They further stated that 'in early adolescence a youngster has relatively long legs, because the bones of the lower extremity experience their growth spurts earlier than those of the upper extremity'. Many coaches have observed this 'long-legged' phenomenon and realize they simply have to wait for the trunk to develop before their athlete has balanced proportions

KINANTHROPOMETRIC ASSESSMENT

Human size and proportions are assessed by the use of anthropometry. The most common anthropometric measures are those which assess the lengths, widths, girths and volumes of body segments, using precision instruments (see Section 3 for further details). Anthropometric variables are often expressed as indices to allow a more meaningful description of physique to be made. For example, the relationship of the length of the leg (foreleg or lower leg) to the thigh, that is the crural index, can be calculated in the following way.

$$\text{crural index} = \frac{\text{(lower) leg length} \times 100}{\text{thigh length}}$$

Similarly, the brachial index, which demonstrates the length of the forearm in relation to the arm (upper arm), may also be calculated:

$$\text{brachial index} = \frac{\text{forearm length} \times 100}{\text{arm length}}$$

When various anthropometric measures have been taken and the indices computed, then it is possible to make meaningful comparisons between individuals.

INDIVIDUAL COMPARISONS OF ATHLETES

For many years individual comparisons have been made by comparing the raw anthropometric scores

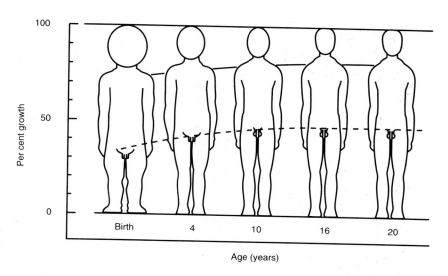

Fig. 7.2 General changes in body proportions with age (adapted from Hills 1991).

of one athlete with those of another, or with one team against another. If coaches are very aware of the significance of the raw measures, for example when comparing the heights and weights of two eight-oared rowing crews or the heights and weights of two rugby packs, then this method of comparison is of value.

The above system, although useful, has a limitation when the magnitude of the differences between individuals, groups, or when data over time, are compared. A number of strategies have been proposed including the somatogram (Behnke & Wilmore 1974) and the unisex phantom (Ross & Wilson 1974; Ross *et al.* 1988), that have enabled sports scientists and coaches to view data from another perspective.

The Somatogram

The somatogram (Fig. 14.19), where the individual's percentage deviation from the mean value of the population is plotted on the gram, is a useful way to compare data. If the anthropometric proportions of an individual conform to the mean of the population, then all the values would fall on the central or zero line. This system however, does not account for variations in body size. (See Chapter 14 for further details.)

The Phantom

Dimensional scaling of anthropometric measures with an adjustment for stature using a 'unisex phantom' (Figs 14.20, 14.21) is a method which can facilitate meaningful comparisons of individual proportions. In this system, raw data are compared with phantom values and the resulting deviations, in the form of Z-scores, are the basis for analysis. The phantom stratagem has been used to compare the growth of individuals over time, as well as comparisons of individuals with specific group data. (See Chapter 14 for further details.)

PROPORTIONALITY APPLIED TO SPORT PERFORMANCE

Lever Lengths

The basic laws of physics as they relate to leverage, play an important part in sport and bone lengths can be either an advantage or a disadvantage depending on the physical demands of the sport in which the individual competes. These lengths are absolute when the individual has reached full maturity and cannot be altered.

In some sports, such as weightlifting, athletes with short levers will have an advantage over those who possess long levers, because the weight only needs to be lifted through a shorter distance (Hart *et al.* 1991). In other sports such as diving or gymnastics, where the body rotates rapidly in a given distance, short levers will also be an advantage to the performer. On the other hand if an athlete requires a long powerful stroke, such as in swimming, canoeing or rowing, then a longer lever, provided it is accompanied by the muscular power to propel it, has an advantage in these types of sports. The same point can also be made in other sports where hitting or throwing are important. For example, velocity generation for a tennis serve, a volleyball spike or a baseball pitch will all be higher for long-levered athletes, if they have the muscle power to rotate the longer segments.

Insertion Point

Although the gross bone length is usually referred to as *the lever*, this is only a general concept in sport to differentiate athletes with long or short levers from one another. However, it is the insertion point of the tendon as it attaches to the bone which is the main determinant of the lever's effectiveness. If this point is further away from the joint (axis of rotation), then it will positively affect the muscle function, giving that person a mechanical advantage, thus making him or her stronger and/or more powerful. Many coaches will have observed two athletes who are similar in size, body shape, lever lengths and muscle mass, yet one is more powerful than the other. This is usually due to the tendon insertion position and/or muscle fibre type.

Trunk and Extremity Indices

In general, individuals with long extremities and relatively short trunks are physically weak types, while people with short extremities and long trunks are usually powerful types.

For decades, coaches have used the above general statement in order to assess the strength, power and speed potential of their athletes and have mostly found it to be a useful guide. However, although it is generally accurate, it needs another

dimension added to it which would enable coaches to make more accurate forecasts of their athletes' potential. This additional factor relates to the indices of the trunk and the upper and lower extremities, as well as the indices of the extremities themselves. This will be fully discussed in the following section.

PROPORTIONALITY CHARACTERISTICS OF ATHLETES

One sometimes hears the statement, that 'athletes are born and not made' and in the case of proportionality or 'lever advantage', this is largely correct. It is very clear to those persons who have carried out research on, or spent a great deal of time with, various types of athletes, that some people are greatly advantaged by their body segment lengths, while others are not.

However, one should not overestimate the importance of this physical capacity, because there are many other important factors that go to make up an optimal performance. If one uses a high jumper as an example to illustrate the above point, it is clear that as well as having the optimal height and body shape, that is long lower limbs compared to the jumper's trunk, and long lower legs in comparison to thighs, the following characteristics will also be necessary:

- Sufficient muscle mass with a high proportion of fast twitch muscle fibre compared to slow twitch fibre and tendon insertion points which give a greater mechanical advantage
- A high level of skill which will enable the jumper to coordinate his or her body segments to 'smoothly' clear the bar
- Psychological control which will assist the athlete to focus on each jump in order to attain the best result

All performances in sport consist of a multiplicity of variables, therefore it is important not to stress any one as being much more important than the others. However, the athlete's proportions are vitally important in ballistic events where explosive power and speed are necessary.

Specific Proportionality Characteristics

RACQUET SPORTS (TENNIS, BADMINTON, SQUASH, RACQUETBALL)

Being agility athletes, *racquet sports* players have variable proportions because of the multifaceted demands of their games. No definitive research has been carried out on these athletes; however, coaches state that they are a variable group of individuals. The shots used in the racquet sports are executed with the upper extremities, and therefore knowledgeable coaches can help a player to compensate for an inefficient lever system. For example, the forearm can be flexed at the elbow to facilitate greater control when volleying, while it must be fully extended to enhance service technique. Two hands may be used for ground strokes to compensate for a lack of strength, but if the athlete is powerful enough, then it may be best to use one hand, because a longer lever, provided enough force can be applied to the stroke, will increase racquet head velocity. This will increase the speed of the ball as it rebounds from the strings of the racquet. Furthermore, while longer levered athletes may structure their basic game on high velocity shots, shorter players must be agile and fast around the court in order to compensate for their lack of power because of their shorter levers.

AQUATIC SPORTS

Swimming

Swimmers, at the highest levels of competition, have been increasing in height and weight for the past 30 years (Carter 1984, Ackland *et al.* 1994). Elite level swimmers are generally heavier, taller and have a more robust upper body (Fig. 7.3), with larger feet than lower level competitors. Even among top level swimmers there are special characteristics which differentiate them from one event to another. If a comparison is made between sprint and middle distance swimmers, the differences are quite marked. For example, sprint swimmers have a higher brachial index than middle distance swimmers because of their longer forearms and shorter upper arms, while sprinters also have low crural indices (i.e. a short lower leg length in com-

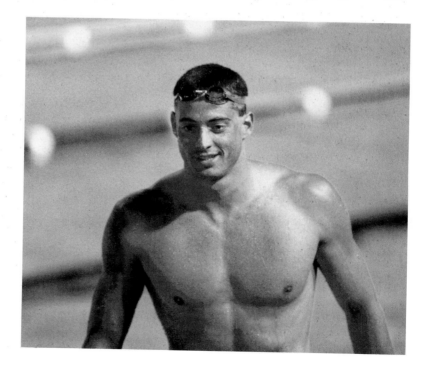

Fig. 7.3 High level swimmers are tall and have powerful trunks as portrayed by this world sprint swimming champion (West Australian Newspapers with permission).

parison to their thigh length) which tends to give them a mechanical advantage over middle distance swimmers for freestyle kicking (Bloomfield & Sigerseth 1965). Within strokes (Ackland *et al.* 1994) the freestyle and backstroke swimmers are taller than those competitors in the other strokes and have longer limbs, while butterfly swimmers were found to have longer trunks than the others. Breast-stroke swimmers on the other hand were very robust and powerful in the trunk region.

Waterpolo

Both male and female world class *waterpolo* players (Ackland *et al.* 1994) are tall and well built, but there are significant proportionality differences within this sport when players in the various positions are compared with one another. Centre forwards and centre backs are larger and more robust than the other players, mainly because their greater size enables them to use their bodies very effectively in both attack and defence. Goalkeepers on the other hand are tall, less bulky and long-limbed compared to the other players. They have a high skeletal mass, with lower upper body girths and are basically more ectomorphic. Ackland *et al.* (1994) state that this attribute gives them a 'reduced upper limb inertia which would facilitate relative quickness of movement to protect the goal'.

Rowing and canoeing

High level *oarsmen*, especially those rowing in eight-oar crews, are tall and heavy with average heights of approximately 189 cm and an average body mass of 91 kg (Railton 1969). Carter's (1984) statistics on oarsmen from four Olympic Games show a continuing trend with increases in both height and body mass. *Canoeists* also display similar developmental trends to rowers, both in height and body mass, but are not as tall nor as heavy as oarsmen (de Garay *et al.* 1974; Carter 1984).

GYMNASTIC AND POWER SPORTS

Gymnasts are relatively short and light (Carter 1984) with long bodies and short legs, giving them a low lower limb/trunk ratio. They also possess a

low crural index (Cureton 1951). *Divers* on the other hand are taller than gymnasts but with similar trunk and leg ratios (Cureton 1951; de Garay 1974; Ackland *et al.* 1994). Male and female world class divers are a reasonably homogeneous group; however, 10 m platform divers are less robust in physique than springboard divers, with relatively longer lower extremities. Ackland *et al.* (1994) state that this characteristic is advantageous to the 10 m diver because the 'decreased moments of inertia are afforded by smaller absolute and proportional limb girths and segment breadths and these may provide an advantage in the performance of aerial manoeuvres'. It may also be possible that a more knife-like entry can be made by a more linear diver.

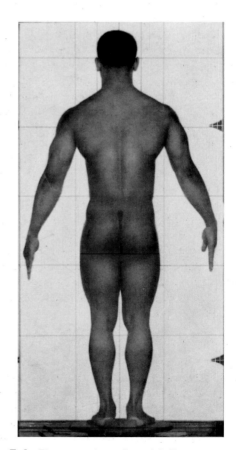

Fig. 7.4 The proportions of a weightlifter (courtesy of Tanner 1964).

When the top 10 m divers were compared with the other competitors in the 1991 World Championships, they were found to be leaner than the other group; however, no other major differences were apparent. *Weightlifters* (Fig. 7.4) have similar proportions to throwers, possessing powerful arms and shoulders. They also have long trunks with short thick and powerful legs, that is, a low lower limb/trunk ratio; and they generally have a low crural index (Cureton 1951; Tanner 1964; Carter 1984).

TRACK, FIELD AND CYCLING

Sprinters

Sprinters are relatively short and muscular (especially in the region of the buttocks and the thighs) compared to middle distance runners, but of medium height (with mean heights of 176 cm for males and 166 cm for females) when compared to other track and field athletes. They have normal trunk lengths with short lower limbs (Fig. 8.9), that is, a low lower limb/trunk ratio (Tanner 1964; Bloomfield 1979). Dintiman and Ward (1988) stated that the champion male sprinter approaches 5 steps/s at full pace, while females average 4.48 steps/s. Such rapid leg movements can only be made by a relatively short limb (a shorter lever generally has a lower moment of inertia or resistance to movement than a longer one), which gives a greater 'ground strike rate' thus giving more propulsive force to the sprinter. It should also be noted that the crural index of sprinters is average. *High hurdlers* (Fig. 7.5) in many respects resemble sprinters, but are taller and possess longer legs (Cureton 1951; Tanner 1964) with proportions similar to 400 m runners.

Middle distance and distance runners

Middle distance runners are tall, linear and long legged with a normal length trunk, that is, with a high lower limb/trunk ratio and an average crural index (Fig. 8.11). This contrasts with *distance runners*, who become progressively shorter as the race distance lengthens (Fig. 7.6). They also have short lower limbs in comparison to their trunks, that is, with a low lower limb/trunk ratio and below aver-

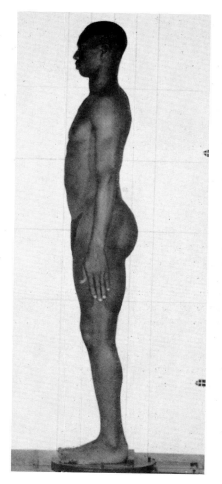

Fig. 7.5 High hurdlers resemble sprinters but are taller and possess longer legs (courtesy of Tanner 1964).

age crural indices (Cureton 1951; Tanner 1964; de Garay *et al.* 1974).

Jumpers

Athletes who take part in jumping events, particularly the *high jump* and the *triple jump*, need to be tall and have long lower limbs relative to their trunk lengths (Fig. 7.7), that is, they should have a high lower limb/trunk ratio (Cureton 1951; Tanner 1964; Eiben 1972; Bloomfield 1979). They also need a high crural index (Cureton 1951).

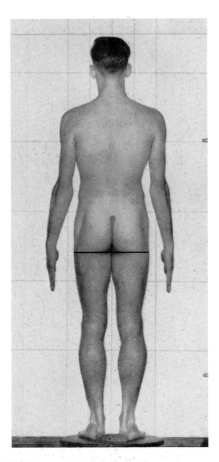

Fig. 7.6 The proportions of an elite marathon runner (courtesy of Tanner 1964).

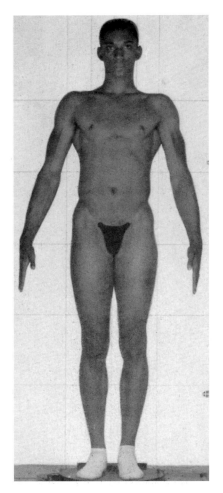

Fig. 7.7 The proportions of a former Olympic high jump champion (courtesy of Tanner 1964).

Throwers

Throwers are tall and heavy with powerful shoulders and arms and they are becoming gradually larger each Olympiad (Cureton 1951; Carter 1984). Their legs and trunks are of normal length for their height; however, many of them have extremely long thick arms, especially the discus throwers (Fig. 7.8). In contrast to the male athletes, Eiben (1972) stated that female throwers had long trunks and a low crural index.

Cycling

Like many other athletes, *cyclists* are steadily increasing their height and weight (Carter 1984). It is well known that track cyclists are more robust and powerful than road cyclists, but they are a reasonably homogeneous group as far as their other proportions are concerned. It should also be noted that anecdotal evidence from coaches indicates that high level track cyclists have short thighs, giving them a high crural index which increases their mechanical advantage while pedalling.

MOBILE FIELD SPORTS (FIELD HOCKEY, SOCCER, LACROSSE)

Individuals in mobile field sports have differing proportions because of the multi-faceted demands

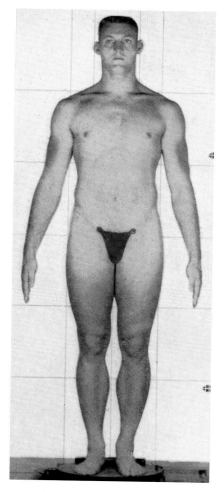

Fig. 7.8 An elite discus thrower with typically long arms (courtesy of Tanner 1964).

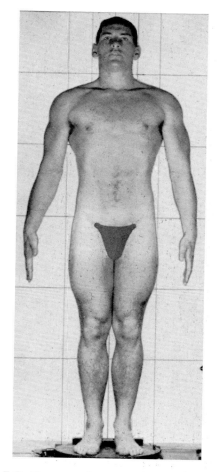

Fig. 7.9 The proportions and body bulk which are needed for a forward in contact football.

of their games. As with racquet sport players, little research has been done on proportionality in mobile field sports and one would not expect that a great deal will be done in the near future because the intelligent coach can use the existing data from agility athletes and sprinters. This can quite easily be applied to athletes in these particular sports, who need speed or power and agility in the various specialized positions.

CONTACT FIELD SPORTS (RUGBY, AUSTRALIAN FOOTBALL, AMERICAN FOOTBALL)

Athletes in contact field sports, because they must be powerful, agile and fast, also need to be classified according to the position they occupy on the field. The winger or backfield player who needs to be very fast should have similar proportions to a track sprinter, while a forward or a lineman will need proportions, bulk and agility similar to that of the field games thrower (Fig. 7.9). Coaches in all games must determine the skills which are appropriate for each specialized position in contact sports at the elite level, then identify the proportionality characteristics which will satisfy them. This is the very essence of intelligent coaching.

SET FIELD SPORTS (BASEBALL, CRICKET, GOLF)

As for the racquet sports and the mobile field sports groups, the proportionality of *cricketers*, *baseballers* and *golfers* is variable. As in racquet sports, intelligent coaches can compensate for an inefficient lever system in these athletes, since many of the skills they use are set or closed, with little or no forward body motion taking place while the skill is being performed. For example, technique modifications in a golf swing or baseball pitch may be made to compensate for an inefficient lever system.

COURT SPORTS (BASKETBALL, NETBALL, VOLLEYBALL)

The games of *basketball*, *netball* and *volleyball* are agility sports which partially rely on leaping skills. To do well in these sports the player must be extremely agile and able to jump, so special proportions are needed to do this. These players must be tall, have long upper limbs, lower limbs and trunks and display a high crural index, that is, long lower legs in comparison to the length of their thighs.

MARTIAL ARTS

Wrestling and judo

Individuals in *wrestling* and *judo* have powerful shoulder girdles and arms, with long bodies and short lower extremities, that is, a low lower limb/trunk ratio. They often have heavy legs and possess a low crural index (Fig. 7.10). All these features combine to give them a low centre of gravity which makes it difficult to force them off balance (Cureton 1951; Tanner 1964).

Boxing

Athletes in *boxing* are variable in their proportions and do not have the same basic lever system as those individuals in the grappling sports. Be-

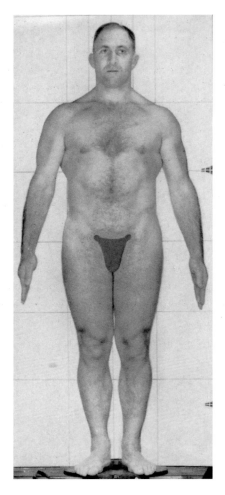

Fig. 7.10 The bulk and proportions which are needed for an international heavyweight wrestler (courtesy of Tanner 1964).

cause there is a high degree of variability in their proportions, especially in the weight classes, it is up to the coach to compensate by modifying the fighter's technique.

RACIAL CHARACTERISTICS

Physical anthropologists and coaches have observed for some time that there are basic differences in the proportionality characteristics of the major races of the world. Africans (currently in or originally from Africa) have longer upper and lower extremities than Europeans (currently in or originally from Europe), while Asians (currently in or originally from the south-east and western Asian regions) have shorter extremities than both Africans and Europeans. It is interesting to note that Europeans cover a greater range of proportions than either of the other groups. In many cases they have proportionality requirements which suit certain sports admirably, but at the extremes of the range there are fewer individuals with the optimal lever systems for some specialized sports. They therefore find it difficult to compete against persons of other races who have larger numbers in their population with more suitable proportions.

More research has been done comparing African Americans and European Americans because of the large population which inhabits the United States of America and as the two racial groups compete in many sports together. Metheny (1939) found that African Americans exceed European Americans in body mass, arm length, forearm length, lower limb length, leg length, shoulder breadth, chest depth and width, neck girth and limb girths, when they were divided by stature. Cureton (1951) made similar observations and further reported the work of Codwell, who compared the vertical jumping ability of both groups of high school boys. He found the African Americans to be superior on this test and one could only assume that their long lower limbs and legs were important factors in this result.

Specific Racial Differences

FIELD AND COURT SPORTS

In the majority of these sports, there are many variables which contribute to high performances and although proportionality is one, this can be partially compensated for by intelligent coaching to

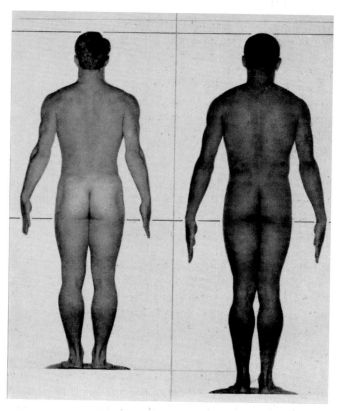

Fig. 7.11 A comparison of a European and an African American sprinter who have identical trunk lengths (courtesy of Tanner 1964).

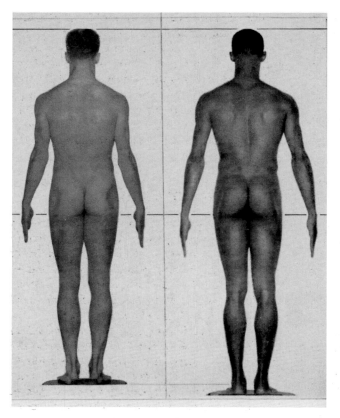

Fig. 7.12 A comparison of a European and an African American 400 m runner who have identical trunk lengths (courtesy of Tanner 1964).

modify the individual's skills. Therefore, except for very specialized positions, racial proportionality differences should not affect performances in these sports a great deal.

TRACK AND FIELD SPORTS

Tanner (1964) in his definitive work on Olympic athletes, demonstrated conclusively that Africans have longer arms and legs (relative to their stature), narrower hips and more slender calves than Europeans competing in the same event (Figs 7.11, 7.12). He also stated that in sprinting the lighter calves of the former group produce 'a lower moment of inertia in the leg, and this would permit a more rapid recovery movement, that is a faster acceleration forwards, of the trailing leg'. Tanner (1964) further suggested that the original East African was more successful in the middle and long distance races, while the West

African performed very well in the sprints. However, he did not point out the reason for this difference, which has become more obvious recently, and this is that the tall slim Nilotic East African is perfectly suited to middle distance and longer events, having the optimal physical proportions for them, and that the shorter, muscular West African is more suited to the power (sprint) events for the reasons given earlier in this chapter.

GYMNASTIC AND POWER SPORTS

Many coaches have pointed out that individuals with long trunks and short upper and lower limbs do well in gymnastics and we are now seeing more gymnasts and divers coming from Asian countries. It would appear that Asians are well suited to these events, as well as to weightlifting. Tanner (1964) also suggested that the proportions of this group are well suited to power sports, especially weight-lifting where the upper and lower limbs are strikingly short in successful competitors of all races.

Body Modification

The specific proportionality requirements for various athletic events have already been discussed in this chapter and they clearly demonstrate the important role of this capacity in high level performance. As a general rule, human proportions cannot be modified in the same manner as the other physical capacities using a simple intervention programme, because the mature athlete's bone lengths are absolute and cannot be changed, and as a result are significant parameters in the process of self-selection for various sports and events.

As a matter of interest, some bodies have been modified either accidentally or by design. However, on both moral and ethical grounds, deliberate changes are not recommended under any circumstances. They are as follows:

- *Growth plate compaction* — anecdotal evidence suggests that pre-adolescent and early adolescent weightlifters were given very heavy weights to lift over prolonged periods of time in the 1970s and 1980s, in some countries in Eastern Europe. It has been reported that this practice compacted the growth plates in the legs, inhibiting the long bone growth and thus shortening their legs. It has also been claimed that prolonged heavy weight bearing exercise may develop thick bones with a high mineral content. If this is the case, a mechanical advantage and a more solid base of support would be obtained

- Tendon insertion — earlier in this chapter in the section on Proportionality Applied to Sport Performance, the subject of tendon insertion was discussed with relation to an individual being more powerful if the distance between the insertion of the tendon and the joint (axis of rotation) is greater than normal. Again, anecdotal evidence suggests that power-lifters who have ruptured a muscle by pulling the tendon off a bone during various lifts, particularly a deadlift, have become stronger in that region of the body where the tendon was reattached to the bone a little further away from its previous position. For example, Bill Kazmair (see Chapter 9), who ruptured his triceps brachii muscle, found he was stronger in forearm extension after the tendon had been reinserted into the ulna further away from its original position

TECHNIQUE MODIFICATION

The only acceptable way in which proportions can be changed is by a process known as technique modification and the coach can play a significant role in this. By altering the individual's technique, it may be possible to modify the lever system, thereby enabling the athlete to perform the skill in a more biomechanically efficient way.

Technique modification, to suit each individual athlete, is the basis of good coaching, so that the skilled coach must know when the individual's proportions are unsuitable and which changes will be needed to improve his or her performance. The following examples from the various sports groups will illustrate this point:

- A *tennis player* (Fig. 7.13) may have the majority of the motor skills and the psychological profile needed to perform well in this sport, but be of tall stature with a relatively weak musculature. As well as a strength training intervention programme which will no doubt assist the overall performance, the player's volleys and ground strokes may need to be modified by the coach. This can be done by flexing the forearm at the elbow, thus shortening the lever to produce a more powerful forehand ground stroke. The player may also adopt a double-handed backhand technique, which not only shortens the striking lever, but may also facilitate greater stability and a better technique to hit a top spin shot (Bloomfield 1979; Ackland & Bloomfield 1992)

- A *swimmer* (Fig. 7.14) may have a large number of the variables which are essential for a cham-

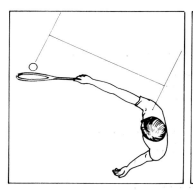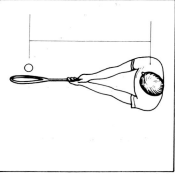

Fig. 7.13 Shortening the effective lever using a two-handed backhand in tennis (from Bloomfield *et al.* 1992).

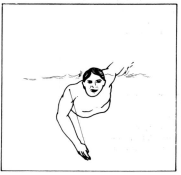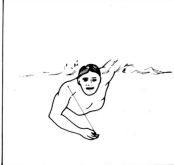

Fig. 7.14 Shortening the effective lever in freestyle swimming (from Bloomfield 1979).

pion, but lack the proportions and strength needed for efficient freestyle pulling. In addition to increasing the swimmer's strength, the propulsive lever can be shortened by flexing the forearm more than is normal for most swimmers (Bloomfield 1979)

- A female *gymnast* in the early stages of adolescence, will undergo a major growth spurt during this time which will increase her linearity, but at the same time decrease her stability. At this stage of her development, the coach will need to compensate for this proportionality change in events carried out on the beam, by having her flex more at the knee joints, thus lowering her centre of gravity in order to increase her stability
- In *contact* and *combative* sports, athletes with long lower limbs should flex them at the knees a little more than shorter-legged athletes, in order to lower the centre of gravity and thus

increase their dynamic stability

- A *baseball* pitcher with a long upper extremity, should flex the forearm more at the elbow than the shorter-limbed pitcher. This is done in order to make it easier to swing the arm forward in the early phase of the pitch prior to extending the forearm near ball release. This will increase the linear velocity of the hand, resulting in a faster ball being thrown
- A *golfer* with long lower limbs should set up to the ball with a wider stance than a shorter limbed player, in order to prevent swaying laterally 'past the ball', which causes the club face to be slightly open at impact and may result in a push–slice being made

CONCLUSION

Human proportions cannot normally be modified using a physical intervention programme because

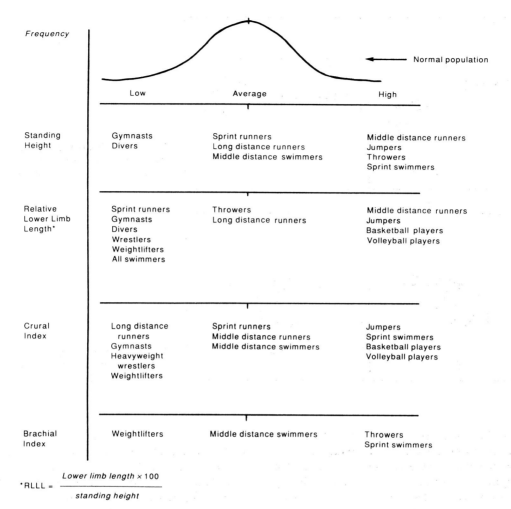

Fig. 7.15 Athletes have proportions which are highly suited to some sports but not to others (from Bloomfield *et al.* 1992).

individual bone lengths are finite, and under normal circumstances, cannot be changed. Proportionality is a self-selector for various sports and events and some athletes are born with proportions which are highly suited to some sports but not at all suited to others (Fig. 7.15). If an athlete has many of the physical characteristics which are suitable for a particular sport, but lacks the leverage capacity to do this, then the intelligent coach can modify his or her technique to partially overcome this physical disadvantage.

REFERENCES

Amar J. (1920) *The Human Motor*, pp. 129–130. E. P. Dutton and Co., New York.

Ackland T. & Bloomfield J. (1992) Functional anatomy. In Bloomfield J., Fricker P. & Fitch K. (eds) *Textbook of Science and Medicine in Sport*, pp. 2–28. Blackwell Scientific Publications, Melbourne.

Ackland T., Mazza J. & Carter J. (1994) Summary and implications. In Carter J. & Ackland T. (eds) *Kinanthropometry in Aquatic Sports*. Human Kinetics Publishers, Champaign, IL, USA.

Arnold A. (1931) *Korperent Kicklung und Leibesubungen*

für Schul und Sportarzte, p. 166. Johann Barth, Leipzig, Germany.

Behnke A. & Wilmore J. (1974) *Evaluation and Regulation of Body Build and Composition*, pp. 75–77. Prentice-Hall, Englewood Cliffs, NJ, USA.

Boardman R. (1933) World's champions run to types. *Journal of Health and Physical Education* **4**, 32.

Bloomfield J. (1979) Modifying human physical capacities and technique to improve performance. *Sports Coach* **3**, 19–25.

Bloomfield J. & Sigerseth P. (1965) Anatomical and physiological differences between sprint and middle distance swimmers at the university level. *Journal of Sports Medicine and Physical Fitness* **5**, 76–81.

Bloomfield J., Fricker P. & Fitch K. (1992) *Textbook of Science and Medicine in Sport*, pp. 10, 15. Blackwell Scientific Publications, Melbourne.

Carter J. (ed.) (1984) *Physical Structure of Olympic Athletes*. Medicine and Sports Science, Vol. 18, pp. 56–63. Karger, Basel.

Cureton T. (1951) *Physical Fitness of Champion Athletes*, pp. 28–50, 379–441. The University of Illinois Press, Urbana, IL, USA.

de Garay A., Levine L. & Carter J. (1974) *Genetic and Anthropological Studies of Olympic Athletes*, pp. 28–48, 83–146. Academic Press, New York.

Dintiman G. & Ward R. (1988) *Sport Speed*, p. 14. Leisure Press, Champaign, IL, USA.

Eiben O. (1972) *The Physique of Women Athletes*, pp. 181–184. Hungarian Scientific Council for Physical Education, Budapest.

Hart C., Ward T. & Mayhew J. (1991) Anthropometric correlates of bench press performance following resistance training. *Sports Training, Medicine and Rehabilitation* **2**, 89–95.

Hills A. (1991) *Physical Growth and Development of Children and Adolescents*, p. 33. Queensland University of Technology, Brisbane, Australia.

Kohlrausch W. (1929) Zusammenlägne von korpenform und leistung — ergebruise der anthropoinetrischen messungen an der athleten der Amsterdamer Olympiade. *Arbeitsphysiologie* **2**, 129.

Malina R. & Bouchard C. (1991) *Growth, Maturation and Physical Activity*, p. 260. Human Kinetics Books, Champaign, IL, USA.

Metheny E. (1939) Some differences in bodily proportions between the American Negro and white male college students as related to athletic performance. *Research Quarterly* **10**, 41–53.

Railton J. (1969) *International Rowing*, p. 64. Amateur Rowing Association Publication, London.

Ross W., De Rose E. & Ward R. (1988) Anthropometry applied to sports medicine. In Dirix A., Knuttgen H. & Tittle K. (eds) *The Olympic Book of Sports Medicine I*, pp. 233–265. Blackwell Scientific Publications, Oxford.

Ross W. & Wilson N. (1974) A stratagem for proportional growth assessment. *Acta Paediatrica Belgica* **28**, 169–182.

Sargent D. (1887) The physical characteristics of the athlete. *Scribners II*, **5**, 541–561.

Tanner J. (1989) *Foetus into Man*, p. 15. Castlemead Publications, Ware, UK.

Tanner J. (1964) *The Physique of the Olympic Athlete*, pp. 65–85, 104–110. George Allen and Unwin, London.

CHAPTER 8

POSTURAL CONSIDERATIONS IN SPORT PERFORMANCE

Some coaches may not be aware that an individual's posture can be very advantageous in many sports. In fact, after proportionality, posture is probably the most important self-selector for various sports and events.

Posture is unique to every individual and no two people have identical postures, although some are very similar. The determinants of an individual's posture are linked to the structure and size of bones, the position of the bony landmarks, injury and disease, static and dynamic living habits and the person's psychological state.

Good posture, both *static* and *dynamic*, is important for an attractive appearance, but more importantly it is essential if the body is to function with an economy of effort. If posture is poor it can lead to fatigue, muscular strain and poor muscle tone, the sagging of some parts of the body and low self-esteem.

EVOLUTION AND DEVELOPMENT OF POSTURE

The evolution of man from quadrupedal to bipedal hominid was accomplished through many adaptations of the musculoskeletal system over millions of years (Krogman 1951; Napier 1967). The four-legged animal possesses a skeletal system similar to a bridge, with an arched backbone to support the internal structures and with the legs acting as stanchions to support it. When primates slowly moved towards an upright posture, the advantages of such a system were lost, as the body was solely supported by the hind legs. The following structural changes and their ramifications occurred during this evolutionary period:

- The vertebrae had to adapt to vertical weight-bearing stress and this was achieved by changing from a curved C-shaped vertebral arch into an S-shaped one. The primary thoracic curvature therefore still exists, but other curvatures have developed
- The erect posture places an extra burden on the pelvis which now has to support the entire weight of the upper body. By standing erect, the whole structure was tilted upward and in so doing additional weight was placed on the pelvic basin. As this occurred the bones in the pelvis changed shape and now resemble a basin which supports the intestines and some organs
- The foot has changed shape to become less of a grasping appendage and more of a weight supporter. This has occurred by a shortening of the toes and a lengthening of the remainder of the foot; these changes place considerable stress on the arches, sometimes causing problems such as pronated feet and functional flat feet
- To permit the bending and twisting movements of the human spine, the vertebrae have changed shape to the point where they are

95

now a partial wedge. This shape, although very good for mobility, has weakened the vertebral column, especially in the lumbar region where the discs may herniate with overstress. Furthermore, the lumbosacral joint must support the total weight of the upper body and the modifications to the articulation, due to the new alignment of bones, have created an area of instability if it is overstressed

CHANGES IN POSTURE DURING GROWTH

At birth the infant has two primary vertebral curves. The major curve is in the thoracic region, while the minor one is in the area of the sacrum. At around 6 months of age, a secondary curve develops in the cervical area and is the result of the infant holding its head up. When the child stands upright, the lumbar curve starts to develop, and by the time the individual reaches 6 years of age there are two definite primary curves and two secondary curves (Fig. 8.1).

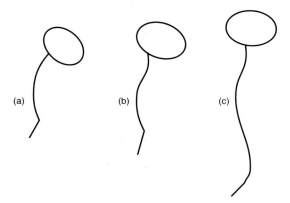

Fig. 8.1 Changes in the spinal curvatures from birth to adulthood: (a) infant; (b) 6 month old; (c) adult. (Adapted from Sinclair 1973.)

When the infant is born, the legs are flexed and the feet are inverted, but as the child stands and the legs develop, the feet become everted. An 18 month old child will have 'bow legs' when standing, but by 3 years of age will develop 'knock knees'. In most cases by 6–7 years of age the legs will have straightened (Fig. 8.2).

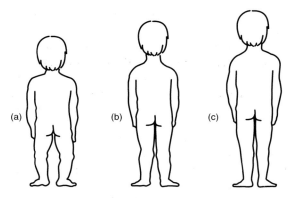

Fig. 8.2 The development of leg posture in the child: (a) 18 months old; (b) 3 years old; (c) 6 years old. (Adapted from Sinclair 1973.)

MAINTENANCE OF POSTURE

The maintenance of posture in an upright position depends upon a series of reflexes which are smoothly coordinated with the nervous system. The reflex which plays the major part in this development is known as the myotatic reflex, which responds to stretch and is described in detail in Chapter 10.

The mechanism that enables humans to assume various postures and maintain them, works in the following way. If a joint starts to flex, the muscle spindles of the major muscle group controlling the joint are stretched and an impulse is generated that goes to the spinal cord, where a synapse is made with a motor neuron. This then innervates the fibres of the controlling muscle group so that they contract and re-extend the joint, thus placing it into a normal position. The reflex only operates in the presence of facilitation by the vestibular nucleus in the medulla through the spinal cord, as well as through the extrapyramidal and autogenetic governor system. These mechanisms enable very smooth and coordinated contractions which maintain normal posture.

ADVANTAGES OF GOOD POSTURE

Posture can be defined as the relative arrangement of body parts or segments, but generally it is the term used to describe the way a person stands.

When considering *good* or *bad* posture, the bones should represent a series of links connected by joints being held together by muscles and ligaments. If these links are arranged in a vertical plane so that the line of gravity passes through the centre of each joint (Fig. 8.3) then the least stress will be placed on the muscles and ligaments. *Good posture* therefore, is a state of muscular and skeletal balance which protects the supporting structures of the body against progressive deformity or injury. *Poor posture*, on the other hand, is the faulty relationship of the various segments of the body, producing increased stress on supporting structures (Fig. 8.4). This type of posture makes it more difficult to maintain efficient balance over the base of support and causes habitual sagging which can permanently stretch some muscle groups and shorten others. The advantage of having good posture is that the least use of energy occurs when the vertical line of gravity falls through the supporting column of bones, and the body does not have to continually adjust its position to counter the forces of gravity. Good posture, therefore, is both mechanically functional and economical.

POSTURAL DIVERSITY WITHIN INDIVIDUALS

Postural diversity can occur within individuals because they have disharmony between different regions of their body. Sheldon *et al.* (1940) termed this phenomenon *dysplasia* and related it to the person's somatotype, by suggesting that a subject

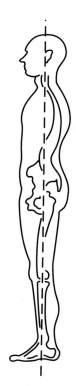

Fig. 8.3 In 'good posture', a vertical line should pass through the anterior portion of the ear and then through the centre of each joint of the lower extremity.

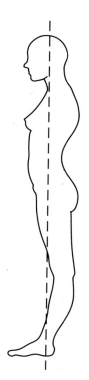

Fig. 8.4 If any segment of the body deviates from its vertical alignment, its weight must be counterbalanced by the deviation of another segment in the opposite direction. Also note the severe genu recurvartum in the legs.

could 'be in proportion' in one region of the body and yet be quite disproportionate in one, or several segments.

One sees dysplasic characteristics in many people, but this does not always mean that they have poor posture, because they have in some cases adjusted it naturally, so that their general postural alignment is quite good. Figure 8.5 gives examples of individuals with dysplasic characteristics such as small hips and a large head, or heavy legs and buttocks, or large breasts. These subjects certainly have dysplasia but their posture is basically good.

POSTURE AND ITS RELATIONSHIP TO SOMATOTYPE

There is a strong postural relationship with body type, especially among ectomorphs and endomorphs. The *ectomorph* has more postural deformities than the other groups, especially as these relate to the vertebral column. Such defects as a poked or forward head, abducted scapulae or round shoulders, kyphosis or round back, lordosis or hollow back and scoliosis or lateral curvature of the spine, are common with primary ectomorphs, and at times two of the above problems can be combined. *Endomorphs* suffer mainly from

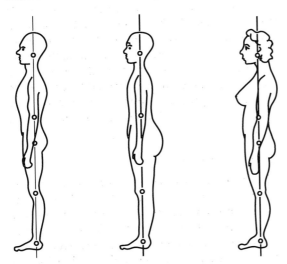

Fig. 8.5 Examples of individuals with dysplasic characteristics.

leg deformities, due to the added burden of additional weight and such problems as genu valgum or knock knees, flat feet, and everted or duck feet are common. *Mesomorphs* are generally free from major postural defects but may develop minor problems as they grow older, especially if they increase their body mass (weight).

POSTURAL DEFECTS

Causes of Postural Defects

Ackland and Bloomfield (1992) stated that there were several factors causing postural defects, some of which are genetic while the others are environmental. These were reported as follows:

- '*Injury* — when a bone, ligament or muscle injury occurs, it may weaken the support normally provided to the total framework. Therefore as long as the condition is present, good posture may not be attainable
- *Disease* — diseases often weaken bones and muscles or cause joints to lose their strength, thus upsetting posture. Examples of such diseases include arthritis and osteoporosis
- *Habit* — postural habits are acquired by repeating the same body alignment on many occasions, such as when leaning over a desk or slouching in a chair. If body segments are held out of alignment for extended periods of time, the surrounding musculature rests in a lengthened or shortened position
- *Skeletal imbalance* — the most familiar imbalance of skeletal lengths is seen in the lower limbs, and in extreme cases this causes a lateral pelvic tilt and may result in the development of scoliosis. However, more subtle skeletal differences such as the location of the acetabulum (Fig. 8.6) and length of the clavicle provide equal potential for defective posture'

Postural defects can also be caused by such variables as an individual's mental attitude over a prolonged period of time, or the wearing of high-heeled shoes, which shift the centre of gravity forward.

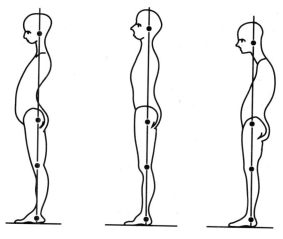

Fig. 8.6 The effect of the location of the acetabulum on back posture.

Interrelationships of Postural Defects

Although postural defects are treated segmentally, it must be stressed that these abnormalities are usually associated with other changes within the body. Normally the downward gravitational pull on any part of the body is borne by the segment below, but if any segment deviates from its vertical alignment, its weight must be counterbalanced by the deviation of another segment in the opposite direction. Therefore postural defects must be seen from a total body perspective. Figure 8.4 illustrates this phenomenon in the following way. The subject, by standing in a tense position increases the pelvic tilt so that the pelvis rotates forward on the femur, carrying the lumbar spine forward and with it the body's centre of gravity. To compensate for this position two additional actions occur. First the legs tend to adopt a hyperextended position (genu recurvartum), while the upper part of the body is thrust backwards, thus increasing the lumbar and dorsal curvatures.

Specific Postural Defects

The following defects range from those which are only just visible to the trained eye, to those which are very extreme. Individuals with minor defects may not need a corrective programme because their bodies have gradually adapted to them; however, those with moderate to severe postural deviations will need various levels of remediation and in extreme cases surgery.

ANTEROPOSTERIOR DEFECTS

Poked or forward head

This is a defect in which the neck is slightly flexed and the head is partially tilted forward. It is often associated with abducted scapulae (round shoulders). To correct this defect the anterior muscles of the neck must be stretched and the posterior muscles strengthened (Mueller & Christaldi 1966).

Abducted scapulae (round shoulders)

This debilitating defect occurs when the scapulae assume an abducted position due to a weakened condition of the trapezius and rhomboid muscles and the medial borders protrude from the individual's back. To correct this condition the adductors of the scapulae need to be strengthened and the anterior thoracic muscles of the upper trunk stretched (Mueller & Christaldi 1966).

Kyphosis (round back or Sheuermann's disease)

This defect increases the convexity of the thoracic curve and is caused by wedging of the thoracic vertebrae (Fig. 8.7). Treatment in mild cases consists of exercises designed to stretch the upper anterior thoracic region and strengthen the muscles of the posterior thoracic area. If the condition is severe, a brace should be considered in order to produce extension of the thoracic spine and decreased lordosis in the lumbar spine (Watson 1992).

Lordosis (hollow back)

Lordosis is characterized by an exaggerated lumbar curve, usually caused by the pelvis tilting too far forward (anterior pelvic tilt; APT). In this condition, the abdominal muscles become stretched and weakened and need to be strengthened along with the extensor muscles of the thigh, while the erector spinae and the flexor muscles of the thigh should be stretched (Ackland & Bloomfield 1992).

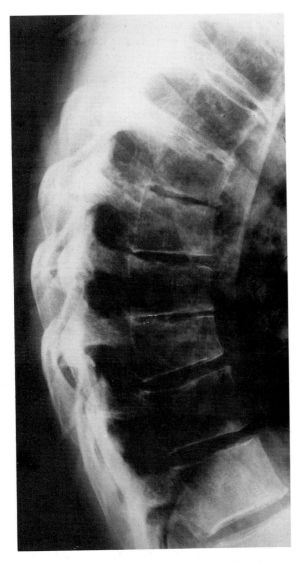

Fig. 8.7 A radiograph of severe kyphosis of the lower thoracic spine depicting vertebral wedging (from Bloomfield *et al.* 1992).

Visceral ptosis (protruding abdomen)

This condition is characterized by the sagging of the abdominal organs and often accompanies lordosis. The downward drag upon the mesenteries occurs when there is not sufficient tension in the abdominal wall to hold them in place. Exercises which strengthen the abdominal muscles are nec-

essary to alleviate this condition (Rasch & Burke 1978; Hills 1991).

Kypholordosis

This defect is a combination of kyphosis and lordosis and as a result places a great deal of stress on the trunk, because the anti-gravity muscles are forced to contract vigorously in order to balance the body segments. It is a condition where the individual is often in a state of chronic fatigue. Exercises which have been recommended for both kyphosis and lordosis should be carried out to alleviate this condition.

Genu recurvartum (leg hyperextension)

This defect is characterized by a backward curve of the legs which creates an unstable knee joint for agility sports (Fig. 8.4). The causes of this condition are basically related to the structure of the femur, the tibia and the cruciate ligaments in the knee joint, and therefore only general strengthening exercises of the musculature surrounding the knee joint should be carried out. It is important to keep the hamstring muscle group almost as strong as the quadriceps (Hills 1991).

LATERAL DEFECTS

Scoliosis

This common defect manifests itself in a lateral curvature of the spine and in many severe cases is accompanied by a longitudinal rotation of the vertebrae (Rasch & Burke 1978). Scoliosis usually begins with a C-shaped curve (functional scoliosis) but over a period of time a righting reflex creates a reversal of the C at the upper spinal levels, producing an S-shaped curve (structural scoliosis). This defect can be caused by uneven leg lengths, muscle imbalance and ligament lengthening.

Functional scoliosis, if identified early, can be corrected or greatly improved by using an orthotic device in a shoe, which will increase the functional leg length of the individual. Exercises which develop general flexibility in the thoracic and lumbar regions of the spine are necessary for individuals with functional scoliosis, but in cases of structural scoliosis medical assistance must be sought.

Genu varum (bow legs) and genu valgum (knock knees)

These conditions are genetic and individuals may need medical attention early in their life if they appear to be serious, as there are at times knee joint irregularities or partial deformities of the femur or tibia bones. Apart from general strengthening exercises for the various muscle groups of the leg, the coach can do little with these defects if they appear to be extreme.

Tibial torsion ('pigeon toes')

Often referred to as *inverted feet*, this condition is characterized by internal rotation at the hip joints. This in turn causes the knees to inwardly rotate ('crossed knees or squinting patellae') so that the feet become inverted. Although it is a structural defect, it can be alleviated by stretching the medial rotators of the hip joint and strengthening the lateral rotators (Rasch & Burke 1978).

Pronated feet ('duck feet')

This defect is also known as *everted feet* and is characterized by a protruding medial malleolus and pseudo flat feet caused by the rolling inward of the ankles. The best treatment for this defect is the use of an orthotic device from an early age and a series of exercises involving toe flexion, foot plantar flexion and supination (Rasch & Burke 1978).

Flat feet

There are several classifications of flat feet and these are as follows:

- *True flat feet* (pes planus) — this is the most serious of the foot defects in which the longitudinal arch is flat. The condition may be accompanied by discomfort and interference with the foot's normal function. Medical treatment should be sought for this defect
- *Functional flat feet* — this is a defect which is caused by weakened and stretched muscles, ligaments and fascia in the foot. If it is not corrected it can distort the mechanical relationships in the ankle, knee, the hip joints and the lumbar spine. Medical treatment should also be sought for this defect

- *Flexible flat feet* — this condition is characterized by a loss of the arches of the feet during weight bearing, but when there is no weight on the feet they appear normal. It is not regarded as pathological, unless it interferes with normal function or becomes painful
- *False flat feet* — this is not a true postural defect but a condition which results from the presence of a fat pad on the plantar surface of the feet. From time to time one hears of elite athletes who have this condition, yet are able to function quite normally with it (Rasch & Burke 1978)

STATIC AND DYNAMIC POSTURE

Posture is static when a person is in equilibrium or motionless. In sport science we are much more interested in *dynamic* posture, that is, when an individual is in motion. Generally there is a high positive correlation between static and dynamic posture, a phenomenon that has been observed by high level coaches for many years. However, a further item of interest when one compares static and dynamic posture relates to injuries that can be the result of postural defects. The following section briefly examines this:

Injuries Resulting from Static Postural Defects

Lorenzton (1988) reported in a study of injured runners, that 40% of them had a variety of postural defects, muscle weakness and imbalance, or decreased flexibility. Malalignment problems of the following types were involved:

- Pronated feet or flat feet, which caused excessive pronation during running, resulted in injury
- During the running cycle, it is necessary to have the correct alignment of the feet and the leg. Runners who did not possess this characteristic, or who had eversion of the heel, predisposed themselves to injury
- Runners with flat feet (pes planus) were liable to develop a further depressed longitudinal arch

without eversion, while those with high arches (pes cavas) suffered from injuries attributed to excessive motion of the subtalar joint

- Individuals with a wide Q-angle (i.e. a measure obtained by connecting the central point of the patella with the anterior superior iliac spine and the tibial tuberosity) or genu valgum (knock knees), experienced injuries to the patellofemoral joint and the patella itself. Athletes with genu varum (bow legs) also predisposed themselves to injuries in the patella region as well as iliotibial band friction syndrome

- Athletes with leg length discrepancies accompanied by a pelvic tilt developed trochanteric bursitis and iliotibial band friction syndrome, as well as intervertebral compression on the concave side of the lateral lumbar curve

The above injuries can be partially eliminated if coaches and sports medicine specialists become more aware of the increased risk of injury among athletes with the above postural defects. Astute observation can often save an athlete from developing a chronic and debilitating injury which could have been avoided.

Prevention of Postural Defects

In order to prevent minor postural defects occurring, most athletes should, as part of their flexibility and strength training programmes, carry out a pro-active exercise routine designed to assist in the maintenance of good posture. Many postural defects can develop from the overuse of one or several regions of the body and they can cause physical discomfort and injury in the more mature athlete. Figure 8.8 shows the overdevelopment of the left side of the upper body of a high performance left-handed fast bowler in cricket and the accompanying scoliosis which developed over several years. This can occur with all unilateral athletes if it is not guarded against, while bilateral athletes such as swimmers, cyclists, wrestlers and boxers, can develop various anteriorposterior curvatures, the most common of these being round shoulders resulting from their

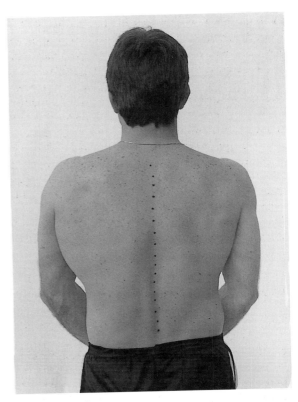

Fig. 8.8 Overdevelopment of the left side of the upper body with an accompanying scoliosis, of a high level cricketer.

intensive sport-specific training programmes. There are however some postural characteristics, which if not too extreme, are a definite advantage to the athlete and these are explained in the section on posture modification later in this chapter.

POSTURE ASSESSMENT

Static posture is usually assessed subjectively in the standing position using a rating chart as a guide for the observer. The alignment of body segments when viewed from the posterior and lateral perspective is thus examined. More objective tests which focus on a particular postural deformity rather than mass screening, include medical imaging techniques using radiography and computerized tomography. In addition, special photographic techniques such as Moiré Topology have been developed for the accurate assessment of scoliosis and other spinal postural disorders.

Instrumentation and methodologies for measuring dynamic posture are not generally available; however, these may eventually be developed in association with the biomechanical techniques of cinematography and electrogoniometry (Marshall & Elliott 1992). In the field of occupational biomechanics, several quasi-static techniques have been used to quantify dynamic postures in the work environment and these have been reviewed by Chaffin and Andersson (1984). Section 3 discusses posture assessment in more detail.

DESIRABLE POSTURES FOR HIGH LEVEL SPORT PERFORMANCE

There are various minor postural deviations which are well suited to different sports and events, because the alignment of the bones and the muscles covering them produce a mechanical advantage, either with speed and/or power or balance (Bloomfield 1979). Posture has a marked effect on performance, but little research has been carried out on its advantages or disadvantages. The following application of various postural phenomena to the major sports groups has been mainly done by coaches, who by trial and error have made the following observations.

Racquet Sports (Tennis, Badminton, Squash, Racquetball)

Competitors in racquet sports have variable postures; however, those with inverted feet (pigeon toes) have a speed advantage over a short distance such as on small courts, because they automatically take short steps which are usually very rapid. There has been some debate as to why this postural characteristic enables them to move fast over a limited distance and the most quoted theory is that tibial torsion tends to shorten the hamstring muscle group, preventing the individual 'striding out' and taking long steps. This charac-

teristic is of little value to athletes who wish to move very fast over any distance more than 15–20 m because to attain very high speeds one needs both a fast stride rate and a reasonably long stride. Furthermore it is also thought that by cutting down the player's stride length, the dynamic balance is improved, because there is more ground contact while moving.

It is also important to reinforce the point which was made earlier in this chapter relating to unilateral athletes, and many racquet sports players fit into this category, especially mesomorphic males. Such players should have compensatory strength and flexibility training on the opposite side of their body to their preferred side, in order to prevent muscle overdevelopment and in some cases scoliosis from occurring.

Aquatic Sports

SWIMMING AND WATERPOLO

Swimmers with square shoulders and upright trunks, who possess long clavicles and large scapulae appear to have lower levels of shoulder flexion–extension than those with sloping shoulders. If square-shouldered swimmers need high levels of flexibility, then they must undergo a particularly intensive programme to improve this physical capacity. Swimmers with inverted feet (pigeon toes) are admirably suited for back and front crawl or butterfly kicking, while those with everted feet (duck feet) are very well suited to breast-stroke kicking. Brodecker (1952) suggested that leg hyperextension is very prevalent in swimmers and some sports medicine doctors have suggested that it occurs because the cruciate ligaments of the knee slowly stretch from constant kicking, thus allowing more recurvartum to develop. High level coaches and biomechanists however do not seem to have reached a consensus as to whether it is an advantage to the swimmer or not, with some stating that it makes little difference in kicking, while others suggest that this posture gives a greater range of anterior and posterior motion at the knee joint.

ROWING AND CANOEING

Rowers and *canoeists* do not appear to need any inherent postural characteristics in order to gain an advantage over other competitors in their sports. It is true that many of them have a slightly rounded back, but this phenomenon is thought to be the result of intensive training with slightly hunched shoulders, rather than being a contributing factor to their self-selection for these two sports.

Gymnastic and Power Sports

GYMNASTICS

Female *gymnasts* with lordosis and an APT are able to hyperextend their spine more easily than those who are more flat backed. If they have protruding buttocks with the above characteristics, they will possess hip extension advantages over flat-buttocked competitors and will also be able to spring very effectively in the floor exercise part of their programmes.

WEIGHTLIFTING

These athletes do not appear to need any one major postural characteristic in order to gain a distinct advantage over their fellow competitors. From a postural perspective they are a very variable group of individuals.

Track, Field and Cycling

SPRINTING

Athletes with APT as well as protruding buttocks (provided they have all the other necessary physical capacities) are usually excellent *sprinters* (Fig. 8.9). This postural phenomenon is commonly found in Africans (currently in or originally from Africa) and is less common in Europeans, while Asian males very rarely possess it. It should be noted however that this characteristic is more common among European females and is sometimes found in Asian women. Webster (1948) appears to be the first coach to have commented on it when he stated that 'actual dissection of negroes has

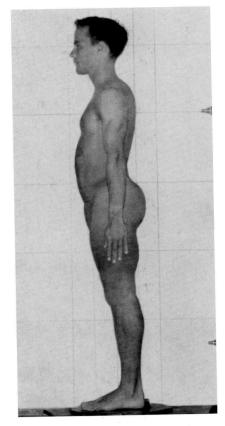

Fig. 8.9 This sprinter demonstrates an anterior pelvic tilt and protruding buttocks (courtesy of Tanner 1964).

shown that they have a more forward pitch of the pelvic bones and consequently a more forward hang of the thigh'. Brodecker (1952) supported this observation and linked it to protruding buttocks. He further stated that many African American athletes possess APT and that it is also 'typical of the female'. He also suggested that the 'overhanging knee joint' (overhanging thigh), where the patella is well forward of the junction of the anterior part of the ankle joint when viewed laterally (the exact anatomical position is with the patella vertically above the tarsometatarsal joint), occurs in individuals with a tilted pelvis (Fig. 8.10). This is a contrasting leg posture to that of swimmers, who generally have little pelvic tilt, relatively flat buttocks, and almost no overhanging

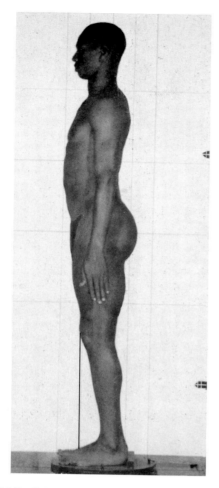

Fig. 8.10 This high hurdler, although taller than the majority of sprinters, has an almost identical posture to them and as well displays an overhanging thigh (courtesy of Tanner 1964).

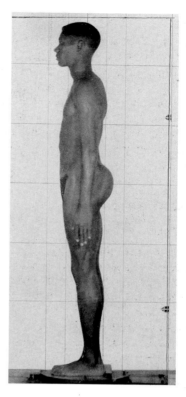

Fig. 8.11 This 400 m runner has a similar buttock posture to sprinters (courtesy of Tanner 1964).

thigh. Brodecker (1952) suggested that individuals with APT and protruding buttocks are able to exert more force in running as the leg is extended back. This is in agreement with many sprint coaches, who believe that the above posture gives the sprinter an optimal driving angle in the extension phase of the running cycle. The high hurdler, although taller, has an almost identical posture to the sprinter and Fig. 8.10 illustrates this phenomenon.

The above postural characteristics in very fast runners are accompanied by large and powerful buttocks (gluteus maximus muscle) and thighs, particularly the hamstring muscle group (biceps femoris — long head, semitendinosus, semimembranosus) which, with the gluteus maximus, extend the thigh with a powerful 'driving action'.

MIDDLE DISTANCE RUNNING

Athletes in middle distance running events, particularly those in the 400 m, and some in the 800 m events, have a similar buttock posture, although usually not as extreme, to that of sprinters (Fig. 8.11). As the races get longer, the protruding buttocks characteristic disappears, with long distance runners having reasonably flat backs and buttocks (Fig. 8.12).

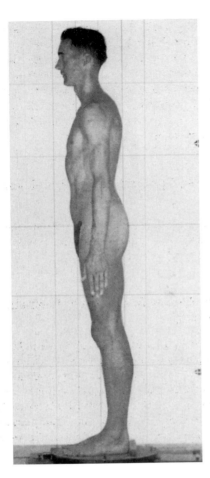

Fig. 8.12 This distance runner displays the flat back and buttocks of the majority of the athletes in his group (courtesy of Tanner 1964).

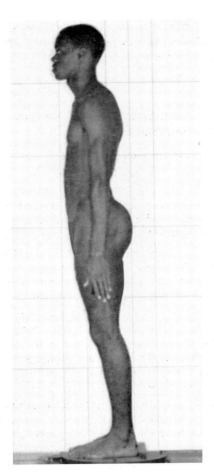

Fig. 8.13 This jumper has a similar hip and buttock posture to sprinters (courtesy of Tanner 1964).

JUMPING

The group of *field athletes* who compete in jumping, although different to sprinters in their proportions, have almost identical postures to them. Figure 8.13, which shows an outstanding long jumper, illustrates this and demonstrates the APT and particularly the protruding buttocks which are accompanied by the overhanging thigh of the vast majority of agility athletes.

THROWING

Elite level *throwers*, like weightlifters, have no single postural characteristic that is obvious.

Their performances are related more to body bulk, proportionality and explosive power.

CYCLING

Cyclists have definite postural characteristics but these are thought to relate more to their heavy training routines over prolonged periods of time than to their constitutional bone shape. They tend to have slightly rounded backs and possess the overhanging thigh phenomenon. It is thought that the latter posture is caused more by the heavy musculature in the thighs and buttocks, particularly in sprint cyclists, than by natural APT and protruding buttocks, which the majority of sprint and agility athletes display. In other words, their very heavy power training has influenced their posture.

Mobile Field Sports (Field Hockey, Soccer, Lacrosse)

Athletes in mobile field sports are usually a varied group with no rigid postural requirements. Players in positions where they have limited territory to cover may have a specialized posture such as inverted feet. Where a high level of speed is needed for a reasonable distance, for example in wing positions in various sports, APT and protruding buttocks can be of value, provided however that the player has the necessary skill and other physical requirements to be a valuable team member. In these sports a non-rigid or non-upright spine is an advantage, because the player is in a slightly flexed position for a reasonable period of time during the game. It is an advantage therefore for these athletes to have at least moderate lumbar and dorsal curves. As for all agility sports, genu recurvartum (Fig. 8.4) is an inferior leg posture in comparison to the overhanging thigh posture (Fig. 8.10), not only because the knee joint is already hyperextended and takes a longer time to straighten than the slightly flexed knee joint, but also because the genu recurvartum posture creates an unstable knee joint for twisting and turning movements.

Contact Field Sports (Rugby Codes, Australian Football, American Football)

Players in contact field sports are posturally similar to the former group but generally have more body bulk. Postural characteristics which are advantageous are those with a reasonable degree of spinal curvature rather than a rigid upright posture; inverted feet, where quick stepping and elusive running are needed for short distances; and APT, protruding buttocks and an overhanging thigh for players who need

bursts of speed. Genu recurvartum is a poor posture for contact sport, therefore any swimmers who have this characteristic and who also play contact sports should be advised against doing very much front or back crawl kicking, which accentuates the problem, making the knee joint more unstable and less functional for agile movement.

Set Field Sports (Baseball, Cricket, Golf)

One sees a wide variety of postures in set field sports and no one posture seems to give any advantage to players in them.

Court Sports (Basketball, Netball, Volleyball)

Basketball, volleyball and *netball* are agility sports where superior height, reflexive movement and jumping ability are important. Inverted feet, which promote fast steps and good balance are desirable, as are the APT and protruding buttocks, accompanied by an overhanging thigh, along with reasonable spinal curvatures both in the lower and upper back.

Martial Arts (Judo, Wrestling, Boxing)

In the grappling sports good balance is important, therefore inverted feet could be advantageous. To have reasonably accentuated spinal curves will also give the competitor more trunk mobility, which should be an advantage.

MODIFYING POSTURE AND TECHNIQUE TO IMPROVE PERFORMANCE

It will be quite obvious to the reader by now that there are several postures which, if not too extreme, may be advantageous to top athletic performance and that posture is another way in which self-selection can occur for various sports or events. Therefore, there should be no attempt to modify these characteristics in any way, even though at first glance they may appear to be partially defective. Other postures however may be detrimental to performance, so that a strategy should be worked out to modify them.

A decision therefore must be made by the coach as to whether the athlete should undergo a modification programme or not. In many cases this will not be necessary, but should be considered if it is felt that a high level athlete can benefit from it, particularly in sports where winning margins are very small. The following actions can be taken:

- The first approach should be to modify any *static* defects which may need correction, using a series of exercises which will stretch tight muscles and strengthen those which have become slack. This corrective programme should be undertaken if at all possible in pre- or early adolescence. In post-adolescence it will take longer, but reasonable results can still be obtained at this time if the programme is intensive enough. It must always be kept in mind that static defects which are evident just prior to and in adolescence will become more extreme as the individual ages and that physical discomfort and the incidence of injury will probably increase as time goes on

- The second action is one which only a few enlightened coaches have used thus far, but it will become more popular in the future. This is to accentuate those postures which are known to be advantageous for various sports. This is particularly important for individuals who appear to have almost all of the other necessary physical capacities for optimal performance, but who lack the postural characteristics needed for highly specialized events. The following two examples will illustrate this point. If a sprinter has all the other characteristics to run very fast, but does not have enough APT, then a minor postural modification may

be made, so as to enable a slightly better 'driving angle' during the thigh extension phase of the running cycle, by tilting the pelvis forward. To do this the trunk extensor and thigh flexor muscles must be strengthened and at the same time the abdominal and thigh extensor muscles stretched. Also, agility athletes who need speed over a short distance can slightly increase their level of tibial torsion (inverted feet or 'pigeon toes') by strengthening the medial rotators of the hip joint and stretching the lateral rotators. It should be stressed again that posture modification will only occur with an *intense* intervention programme taking place, often over several years

- *Dynamic* posture can also be changed with good skills coaching, and this has been done by enlightened coaches for the past half century in technique-oriented sports such as track and field, gymnastics, diving, rowing, golf and swimming. These coaches know how to incorporate various postural positions into their athletes' techniques such as tilting the pelvis, rounding the back, tucking in the chin, squaring the shoulders, everting the feet and so on. However, less attention has been paid to dynamic posture in team sports where agility is an important factor in the game and more specialization in various positions is becoming necessary. For example, the footballer who is straight backed with little mobility in his spine has a poor posture for collision sports, where players are running into rucks, mauls and packs; or for closed field running, where tacklers are able to hit the ball carrier with little notice. The round-shouldered player has a natural advantage in this situation, because he is able to 'tuck in' or 'cover up' very quickly, whereas the straight-backed player is not in as good a natural position to take the heavy contact and can easily become injured. Well-informed coaches can develop this dynamic characteristic with intensive practice in the correct postural position, thereby making their players more physically effective and less prone to injury

CONCLUSION

To conclude this chapter, it must be stressed again that there is a large number of physical, physiological, psychological and skill factors that contribute to top sports performance and that posture may only play a small role in some sports, or almost none in others. It is important, however, for coaches to be aware of the situations where posture is very important and to be able to appreciate its value in their athletes. If a particular posture appears to be an essential characteristic for a highly specialized sport, then coaches need to have enough knowledge in order to better select their athletes, or to at least modify their postures so that they can improve their performance.

REFERENCES

Ackland T. & Bloomfield J. (1992) Functional Anatomy. In Bloomfield J., Fricker P. & Fitch K. (eds) *Textbook of Science and Medicine in Sport*, pp. 9–12. Blackwell Scientific Publications, Melbourne.

Bloomfield J. (1979) Modifying human physical capacities and technique to improve performance. *Sports Coach* **3**, 19–25.

Bloomfield I., Fricker P. & Fitch K. (eds) (1992) *Textbook of Science and Medicine in Sport*, p. 456. Blackwell Scientific Publications, Melbourne.

Brodecker P. (1952) *Physical Build vs Athletic Ability in American Sports*, pp. 55–59. Athletic Ability Publications, Chicago.

Chaffin D. & Andersson G. (1984) *Occupational Biomechanics*. John Wiley, New York.

Hills A. (1991) *Physical Growth and Development of Children and Adolescents*, pp. 73–84. Queensland University of Technology, Brisbane.

Krogman W. (1951) The scars of human evolution. *Scientific American* **185**, 54–57.

Lorenzton R. (1988) Causes of Injuries: Intrinsic Factors. In Dirix A., Knuttgen H. & Tittle K. (eds) *The Olympic Book of Sports Medicine I*, pp. 376–389. Blackwell Scientific Publications, Oxford.

Marshall R. & Elliott B. (1992) Biomechanical Analysis. In Bloomfield J., Fricker P. & Fitch K. (eds) *Textbook of Science and Medicine in Sport*, pp. 47–64. Blackwell Scientific Publications, Melbourne.

Mueller G. & Christaldi J. (1966) *A Practical Program of Remedial Physical Education*, pp. 65–73, 121–170. Lea & Febiger, Philadelphia.

Napier J. (1967) The antiquity of human walking. *Scientific American* **3**, 38–48.

Rasch P. & Burke R. (1978) *Kinesiology and Applied Anatomy*, pp. 361–387. Lea & Febiger, Philadelphia.

Sheldon W., Stevens S. & Tucker W. (1940) *The Varieties of Human Physique*, p. 7. Harper and Brothers, New York.

Sinclair D. (1973) *Human Growth After Birth*, pp. 113–118. Oxford University Press, London.

Tanner J. (1964) *The Physique of the Olympic Athlete*, pp. 103–113. George Allen and Unwin, London.

Watson A. (1992) Children in sport. In Bloomfield J., Fricker P. A. & Fitch K. D. (eds) *Textbook of Science and Medicine in Sport*, p. 456. Blackwell Scientific Publications, Melbourne.

Webster F. (1948) *The Science of Athletics*, p. 331. Nicholas Kaye, London.

CHAPTER 9

STRENGTH AND POWER IN SPORT

By Greg J. Wilson

Athletes for thousands of years have used various forms of resistance training to enhance their sporting performance. The tale of Milo of Crotona, who as a young man lifted a calf onto his shoulders and carried it around his yard, is legendary. As the calf grew to become an adult bull young Milo grew to be a large strong man and become one of the greatest athletes in ancient Greece. Even in those early days of resistance training the Greeks were reported to use detailed periodization strategies based on a 4-day training cycle with a varied training intensity, so that there was only one intensive training session every 4 days (Sweet 1987). Such programmes are commonly performed 2000 years later.

The use of resistance training is thousands of years old, but it is only during the past 20 years that it has been transformed from the pursuit of a relatively small number of strength athletes into an integral part of the training routine of most athletes. While resistance training has historically been seen as a means to enhance muscular strength and size, it is currently used by a variety of individuals to also increase power, speed and endurance, enhance muscle tone, assist in rehabilitation and injury prevention and to aid in the maintenance of muscular function into old age.

This chapter reviews the current use of resistance training in the development of the muscular functions of strength, explosive power and endurance, from a performance enhancement perspective. It outlines the latest developments in resistance training and compares various optimal training strategies. Sport-specific training routines will be outlined in detail and new training techniques and equipment discussed. A great deal of research has been performed on the effects of resistance training, in particular strength training; however, little of this research has been applied to enhance the day to day practices of the many athletes who currently use such programmes. In fact while literally thousands of research papers have been published in the area over the past 20 years, the resistance training routines currently adopted by athletes have changed little during this time. This chapter therefore, while relying heavily on both research findings and theory, is written from an applied perspective which can be easily understood by both the athlete and coach.

VALUE OF STRENGTH AND POWER IN SPORT

Muscular strength can be defined as the amount of force (or torque) a muscle group can exert against a resistance in one maximal effort. Power can be defined as the ability to produce high levels of work (the product of force and the distance through which the force acts) quickly. Power is the result of speed and strength and is often expressed as:

power = strength × speed (force × velocity)

The physical capacities of strength and power are important qualities for many sports. Maximum strength and/or power can clearly discriminate between athletes of different performance levels within sports such as American football (Fry & Kraemer 1991), volleyball (Fry *et al.* 1991), rowing (Secher 1975), swimming (Rohrs *et al.* 1990), sprint running (Mero *et al.* 1981) and kayaking (Fry & Morton 1991). In fact Miyashita and Kanshisa (1979) have reported a strong relationship between sprint swimming performance and strength, while Sharp *et al.* (1982) have reported an even stronger relationship between swimming performance and power.

The importance of resistance training to sports performance has been supported by studies which have demonstrated that resistance training in the form of weight training and, more recently, plyometric training, have enhanced some competitive performances. Most typically this has been reported as an improvement in vertical jumping ability. Adams *et al.* (1992) reported that a 6 week period of weight training resulted in a 3.3 cm increase in the vertical jump, as compared to a 3.8 cm increase achieved from plyometric training, and a 10.7 cm increase from a combined strength training–plyometric routine.

However, there are many studies which have reported that resistance training has enhanced muscular strength, but failed to induce changes in dynamic sporting performance such as sprint running (Fry *et al.* 1991). For example, Bloomfield *et al.* (1990) observed a significant relationship between strength and throwing velocity in elite waterpolo players. However, when these athletes were placed on a resistance training programme which resulted in significant improvements in strength, throwing velocity did not vary as a consequence of the training. Rutherford *et al.* (1986) reported that 12 weeks of weight training increased the weights lifted in a leg extension task by 160–200%, however peak power output in a cycle test was unchanged by the training. Wilmore and Costill (1988) claimed that although strength training had been a part of the conditioning programme of competitive swimmers for the past 50 years, it did not appear to significantly improve swimming performance. In many sports there appears to be a minimum level of strength that is required for

high level performance; however, additional strength above this minimum does not necessarily improve it.

Thus while traditional heavy weight training results in large changes in strength in previously untrained subjects, and strength appears to be an important physical capacity in most sports, whether standard strength training methods can enhance sporting performance appears to depend upon the sport. Strength-dominated sports that involve the production of large forces over relatively long time periods (such as weightlifting, wrestling, rugby and American football) would appear to be readily improved by strength training. However, more speed-oriented activities such as throwing, hitting, punching and kicking seem less responsive to traditional strength training techniques.

RELATIONSHIP BETWEEN STRENGTH, POWER AND STRENGTH–ENDURANCE

Strength versus Power

If an individual is asked to exert maximum force against a resistance it takes time to develop this level of tension. For an isometric task involving the forearm flexors it has been reported to take up to 1.6 s to develop maximum tension; for the leg extensors the time taken is even longer (Atha 1981). This delay occurs because prior to the achievement of maximum tension the following actions must take place:

- All the muscle fibres for the appropriate muscles must be recruited and fired at their maximal rate
- The muscles and tendons may need to be stretched prior to force development, in order to extend the elastic components of the musculature

In many sports however, the time over which the force can be exerted is very limited. For example, the foot contact time in sprinting or jumping is very brief, being in the order of approximately

100–150 ms. Thus the ability to quickly produce force is of paramount importance.

Three force–time curves are depicted in Fig. 9.1. These theoretical curves represent the force-generating capacity of differing athletes when performing a maximal contraction. Curve 1 represents the force–time characteristics of an individual who is very strong but not very powerful, for example, a power-lifter. These individuals would be effective in performing strength movements, such as a squat or bench press lift, but less effective in a power event like a high jump or shot put, as they are unable to produce relatively high force levels quickly. Curve 2 represents an individual who has less absolute strength than the athlete in Curve 1; however, this competitor is able to generate a greater force over a brief period (i.e. 150 ms). Although not capable of lifting as much weight, this individual may outperform the athlete in Curve 1 in a dynamic power event such as a high jump. Indeed Hakkinen *et al.* (1984) have reported that elite wrestlers developed force significantly more rapidly when compared to elite power-lifters. Curve 3 represents an athlete who can produce the available force very rapidly but does not have a high strength level. Consequently this individual is ineffective in both strength and power dominated events.

Curve 3 demonstrates the fact that the *level of maximum strength of an athlete places an upper*

limit on the performance of power events; thus power athletes must be strong. There is little value in having the capacity to develop force quickly if the overall level of force is particularly low. Consequently some researchers have reported strong relationships between maximal strength and power (Rutherford *et al.* 1986). However, in comparing Curves 1 and 2, it can be seen that simply being strong does not necessarily make an individual powerful. *Thus power athletes must be strong and also able to generate high levels of force over relatively short periods of time.*

The above analyses clearly demonstrate that although strength and power are related, they are different capacities. This is one of the reasons why the strongest man or woman in the world is not necessarily the best javelin thrower or shot putter. It is not just that they do not have the appropriate technique, but their muscles may not be capable of generating the applied force rapidly, as is required in most dynamic sporting performances. It is also one of the reasons why athletes may increase strength in the gymnasium but not alter their competitive performance. The realization that *strength and power are different qualities* is very important in the correct formulation of resistance training for athletes and this has often been misunderstood by coaches. Research from Hakkinen *et al.* (1985a,b) has shown that while heavy weight training results in increases in the maximum force, the rate of force development remains unaltered. That is, the force–time curve is extended so that higher forces are generated over the long time periods (Fig. 9.2). Explosive resistance training, in the form of traditional plyometrics, tends to have the opposite effect. There is a smaller change in maximal strength, but a greater increase in the rate of force development. This is observed as a shift in the force–time curve in order that greater forces are produced over shorter periods of time (Fig. 9.2).

Strength versus Endurance

All other factors being equal, a stronger muscle will have greater endurance when it is compared to a weaker muscle, as it uses a smaller percen-

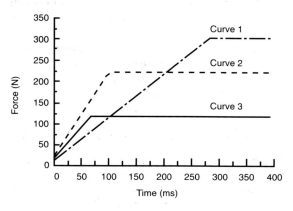

Fig. 9.1 Hypothetical force–time curves for individuals of differing strength and power capacities.

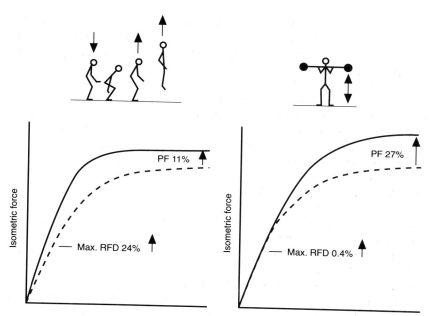

Fig. 9.2 Changes in the force–time curves in response to plyometric and strength training (adapted from Hakkinen et al. 1985a,b).

tage of its maximum strength in performing a given task, thereby delaying the onset of fatigue (Tuttle *et al.* 1950). For example, if at a given velocity a rower is required to produce a mean force against the oar of 500 N per stroke and has a maximum strength capacity of 1000 N, then the rower is working at 50% of his or her maximum during each stroke. If the rower's maximum strength capacity is only 750 N, then the athlete will be working at 67% of maximum and thus may fatigue more quickly.

The proportional relationship between strength and endurance has been rationalized differently by Counsilman (1986) who stated that: 'If you have to use every motor unit to pull your arm through the water at the desired speed to swim fast you'll tire quickly. But if you can improve your strength to the point where you only need to use a portion of the motor units, you can alternate motor units and thereby improve your strength endurance.'

A similar example of the importance of strength to endurance is seen by the inverse relationship between the load used in a lift and the maximum number of repetitions that can be achieved, as illustrated in Fig. 9.3. Using data provided by McDonagh and Davies (1984), an individual with a maximal bench press of 100 kg should be capable of performing six to seven repetitions (Fig. 9.3) at a load of 75 kg (i.e. 75% of maximum). If, however, the individual's maximum was 150 kg, the 75 kg load will only represent 50% of maximum and thus 12–13 repetitions should be performed (Fig. 9.3). Consequently through a 50% increase in maximal strength (100–150 kg) a 100% increase in endurance is realized (6–12 repetitions). The importance of strength and power to endurance can also be seen in the relatively high relationships recorded by Sharp *et al.* (1982) between arm power and swimming performance over 500 m. Therefore, *the physical capacities of strength and endurance are closely related and hence strength–endurance athletes, such as 400 m runners, need to have relatively high levels of absolute strength*.

MUSCLE STRUCTURE AND FUNCTION

Muscular Components

A single muscle is composed of a number of individual muscle fibres whose number vary considerably, depending on the size and function of the muscle. Each muscle fibre is between 1 and

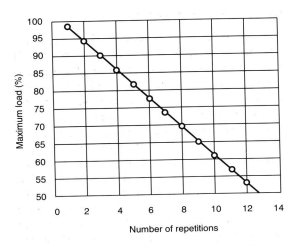

Fig. 9.3 Relationship between number of repetitions and load (adapted from data reported in McDonagh & Davies 1984).

40 mm in length and is 10–100 microns (μm) in diameter. Inside the muscle fibres are numerous myofibrils which range in diameter from 1 to 2 μm. These myofibrils are aligned in columns and have distinctive markings. The repetitive markings define the contractile unit of muscle, the sarcomere, which is bound on each end by a Z-line. Each myofibril is composed of numerous sarcomeres which are joined end to end (i.e. in series) at the Z-lines. Each sarcomere is approximately 2.3 μm in length and composed of a number of microscopic myofilaments called actin and myosin. The thinner of the two small filaments is the protein actin, while the protein myosin forms the thicker filament (Fig. 9.4).

Sliding Filament Theory

In developing force a muscle contracts and thus shortens. The precise mechanism used to shorten the sarcomere is not fully understood, but there is evidence to suggest that when stimulated the actin and myosin filaments slide past one another. This motion is accomplished by the pulling action of cross-bridges that reach out from the myosin filaments and attach themselves to the actin filaments. After binding, the cross-bridges suddenly shorten, drawing the two protein threads past one another and reducing the length of the sarcomere by 20–50%. This action takes place simultaneously in millions of muscle fibres, resulting in a forceful pull on the tendons (Fig. 9.4).

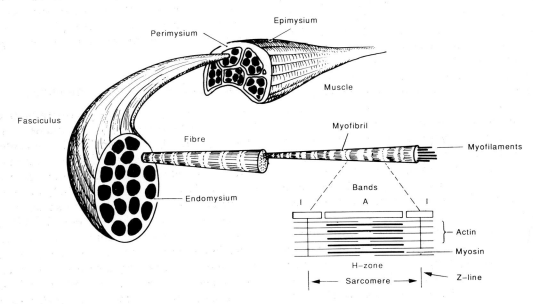

Fig. 9.4 Structural design of human skeletal muscle (from Bloomfield *et al.* 1992).

Muscle Fibre Types

Two discrete categories of muscle fibre types, slow and fast twitch, have been identified based on their histochemical staining qualities as well as their physiological characteristics. The *slow twitch* (ST or Type I) fibres account for approximately 50% of normal human skeletal muscle fibres and are characterized as possessing an aerobic endurance quality. *Fast twitch* (FT or Type II) fibres may be further divided into three categories based on their stained appearance, as well as their propensity for recruitment. Fast twitch type 'a' (FTa or Type IIa) constitute about half the FT muscle fibres, with the remainder predominantly fast twitch 'b' (FTb or Type IIb). Only a very small number of fast twitch 'c' (FTc or Type IIc) have been identified. The FT fibres produce more force than ST fibres but they fatigue more rapidly. For this reason, ST fibres are preferentially recruited during low intensity activities and as the tension requirements increase, more FT fibres are activated.

RATE OF CONTRACTION

The rate at which a muscle can contract and develop force is dependent on the number of sarcomeres in series that the muscle possesses. The greater the number in a given length of muscle, the more actin and myosin will be simultaneously sliding past one another and thus the greater the rate of muscle contraction. Fast twitch fibres have relatively short sarcomeres, being 2.4 μm in length, as compared to ST fibres, whose sarcomeres are 6.0 μm in length. Thus with all things being equal, there are more FT sarcomeres in series for a given length of muscle in comparison to ST, and therefore FT fibres have a higher rate of contraction. Further, FT fibres have cross-bridges whose actions are very rapid, enhancing the development of force production, whereas ST fibres contain cross-bridges whose actions are relatively slow, thus reducing their rate of contraction. Consequently, it is not surprising that researchers have reported that the maximum shortening velocity of bundles of FT fibres are three times greater than equivalent bundles of ST fibres (Edman 1979; Faulkner *et al.* 1986).

MUSCLE FIBRE CHARACTERISTICS

In general, ST muscle fibres are characterized as having good aerobic endurance, whereas FT muscle fibres develop more force but fatigue more quickly. Indeed Faulkner *et al.* (1986) reported that the peak power output of FT fibres was four times that of ST fibres. The differing capabilities of these muscle fibres mean that the relative percentage of FT and ST fibres is important in elite sport performance. Mero *et al.* (1981) performed a study on 25 male sprinters who had recorded 100 m sprint times that varied between 10.4 and 11.8 s. These investigators reported that the percentage of FT muscle fibre was positively related to maximal running speed, vertical jump height and strength, and negatively associated with endurance. Further, the faster sprinters (mean 100 m time of 10.7 s) had a mean percentage of FT fibres of 66.2%, which was significantly higher than the 50.4% recorded by the slower sprinters (mean 100 m time of 11.5 s). Similarly, the group with the higher percentage of FT fibres was also significantly stronger and more powerful than the group with a higher percentage of ST fibres. However, in an endurance test the FT group performed poorly when compared to the ST group. Thus *a high percentage of FT fibres tends to be associated with good performance in strength, speed and power, but with relatively poor endurance performance.*

CHANGES IN FIBRE TYPE WITH TRAINING

The vast majority of research has demonstrated that the relative percentage of FT and ST muscle fibres is genetically determined and varies little in response to training. With endurance training, FT fibres may enhance their endurance capacity; however, they will not turn into fully functional ST muscle fibres, and the reverse situation also applies. Hakkinen *et al.* (1988) reported the performance and muscular changes in nine elite weightlifters over a 2 year training period. Despite these athletes performing intense long-term resistance training, the percentage of FT fibres did not significantly vary over the 2 year period of the study (57.1±9.6%–55.4±9.2%). Thus *the relative*

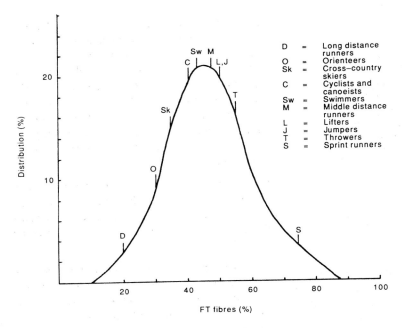

Fig. 9.5 The relative distribution of fibre types in the vastus lateralis muscles of sportspersons (from Bloomfield *et al.* 1992).

percentage of FT and ST fibres appears to present a genetically imposed limitation to performance. The existence of such a performance limitation supports the notion that elite athletes are born and not made. Figure 9.5 outlines the typical fibre type composition of elite athletes in different sports. As is apparent from this figure, endurance-based athletes, such as long distance runners, cyclists, rowers, orienteers and cross-country skiers, possess a greater proportion of ST fibres compared to the normal population, whereas power athletes such as throwers, sprinters and jumpers have proportionally more FT fibres.

While the various muscles in the body can have differing relative percentages of FT and ST muscle fibres, generally individuals will have similar fibre type proportions in their legs to those in their arms.

Size Theory of Motor Unit Recruitment

Individual muscle fibres do not operate independently but are innervated by motor neurons or nerves which originate in the spinal cord. A motor unit includes the motor neuron and all the fibres it innervates. Each muscle has 100–1000 motor units which control the firing of the individual muscle fibres. A single motor unit may innervate as few as three muscle fibres in small muscles that require fine precision such as those controlling the eyes. In larger muscles such as gluteus maximus, as many as 800 muscle fibres may be controlled by one motor unit.

All muscle fibres within the same motor unit will consist of the same fibre type, thus FT and ST motor units exist. Typically ST motor units innervate between 10 and 180 fibres, while FT motor units are larger and innervate 300–800 fibres. As muscular tension is developed motor units are recruited on the basis of their size (Henneman *et al.* 1974); initially the smaller, ST motor units are recruited, followed by the larger, FT motor units (Fig. 9.6). Increases in tension will, at first, be produced by increasing the firing rate of the ST motor units. Greater tension is developed by the additional recruitment of progressively larger FT motor units and by increasing their firing rate. This process continues until maximal force is achieved when all of the available motor units are recruited and fired at their maximal rate.

Based on the size theory of motor unit recruitment, the large FT motor units, which are predominantly responsible for the production of power-

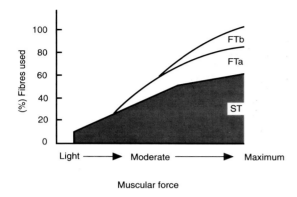

Fig. 9.6 The recruitment of differing muscle fibre types as a function of muscular force (adapted with permission from Wilmore & Costill 1988).

ful movements, will only be recruited if relatively large forces are required. This theory is often used as a rationalization for the use of heavy training loads in the development of muscular power and athletic performance (Schmidtbleicher 1988). It is suggested that training with light loads does not allow for the recruitment of FT muscle fibres, as the force requirement is simply too low. In contrast, heavy load training requires near maximal forces to be developed and thus all motor units, fast and slow, must be used.

Muscle Actions

Once activated, a muscle will attempt to shorten and exert a force on the tendon which is transferred to the skeletal structures. The actual resistance encountered during the muscle action will determine the resulting movement. There are three types of muscular actions:

- *Concentric contraction* — this results when the tension developed is greater than the resistance and thus the musculature shortens. Such an action is produced in the lifting (concentric) phase of most resistance training exercises such as a bench press, squat and arm curl
- *Eccentric contraction* — this results when the tension developed is less than the resistance and the muscle attempts to shorten but is actually lengthened. Such a muscular action is

produced in the lowering (eccentric) phase of most resistance training exercises such as a bench press, squat and arm curl
- *Isometric contraction* — this results when the tension developed is the same as the resistance encountered and the length of the musculature remains essentially unaltered. Such a muscular action is observed when attempting to exert a force against an immovable object such as a wall

The action that a muscle group engages in during an activity is used to define the role played by that muscle. There are basically three differing roles which muscles can play during the performance of an activity.

- *Agonist or prime mover* — when the muscle or muscle group causes the activity to occur; for example, the biceps brachii during the performance of an arm curl exercise
- *Antagonist* — when the muscle or muscle group located on the opposite side of the joint acts to resist the activity; for example, the triceps brachii during the performance of an arm curl exercise
- *Stabilizer or fixator* — when the muscle or muscle group action serves to stabilize the skeletal structures so that tension can be effectively developed by the prime mover. For example, the musculature about the wrist and shoulder joints will isometrically contract during the performance of an arm curl exercise to stabilize

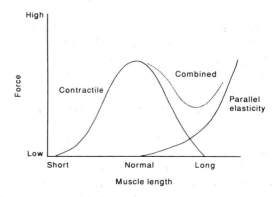

Fig. 9.7 The length–tension curve for an isolated muscle (from Bloomfield *et al.* 1992).

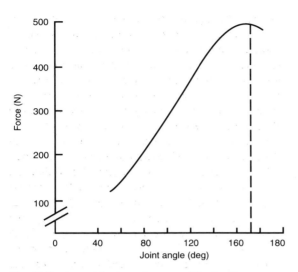

Fig. 9.8 Isometric strength curve of the leg flexors over the full range of leg flexion (adapted with permission from Sale 1991).

the skeletal structures, so that the biceps brachii muscle group can effectively generate force

MUSCLE MECHANICS AND NEUROMUSCULAR CONSIDERATIONS

Length–Tension Relationship

Muscular tension is most effectively achieved at the normal resting length of muscle, as this enables maximum binding of actin and myosin protein filaments (Fig. 9.7). As muscle contracts, its filaments become overlapped and cross-bridge linkages cannot bind completely, with the result that the contraction becomes less effective. Similarly, if the muscle is extended beyond resting length, the overlap between filaments is reduced, not all of the filaments can bind and therefore the muscular force capability is reduced. However, if a muscle is stretched beyond its normal resting length, even in an inactive state, some additional tension is produced as a result of the elasticity of passive structures (e.g. connective tissue) that lie in parallel with the contractile elements. The combined effect of the muscular and elastic factors is depicted in Fig. 9.7, which illustrates the classic length–tension curve of isolated skeletal muscle.

FORCE–POSITION RELATIONSHIP

In any movement range the musculature will possess varying degrees of strength. This is depicted in Fig. 9.8, which illustrates the strength curve for the hamstring muscle group. Such variation in the musculature's ability to produce force at varying positions occurs due to the combined effects of muscle length and the mechanical advantage of the lever system. This latter point relates mainly to the tendon's angle of insertion with respect to the bone at varying positions throughout the movement.

Force–Velocity Relationship

All other factors being equal, high force capacity of a muscle will be realized during an isometric contraction and the muscle's capacity to exert tension will decrease as a function of increased speed of concentric movement (Fig. 9.9). This is due, in part, to the viscous fluid in the muscles which resists motion in proportion to the magnitude of velocity. Furthermore, the cross-bridges break and rejoin more often at higher velocities, resulting in reduced tension, since at high contraction speeds there is not enough time to generate maximum force. As observed in Fig. 9.9, maximum force is realized in rapid eccentric movements. In fact maximal eccentric force is approximately 1.3 times

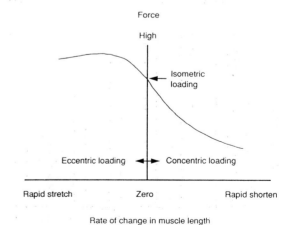

Fig. 9.9 The force–velocity relationship for muscle (from Bloomfield *et al.* 1992).

higher than maximal concentric force (Griffin 1987). This fact is often used to justify the performance of heavy eccentric training as an effective method of enhancing strength, as more force can be developed in the eccentric phase than in the isometric or concentric phases.

Power–Load Relationship

Given the force–velocity relationship of muscle it is evident that, for concentric activities, force and velocity are inversely related. Thus one cannot maximize both qualities at the same time. Therefore maximal power, which is the product of force and velocity, could conceivably be achieved through the following methods:

- High force and low speed
- High speed and low force
- Moderate force and velocity

The last option appears to allow for the maximization of power, as many researchers have reported that peak power occurs at a load of approximately 30–45% of maximum (Kaneko *et al.* 1983, Moritani *et al.* 1987; Fig. 9.10).

Muscle Mechanics

FORCE PRODUCTION

The musculoskeletal system represents a lever system where force is generated by the muscles and

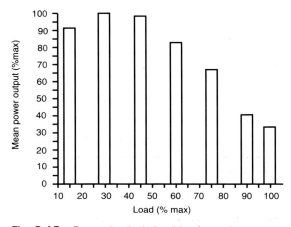

Fig. 9.10 Power–load relationship of muscle.

applied through the tendons to the bone, which consequently attempts to rotate about its axis of rotation, called the joint. This rotatory tendency, termed torque, is a product of the applied force and the perpendicular distance from the force to the axis of rotation. The torque exerted is proportional to the force of muscular contraction and the distance of insertion of the tendon from the joint (axis of rotation) and determines the strength of the individual muscle group(s). Further, the torque will be determined by the angle of pull that the tendon has with respect to the bone. The optimal angle of pull is 90° and the torque effect will reduce as the angle becomes progressively larger or smaller from this optimal value. The angle of pull of the tendon and the muscle's ability to produce force vary with differing positions and thus it is not surprising that the maximal force that can be produced throughout a range of motion will vary quite considerably, as demonstrated in Fig. 9.8.

Often people presume that the strength displayed by individuals is determined entirely by the contractile ability of their muscles; however, the location of the insertion points of the tendons in the bone assumes great significance. Individuals who are fortunate enough to have relatively large distances between the insertion of the tendon and the axis of rotation (the joint), will be capable of producing more torque and hence display greater strength than the average individual. The insertion points of tendons into the bones are not subject to change and represent a genetically imposed limitation to performance that is perhaps as important as the relative proportions of various limbs and the percentage of FT and ST muscle fibres.

EFFECT OF RESISTANCE

The weight of the limb and any additional load on the system will also cause a torque effect about the joint which is generally opposite to that developed by the musculature. The rotatory tendency will be dependent on the load applied and the perpendicular distance that the load is located from the axis of rotation. Thus the torque effect of load on the system will also vary throughout the range of motion. For example, during an arm curl exercise (Fig. 9.11) the torque effect of the load acting about the elbow axis will be greatest at an elbow angle of approximately 90°, when the perpendicular distance from the load (located in the hand) to the axis of rotation (i.e. elbow joint) is greatest. At higher or lower elbow angles the perpendicular distance from the load to the elbow axis is reduced and thus the torque applied by the load about the joint is lower.

EFFECT OF POSTURE ON LOADING

The effect of load on the joints throughout a movement will vary depending on the posture adopted by the athlete. For example, during an arm curl exercise performed in an upright posture (Fig. 9.11), the load will have its greatest effect at an elbow angle of approximately 90° and will have a much reduced effect towards the beginning and end of the range of motion (elbow angles 150–180° and 30–50°, respectively). However, these positions of high and low resistance can be modified by simply altering the posture of the exercise. For example, if the arm curl exercise is performed in a horizontal position, that is, lying face down on a bench (Fig. 9.12), the mechanics of the lever system are altered so that the torque effect of the weight is maximized towards the end of the movement range as opposed to the mid-range of the movement. This is the main reason why bodybuilders perform essentially similar exercises using differing body postures, as each variation in posture will alter the mechanical lever system and allow the muscle to be maximally stressed over different ranges of motion. It is also one of the reasons why *it is important to train the musculature using a posture similar to that which is adopted during the actual competitive performance.*

MUSCLE FIBRE ORIENTATION

The orientation of fibres with respect to the tendon is an important consideration in the ability of the musculature to produce force. If the muscle fibres are oriented longitudinally with respect to the tendon, then the muscles are capable of producing low force but shorten over a relatively long range. These are referred to as *fusiform* muscles. There are relatively few fusiform muscles in the human body and most are located in the extremities, for example, the brachioradialis muscle. If the muscle fibres are oriented so that they are at an angle to the tendon they are termed *penniform*. These muscles produce larger forces but do so over a shorter range than fusiform muscles. They are common within the human body and account for approximately three-quarters of all

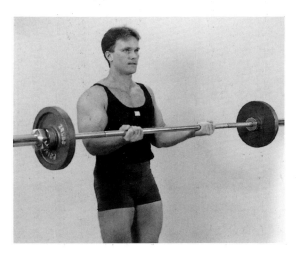

Fig. 9.11 Barbell arm curls.

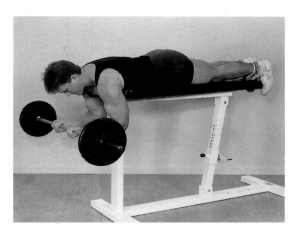

Fig. 9.12 Lying barbell arm curls.

skeletal muscle. There are three types of *penniform* muscles:

- *Unipennate muscles* — which have muscle fibres on one side of the tendon only, for example the semimembranosis muscle
- *Bipennate muscles* — which have muscle fibres on both sides of a central tendon, for example, the rectus femoris muscle
- *Multipennate muscles* — which have muscle fibres on both sides of a number of tendons, such as the deltoid muscle

An example of each of these muscle types, and the orientation of their fibres to the tendon, is presented in Fig. 9.13.

Adaptation of the Neural System in Response to Resistance Training

Training-induced neural adaptations are perhaps best illustrated by the fact that unilateral strength training has been consistently observed to produce strength increases in the untrained contralateral limb (Rasch & Morehouse 1957; Moritani &

DeVries 1979). These neural adaptations are believed to occur through a number of processes, such as disinhibition, motor unit synchronization and the effect of learning.

DISINHIBITION

At all times the nervous system is bombarding the motor units with excitatory and inhibitory impulses. If the excitatory impulses exceed the inhibitory impulses the motor unit will 'fire', but if the opposite occurs it will not. During the process of increasing force production, the human body has in-built feedback mechanisms which can operate as safeguards to protect itself from injury. For example, the Golgi tendon organs, which are located in the musculotendinous junction in series with the muscle fibres, are sensitive to the level of tension in the muscle. If the body produces very high forces, these organs have the capacity to send inhibitory signals to the motor units and thereby prevent the body from recruiting further motor units and/or firing these units at their maximal rate, limiting the force applied. Consequently in some individuals, depending on the sensitivity of these

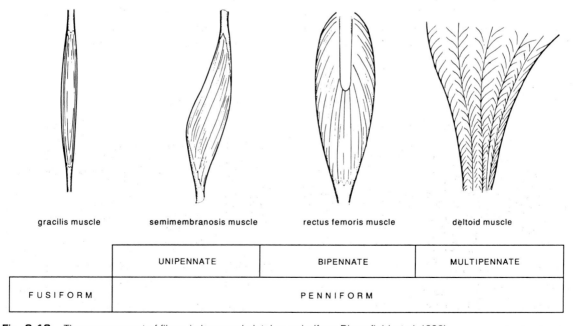

| gracilis muscle | semimembranosis muscle | rectus femoris muscle | deltoid muscle |

	UNIPENNATE	BIPENNATE	MULTIPENNATE
FUSIFORM	PENNIFORM		

Fig. 9.13 The arrangement of fibres in human skeletal muscle (from Bloomfield *et al.* 1992).

organs, a considerable amount of potential force may not be used in maximal activities. However, by continually exposing the body to high levels of tension, the sensitivity of these organs may be reduced through a process known as *disinhibition*, allowing the individual to get closer to the absolute maximum force-producing capacity of the body. One of the benefits of resistance training is to reduce the inhibitory impulses that are produced at high levels of muscular tension. This allows for a greater number of motor units to be recruited and for the activated motor units to be fired at higher rates. *The process of disinhibition allows for increases in strength without muscular hypertrophy.*

STRENGTH DEFICIT

The difference between the maximum voluntary force that the body can exert and the absolute maximum capacity of the system has been termed the strength deficit (Tidow 1990). The maximum voluntary force can be determined in a maximal isometric contraction, while the absolute force capacity of the system has been estimated from the maximum eccentric force produced resisting a load of 150% of maximum. Tidow (1990) reported strength deficits in untrained individuals of up to 45%, while in elite athletes, due to the process of disinhibition, the calculated strength deficits were only 5%. This disparity suggests that elite athletes are able to utilize a greater proportion of their total strength reserves. The value of the strength deficit has been used as a variable to determine what type of training will best enhance performance. If the strength deficit is high, indicating that athletes are not using the full potential of their musculature, then heavy strength training is recommended (loads 90–100% maximum). Such training is seen to promote the process of disinhibition and thus allows athletes to access more of their true strength potential, reducing their strength deficit. If the strength deficit is low, then further improvements in strength will only occur through increased muscle size, and bodybuilding type training methods must be employed to achieve this (8–12 repetitions using a load of approximately

70–80% of maximum). Unfortunately the process of determining the actual strength deficit is very stressful and can sometimes result in injury. Thus its use in practical situations with athletes has been fairly limited; however, recently a field test for the assessment of the strength deficit has been developed, and this is discussed in Section 3.

MOTOR UNIT SYNCHRONIZATION

A single muscle group consists of 100–1000 motor units. Generally when a muscle is activated, the motor units are fired in a random asynchronous manner. This simply means that the actions of differing motor units within the same muscle are independent of each other. However, Milner-Brown *et al.* (1975) reported that synchronization in motor unit firing was a characteristic of strength-trained athletes and that the strength training process enhanced motor unit synchronization. This means that a consequence of strength training is that different motor units within the same muscle can coordinate their actions so that they fire at the same time. This is a further neural adaptation that can contribute to the enhancement of strength.

EFFECT OF LEARNING

A final neural adaptation in response to resistance training is the effect of learning. When first performing a resistance exercise the task is novel and suboptimal coordination between the relevant prime mover, stabilizer and antagonist muscle groups may occur. For example, during an arm curl exercise the triceps brachii muscle (antagonist) may be activated and this tends to retard performance. However, as the neuromuscular system becomes increasingly proficient with the performance of an exercise, the coordination of the muscles improves, facilitating performance. The effect of learning on strength development was investigated by Rutherford *et al.* (1986). These researchers reported that 12 weeks of weight training resulted in a 160–200% increase in the weight lifted during the leg extension training exercise; however, maximum isometric force increased by only 3–20% over this same period. The large disparity between the two measures of strength was largely attributed to learning effects.

The adaptations of the neural system are dominant in the early stages of training and represent the main cause of strength increase over the first 6–8 weeks of resistance training. After this period, neural adaptations still form an important part of the adaptation process; however, they become less important than morphological adaptations in the musculature itself (Moritani & DeVries 1979).

Adaptation of the Muscular System in Response to Resistance Training

The dominant mechanism sustaining long-term enhancement in muscular strength is an increase in the size of the muscle. *A muscle can develop a maximum force of approximately 50 N/cm² of muscle cross-sectional area* and there is a very high relationship between the size and the strength of muscle, in both males and females. Hence to a large extent, the long-term development of strength is dependent on the continual increase of muscular size. Two mechanisms have been proposed which result in increases in muscular size and these are as follows:

- *Muscular hypertrophy* — where the individual muscle fibres increase in size
- *Muscular hyperplasia* — where the individual muscle fibres split and as a result the number of muscle fibres increases

Research indicates that muscle hypertrophy is the dominant mechanism underlying the increase in muscular size. Muscle hypertrophy is attributable to the following changes in the muscle:

- Increased number and size of myofibrils per muscle fibre
- Increased amounts of protein filaments, particularly the myosin filaments
- Increased size and strength of tendons, ligaments and connective tissue

It is interesting to note that most muscle hypertrophy that occurs in response to high intensity resistance training tends to be in the FT muscle fibres (MacDougall *et al.* 1979; Roman *et al.* 1993).

ELASTIC PROPERTIES OF MUSCLES AND TENDONS

The majority of human movements are the result of eccentric contractions, where the musculature lengthens under tension (often referred to as a back-swing, wind-up or counter-movement), followed by a concentric contraction, where the musculature shortens under tension (often referred to as the forward-swing or upward movement). The occurrence of such movement sequences are seen in activities such as running, jumping, throwing, hitting and in most resistance training exercises. This movement sequence is commonly referred to as a *stretch–shorten cycle* (SSC), as the musculature is stretched prior to being shortened. For example, prior to throwing a ball an individual will extend the arm backwards, thereby stretching the musculature around the shoulder girdle and then the musculature shortens to bring the arm rapidly forward.

Movements with a prior stretch augment the concentric phase of the activity, resulting in an increase in work and power or enhanced movement efficiency when compared to similar movements performed without stretch. The ability of the SSC to enhance physical performance has been known since the pioneering research of Marey and Demeny (1885), who observed that in two successive jumps the second was higher than the first because it involved a more intense eccentric muscular action than the first. The augmentation to performance derived from use of the SSC is ascribed to a combination of the recovery of stored elastic energy from the musculature and additional, reflexively induced, neural input due to the stretch reflex.

The mechanics underlying the use of elastic strain energy in SSC activities is a relatively simple process. During a resisted eccentric contraction, or counter-movement, the elastic regions of the musculotendinous unit are minutely stretched and consequently store elastic energy. On movement reversal (i.e. the concentric contraction) the extended regions recoil to their original form and in so doing, a portion of the stored elastic energy is recovered to produce kinetic energy that may augment the performance of the activity. The elastic regions of the musculotendinous unit include the tendon, epi-, peri- and endomysium and the cross-bridge linkages between the actin and myosin filaments of muscle. Of these elastic regions the tendon has been shown to be the dominant site for elastic energy storage (Alexander 1987).

The significance of the SSC to the enhancement of human performance has received various estimates from researchers. Cavagna *et al.* (1964) and more recently Alexander (1987) calculated that the recovery of stored elastic energy from the musculature and foot arches accounted for approximately 50% of the total energy requirement in running. Asmussen and Bonde-Petersen (1974) observed an 11.5% increase in total height jumped due to the use of the SSC. Wilson *et al.* (1991a) reported a mean increase of 14.5% in the maximum weight lifted in a bench press when using a SSC movement, as compared to a lift performed without an eccentric (i.e. downward) phase. This latter finding has important implications for resistance training. When performing some resistance training exercises the first repetition may be performed without a prior eccentric phase, for example, in most exercises using weight machines. The first repetition is often very difficult, as the musculature cannot utilize the elastic and neural benefits of prior stretch; however, subsequent repetitions tend to be more easily performed as they involve a SSC movement. If such activities are to be carried out with near maximal loads, it is often necessary to obtain assistance for the initial repetition, with subsequent repetitions being performed unaided.

Most sporting activities involve the use of a SSC movement sequence. This allows for the use of elastic energy and the stretch reflex to contribute to performance. In maximizing the use of elastic energy and the contribution of the stretch reflex in SSC movements, the following points need to be considered:

- If a delay period is imposed between the eccentric and concentric phases of a SSC movement, the use of elastic energy in the movement will be reduced. In fact stored elastic energy dissipates as an exponential function of delay time with a 0.85 s half-life of decay (Wilson *et al.* 1991a). To maximize the use of elastic energy in SSC movements, such delay periods should be eliminated or at least minimized and the movement should rapidly proceed from the eccentric to the concentric phase (Wilson *et al.* 1991a)

- Elastic energy stored in the muscles and tendons is rapidly released during the concentric phase of motion and contributes for only the initial few tenths of a second of the movement (Wilson *et al.* 1991a)

- The elasticity of the musculotendinous unit is a very important determinant of how much elastic energy is used in SSC movements. For relatively slow SSC movements, such as heavy bench press lifts, it is evident that an elastic musculotendinous unit maximizes the use of elastic energy in the movement (Wilson *et al.* 1991b)

- Wilson *et al.* (1992) have demonstrated that flexibility training increases the elasticity of the muscle and tendons, which serves to enhance the performance of SSC movements by increasing the contribution of elastic energy to the movement. These researchers reported that 8 weeks of flexibility training resulted in a 5% increase in the maximum weight lifted by experienced weight trainers in a bench press exercise

- Pousson *et al.* (1990) reported that strength training tended to increase musculotendinous stiffness, while Wilson *et al.* (1992) reported that flexibility training tended to reduce the stiffness of the muscles and tendons. *These findings strongly suggest that athletes should perform flexibility exercises in conjunction with their strength training to maintain the elasticity of their muscles and tendons*

- At maximal levels of muscular contraction the benefits derived from the use of the SSC appear to be mainly due to the use of elastic energy, with reflex mechanisms contributing little to performance (Wilson *et al.* 1991c)
- A body of research exists that suggests the effectiveness of SSC movements is enhanced if the eccentric (stretching) phase of movement involves relatively high levels of muscular activity (Funato *et al.* 1985)

Wilson (1991) has studied in depth the implications of SSC movements in sport and readers should refer to his work for further information.

TRAINING PRINCIPLES

Progressive Overload

The principle of overload refers to the fact that to force the musculature to adapt and become stronger, it is necessary to expose it to a level of stress beyond the point to which it is accustomed. Stress or overload in training can be modified by altering the following training variables:

- The volume of training, that is, the number of repetitions, sets and training days
- The intensity of training, that is, the load used
- The speed at which the exercises are performed
- The rest interval between repeated sets and exercises

In order to enhance strength, the intensity of the training appears to be the most important factor. Research has shown that strength gains are maximized when loads of approximately 80–90% of maximum are used in training (Atha 1981). For the enhancement of power and strength–endurance, intensity is also important due to the relationship between strength, power and endurance, as outlined previously. However, for the development of power, the speed at which the exercises are performed is also important, while to enhance strength–endurance the volume of training and rest intervals between

repeated sets and exercises are of additional importance.

It is important to emphasize that *the nature of the overload stimulus will determine the training gains that are achieved.* In the introduction the story of Milo of Crotona was outlined. The reason Milo became stronger from lifting and walking with the bull on his back was because the bull became progressively heavier as it matured. Thus the intensity of the training gradually increased, resulting in an enhancement in strength. If Milo had carried the same sized bull, but for progressively greater distances each day, the training stimulus would have been one of volume and the dominant adaptation would have been the enhancement of strength–endurance.

This training principle is referred to as *progressive overload*, for when the musculature adapts to the training stress there is a need to progressively increase the stress to continue the process of adaptation and hence improvement. Such a procedure was outlined in Wilmore and Costill (1988) who stated that:

> ... a young man who initially performs only 10 repetitions of bench pressing using 150 pounds (68 kg) of weight, will, within a week or two of weight training, be able to increase his repetitions to 14 or 15. If he then adds 5 pounds of weight to the bar, giving him a total of 155 pounds (70 kg), his repetitions will drop to between 8 and 10. As he continues to train, the repetitions continue to increase, and within another week or two, he is ready to add an additional 5 pounds of weight. Thus, there is a progressive increase in the amount of weight, or resistance lifted.

Again the important point is that when the adaptations were taking place the intensity of training was increased by the addition of more weight. Had this not occurred and if instead, more repetitions had been performed, the increase in strength would have been reduced. However, when dealing with experienced athletes, the process of adaptation is not quite as simple as that which has been outlined above. As the individual becomes more highly trained, the training gains become progressively harder to achieve. Hakkinen *et al.* (1987) reported no significant changes in strength, muscle fibre area, body mass and muscle girth in elite strength athletes as a consequence of 1 year of strength training. Similar results were also revealed when the athletes were assessed after 2 years of training (Hakkinen *et al.* 1988). This was despite these athletes performing training routines that involved five sessions per week at high training intensities. With such highly trained athletes, it appears either that it is difficult to provide a training intensity that represents an overload, or it is difficult for the body to respond to such an overload and continually adapt. One of the dilemmas facing sport scientists is how to continue the adaptation process for experienced athletes. Some possible answers to this dilemma are discussed in the section on the future development of strength. Sale (1992) suggested that a consequence of the lack of training adaptation in experienced strength-trained athletes has been the use, by some athletes, of anabolic steroids to continue the adaptation process (Fig. 9.14).

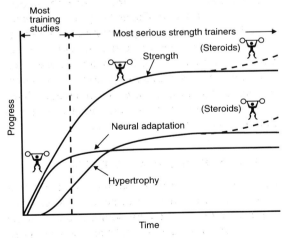

Fig. 9.14 The progress achieved by a typical strength-trained individual. Note that once a highly trained state has been achieved further gains in muscular size and strength are difficult to induce. In such circumstances individuals may be tempted to use anabolic steroids to continue their progress (adapted from Sale 1992).

DE-TRAINING

The human body is an organism that attempts to constantly adapt to its environment in order to meet the demands imposed upon it. Consequently as the body is subjected to high intensity loading, through the use of resistance training, the neuromuscular system will adapt so that it is better suited to tolerate this imposed stress. Conversely if the level of stress is reduced, the body adapts to this lower level of demand. Therefore a cessation of resistance training will result in a reversal of the adaptation process and the skeletal structures and musculature will atrophy and a loss in muscular function will occur.

Hakkinen *et al.* (1985a) reported the effects of weight training and de-training on 11 previously trained male subjects. All subjects trained for 24 weeks using high intensity weight training methods and were then detrained for a period of 12 weeks, during which no weight training was performed. The maximal strength of the subjects increased by 26% in response to the 24 weeks of training and subsequently was reduced by 11.4% in response to the 12 week de-training period. The reduction in strength exhibited during the de-training period was highly related to a reduction in maximal muscular activity, as assessed through electromyography. This relationship suggests that the reduction in strength was, at least to some extent, due to a reversal in the neural adaptations associated with strength training. However, the detraining period was also associated with a significant reduction in muscle fibre area, of both FT and ST fibres, and a reduction in muscle girth. Therefore during detraining, there is a loss in muscular function caused by a combination of neural and morphological changes.

MAINTENANCE OF STRENGTH

Most research tends to indicate that the performance of one high intensity resistance training session per muscle group per week will be sufficient to maintain the muscular functions developed through resistance training. The most important factor in the maintenance of strength is that the training session must be of *high intensity*.

This is very important for the many sports which involve relatively long competitive seasons, for example, team sports such as football, basketball, waterpolo and so on. In these sports the physical capacities of strength and explosive power are developed during the pre-season and maintained throughout the competitive season. Such a strategy will require the performance of at least one high intensity training session per week per muscle group. Some athletes and coaches believe that the regular skill training and actual competition will provide enough stimulus to maintain muscle functioning developed during the pre-season. However, the intensity of such training is typically too low and will result in a loss of muscular function throughout the season.

TAPERING IN SWIMMING

A similar example to this is often seen in competitive swimming, where many swimmers, particularly sprinters, will engage in high intensity resistance training throughout the year. However, 8 weeks prior to a major meet they will commence to taper, which often involves the cessation of all resistance training. Over this period the intensity of swimming training may be quite high, but will not serve to maintain muscular strength. Consequently by the time of the meet some of the strength increases they had trained for during the previous months will have dissipated. To avoid this situation a reduced volume, but high intensity resistance training programme should be adopted during the taper, so that the muscular strength gains can be maintained through to the competition day. Coaches therefore should taper their athletes' resistance training in much the same way as they taper their swimming training, by reducing the volume but maintaining some high intensity work.

Specificity

Specificity is a global concept that relates to the fact that the best gains in performance are achieved when the training is performed in a manner very specific to the competitive action. The more specific the training, the better will be the transfer-ence of the training gains to the competitive performance and this principle has been illustrated on a large number of occasions in many sports. For example, it has been observed that if resistance training is performed at low movement speed, strength and power will tend to increase at the low speeds but there will be little effect at higher speeds. Similarly, isometric strength training at an elbow joint angle of 150° will increase strength at that position, but there will be little improvement at an elbow angle of 60° (Lindh 1979). Isotonic strength training performed in an upright body posture (e.g. standing curls) will result in large strength increases in this position but have little effect on a similar movement performed in a supine position (Rasch & Morehouse 1957). Further examples of the principle of specificity are also seen in endurance training. Long distance running will increase an athlete's aerobic capacity in running; however, it will have less effect on performance in swimming or even cycling.

Therefore to maximize performance gains the velocity of movement, range of motion, movement pattern, body posture and type of contraction used in resistance training should correspond closely to the competitive performance. Given the importance of the principle of specificity, some coaches are reluctant to use strength training as a form of exercise, as it is seen to be non-specific to competitive performance and thus of limited use. Such criticism is not without support and as outlined in the beginning of this chapter, several studies have shown that resistance training enhances strength but not competitive performance.

USE OF OVER-WEIGHT IMPLEMENTS

In an effort to improve strength in a manner specific to competitive performance some coaches are using over-weighted implements, for example over-weight baseballs, softballs and shots in preference to traditional strength training methods. The use of over-weighted implements is seen to allow the musculature to be overloaded in a very specific manner to competitive performance. However, researchers have observed that they are not effective in increasing strength, power or performance when used in isolation. For example, Brylinsky *et al.* (1992) reported that training with a softball that had been modified to increase its mass by 2 ounces resulted in the same improvements in pitching velocity and strength, as compared to a group trained with a normally weighted ball. The use of over-weighted implements is generally not effective at increasing strength, as the level of overload is simply too low to force the musculoskeletal system to adapt and become stronger.

The main reason athletes perform resistance training is to expose their neuromuscular system to a level of overload that cannot be achieved in other activities that more closely resemble the competitive event. To maximize the transference of the gains that are brought about by this overload advantage, one must ensure that the resistance training exercises are performed in a manner *which simulates the competitive performance as closely as possible.*

PRACTICAL EXAMPLE OF SPECIFICITY

In practice, exercises are often selected on the basis of how specific they are to competitive performance. Eppley, a highly regarded American football coach at the University of Nebraska, bases his training programmes on the principles outlined below:

- Exercises must involve ground contact with the feet
- Exercises must involve several joints, that is, be multi-joint exercises
- Exercises must be performed explosively
- Exercises must be specific to competitive events, not only in terms of the movement performed but also the work to rest ratios and dominant energy systems used

In essence, these training principles are simply extensions of the principle of the specificity of training applied to American football. For example, during a football game, all movement occurs when standing on the feet and thus the need to be able to generate force and power in this position is very important. Therefore an exercise such as a bench press would not be seen as particularly specific. To develop upper body strength, standing overhead presses and inclined bench presses are performed. The inclined bench presses are done at a particularly high angle (~60°) so that the athletes are required to exert ground contact with their feet to maintain balance. In this way the athletes enhance their upper body strength and power but do so in a manner that is specific to the way they will need to use this capacity in an actual game situation.

FULL SQUATS VERSUS HALF-SQUATS

Another practical example of the principle of specificity in the selection of exercises, is the use of the squat exercise by track and field athletes. This exercise is very popular for many athletes in sports dominated by lower body strength and power; however, often the actual depth of the squat is a cause of controversy. The load used during a full squat tends to be limited by the force generation capabilities of the body between the knee angles of approximately 95 and 115° (McLaughlin *et al.* 1977). Once through this region, which is commonly referred to as the 'sticking region', the lift is relatively easily completed. In fact towards the end of the exercise, with approximate knee angles of 140–180°, the forces applied by the lifter against the bar are reduced, as the bar simply coasts to the final position. However, the force generating capacity of the body over this range of motion (140–180°) is at least 1.5 times as great as that produced at the more flexed position (95–115°). Consequently, during the top range of motion of the full squat, the leg and thigh extensor musculature are not loaded to anything like their full potential. However, it is during this range of motion (knee angles of 140–180°) that most athletes need to produce high force levels in their events. Therefore, to maximize their training gains, *most athletes should perform a half-squat motion*, preferably in a power rack (Fig. 9.61), with substantially more weight than they can use for a full squat. Therefore, based on the force profiles involved in the movements, full squats cannot be considered specific to the leg action of many athletic events, while half-squats, with substantially more load than that used in full squats, can be considered to be more specific. As an aside to this discussion on specificity, it should be noted that the performance of heavily loaded, deep full squats can stretch the cruciate ligaments of the knee joint, making this joint unstable and hence their use in training should be limited.

The concept of specificity is an integral part of athletic training. However, strength training exercises used to enhance competitive performances are seldom specific to competitive events. Generally strength training programmes used by athletes involve bench presses, squats, power cleans and push presses with some arm curls, sit-ups, calf raises and leg curls as adjuncts. As a result, many athletes train as if they were bodybuilders, powerlifters or weightlifters. However, based on the principle of specificity it would seem logical that *once a sound general strength base has been developed, the use of resistance training exercises that are performed in a manner specific to actual competition, would provide for the best results.*

DEVELOPING SPORT-SPECIFIC RESISTANCE TRAINING PROGRAMMES

To develop effective strength training programmes for sports the competitive activity needs to be biomechanically analysed. From this analysis, exercises which replicate the sporting action should form the basis of the strength training routine. Such exercise selection requires a sound understanding both of the biomechanics of the event and of the exercise potential of gymnasium equipment. One way to develop a sport-specific resistance training programme is to video the sporting action, select the portions of the movement which appear to be the major force producing actions and try to simulate these actions in the gymnasium. Often standard gymnasium equipment is required to be used in ways for which it was not originally intended. For example, the latissimus dorsi muscle group is an important contributor to most swimming strokes and to develop this group many swimmers perform 'lat pull-downs'. However, a more specific freestyle and butterfly arm action can be achieved by using the 'lat pull-down' ma-

chine while standing in front of it, with arms slightly bent and the elbows pointing out to the sides. The bar of the lat pull-down machine should then be pulled down from shoulder height to the thighs (Fig. 9.15). A similar example relates to runners for whom the hamstring muscle group is an important contributor to sprinting performance. Its ability to rapidly accelerate the thigh backwards prior to ground contact is currently seen to be one of the major limitations to sprinting performance. Many sprinters will perform the leg curl exercise on a horizontal leg curl machine to develop their hamstring muscles (Fig. 9.16). However, in order that the exercise be more specific to the actual competitive performance, the athlete should train the hamstrings using a total hip machine as illustrated in Fig. 9.17.

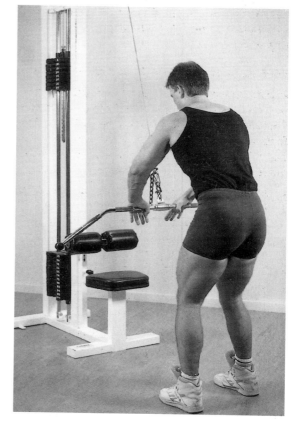

Fig. 9.15 Front pull-downs performed by a butterfly swimmer.

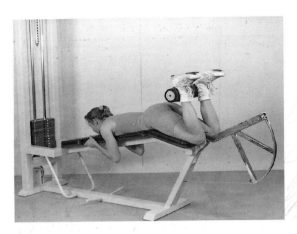

Fig. 9.16 Prone leg curls.

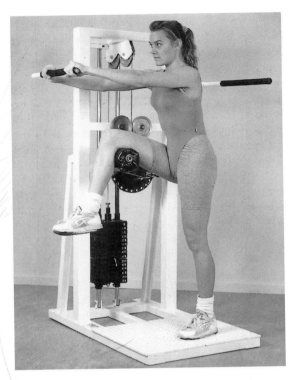

Fig. 9.17 Thigh extensions: training of the thigh extensors in a manner specific to their use in sprint running.

In terms of the specificity of training it is simply not good enough to train those muscles which are used in the activity. One needs to train them so that the exercise is performed in a similar action to the competitive situation. It is from this basis that the exercises outlined later in the chapter are selected (see section on Resistance Training Programmes for Specific Sports). A further point to be aware of is that very few standard pieces of gymnasium equipment are actually designed specifically for athletes, as this market represents a relatively small section of the total fitness industry. Most machines are designed for people who wish to improve their general fitness levels and/or body shape. Consequently it is often necessary to modify these machines or use them in a different manner to that for which they were intended, in an effort to increase the specificity of the exercise to the competitive performance.

Variation

The training principles of overload and specificity are well known and have been extensively researched over many years. The principle of variation is a more recent concept and has been subjected to substantially less scientific scrutiny. This principle relates to the fact that if the training stimulus is consistently presented to the body in exactly the same way, its effectiveness will diminish, the athletes will become stale and their training gains will be reduced (Poliquin 1988a). Variation in training regimens can be achieved by manipulating the variables of overload, such as the number of repetitions, number of sets, load used, speed of performance or the rest interval between sets. Alternatively, exercises can be frequently changed or the order in which the exercises are performed can be altered. *One of the most common training errors is the failure to regularly change the training stimulus.*

PERIODIZATION

Undulating periodized model

The variation of the training stimulus performed in a systematic manner throughout a training cycle is referred to as periodization and there are currently several popular methods in use. The undulating periodized model was advocated by Poliquin (1988b) and in this system the athlete alternates between the use of lighter loads performed for high numbers of repetitions, termed *volume training*, with periods of heavy training where heavy loads are performed with few repetitions, termed *intensity training*. An athlete alternates every 2 or 3 weeks between these phases in an effort to vary the training process. The volume phases are believed to increase muscular hypertrophy, while the intensity phases are thought to promote the neural adaptations to resistance training. By alternating between these phases, optimal strength increases are believed to result. An example of an undulating periodized training routine, used to maximize strength gain over a 12 week training period, is outlined in Table 9.1.

Table 9.1 Undulating periodized training routine

Training week	Sets × repetitions*
1–2	5×10
3–4	5×6
5–6	5×8
7–8	5×4
9–10	5×6
11–12	5×3

* The load used is the maximum possible so that only the nominated number of repetitions can be performed.

The linear periodized model

Another popular periodized form of resistance training was outlined by Stone *et al.* (1981) and is termed the linear periodization model. This method involves a gradual progression from light loads and high volume, to heavy loads with lower volume and greater intensity. This progression is thought to enhance muscular hypertrophy initially and towards the end of the training cycle facilitates the neural mechanisms responsible for strength development. An example of a linear periodized training routine, used to maximize strength gain over a 12 week training period, is outlined in Table 9.2.

At the end of the 12 week training cycle the periodized programmes can be repeated, hopefully commencing with greater loads. These general periodized training routines may be further

Table 9.2 Linear periodized training routine

Training week	Sets × repetitions*
1–2	5×12
3–4	5×10
5–6	5×8
7–8	5×6
9–10	5×5
11–12	5×4

* The load used is the maximum possible so that only the nominated number of repetitions can be performed.

varied by altering the intensity of the training sessions within the week, as outlined in Table 9.3. Thus the linear model will involve a gradual progression towards higher loads and lower repetitions on the heavy training day; however, the light training day may involve relatively light loads throughout the training cycle (Table 9.3).

Comparison between periodized models

In a recent study by Baker *et al.* (1994) the use of the undulating and linear periodized methods resulted in similar improvements in strength over a 12 week training period, when experienced weight trained individuals were used as subjects. Such a result is not surprising and perhaps reflects the principle of variation. Given that a training routine involves sufficient intensity and volume to overload the muscles, and includes variation to continually stimulate the neuromuscular system, the routine should be successful, regardless of the actual periodized model adopted.

Table 9.3 Heavy–light linear periodized training routine

Training week	Sets × repetitions*	
	Heavy	Light
1–2	5×10	5×12
3–4	5×8	5×10
5–6	5×6	5×10
7–8	5×5	5×8
9–10	5×4	5×8
11–12	5×3	5×6

* The load used is the maximum possible so that only the nominated number of repetitions can be performed.

Recovery

Muscle growth and adaptation occur between training sessions and therefore an adequate recovery is essential. As a general rule, a *recovery period of approximately 48–72 h* should occur between intensive resistance training sessions of the same muscle, depending on the intensity of the session, age of the individual and type of contraction. Research has demonstrated that recovery from eccentric muscular contractions takes longer than from concentric contractions and that too little recovery time will result in reduced performance and may also lead to injury.

One of the most common training errors is the failure to provide appropriate recovery between workouts. For example, many people will perform chest exercises such as the bench press, inclined bench press and dips on one day, and deltoid and triceps exercises on the following day. However, these chest exercises are multi-joint and multi-muscle exercises involving most of the upper body muscle groups. Therefore such a training programme requires the deltoids and triceps brachii muscle groups to be trained on consecutive days. Consequently, these muscle groups become overtrained and maximal training gains are not achieved. For many individuals who perform all their resistance training on the one day and have at least one day's rest between repeat sessions, the above represents no problem. However, when more advanced training routines are adopted, which involve resistance training on consecutive days, then the organization of the training week becomes more complicated.

SPLIT ROUTINES

In essence, split routines are adopted when the resistance training session is of such long dura-

tion that a high training intensity cannot be maintained throughout the session. In such instances the workout is partitioned into smaller training sessions. Thus, rather than performing a few large training sessions during a week, the athlete performs many smaller workouts, at higher training intensity. To prevent overtraining when using split routines it is important to *train all muscles that act together in the one training session and have adequate recovery between these sessions*. For this reason it is popular to perform split routines where the upper body (pectorals, deltoids, latissimus dorsi, forearm musculature, biceps and triceps brachii) are trained on one day and the lower body musculature (quadriceps, hamstrings, calf group, erector spinae and the abdominals) are trained on the next training occasion. Similarly push/pull type split routines are also popular, where all the muscles involved in pushing movements (e.g. pectorals, deltoids etc.) are trained in one session and those which pull (e.g. latissimus dorsi, biceps brachii etc.) in the next. Examples of split routines are outlined in Tables 9.4a,b.

One problem that is often encountered when training muscle groups which act together in the same workout is that the muscles trained towards the end of the session are subject to fatigue. For

Table 9.4a Example of a two-way (upper body/lower body) split routine

Monday and Thursday	Wednesday and Saturday
Pectorals	Quadriceps
Deltoids	Hamstrings
Latissimus dorsi	Erector spinae
Biceps brachii	Abdominals
Triceps brachii	Calf group
Forearm musculature	

Table 9.4b Example of a three-way split routine

Monday and Thursday	Tuesday and Friday	Wednesday and Sunday
Pectorals	Latissimus dorsi	Quadriceps
Deltoids	Erector spinae	Hamstrings
Triceps brachii	Biceps brachii	Calf group
Forearm musculature	Abdominals	

example, the fatigue accumulated from exercising the pectorals may impede the training of the deltoid and triceps brachii muscles. This is why exercises for such similarly acting muscle groups are often performed on separate training occasions. To prevent this problem *the muscle groups just trained should be rested prior to the training of subsequent muscle groups that have similar actions.* For example, consider the athlete who has just trained the pectoral muscle group and wishes to train the deltoids in the same session. If the deltoids are trained directly following the pectoral exercises then they will be fatigued and unable to be trained at maximal intensity. To reduce this problem, prior to training the deltoids, one of the following strategies may be used:

- An unrelated muscle group such as the calf group or the abdominal muscles may be trained
- The individual may perform some aerobic training such as riding a bike
- The individual may simply rest for 20 min

After this 'rest period' the deltoid and triceps brachii muscles will have had time to at least partially recover and can be trained with greater intensity.

STRENGTH TRAINING METHODS

There is a variety of methods that can be used to enhance muscular strength. These include the use of free weights, pneumatic resistance systems, variable resistance machines, heavy eccentric training, isometric training and accommodating resistance training. The uses and limitations of each of these training modalities will be outlined in the following section. There are several important factors to consider when attempting to increase the strength of muscle, and these are as follows:

- The intensity of the training, in terms of load lifted, appears to be the most important factor for the development of strength
- The musculature needs to be progressively loaded above the point to which it is accustomed in order to realize continued strength gains

- The development of strength in response to training decreases as a function of the current level of strength, so that initial strength increases for novice subjects will occur with almost any training method, whereas further adaptation in highly trained individuals may not occur even with the adoption of the best training method
- The strength of muscle is closely related to its size

Weight Training

Despite recent advances in the development of exercise equipment and machines, most athletes are heavily reliant on the use of free weight training exercises, in the form of barbells and dumbbells, for their strength training. Free weight training apparatus have the following benefits in that they:

- Are relatively inexpensive
- Are easily maintained
- Allow the load to be readily determined and varied
- Can be used in a variety of exercises
- Involve the use of stabilizing muscles
- Are motivational to use in practice

However, the use of free weights in the development of muscular function and performance has a number of limitations. An understanding of these limitations can enable one to appreciate the value of the new machines and the reasons why they have been developed.

LIMITATIONS OF FREE WEIGHT TRAINING

Sticking region

Perhaps the most universally accepted limitation to free weight training is the fact that the load is limited to the weakest point in the range of motion of the exercise, generally termed the *sticking point*. This is the region throughout the concentric phase of a lift in which it is most difficult to generate force. It is the region in the lift where the force generated by the lifter is lower than the force due to the weight of the bar, and is depicted in

Fig. 9.18. If a lift cannot be completed, it generally fails in this location.

During an exercise the ability of the musculature to develop force is modified by a combination of the length–tension relationship, the force–velocity relationship and the changing mechanics of the lever system. Further, throughout the motion the resistance effect of the load also varies (see section on Muscle Mechanics). Consequently the ability of the musculature to develop force and the load requirement placed on the muscle are rarely matched. In fact during the performance of a maximal set, the musculature is only subjected to a load requirement that matches its capacity to exert force during the sticking region of the concentric phase of the final repetition. In all other instances the musculature can be performing submaximally.

In an effort to overcome this limitation, free weight trainers perform forced repetitions, using spotters or assistants to help them through the sticking region. In this way repetitions can be performed which enable the production of maximal effort throughout a greater range of motion and over a number of repetitions.

Compensatory acceleration training

A method used to overcome the limitation imposed by the existence of sticking regions is termed *compensatory acceleration training*. This training technique is based on the fact that the force produced throughout an exercise will be dependent not only on the load but on the acceleration of the load. That is:

F = acceleration effect + load effect
i.e. $F = m \cdot a + m \cdot g$

where F = force applied, m = mass of the system, a = acceleration of the system and g = acceleration due to gravity.

This training technique involves an acceleration of the load during those ranges of motion in which the applied load is less than the musculature's capacity to generate force. For example, during the initial portion of an arm curl exercise, the muscle's ability to produce force is often greater

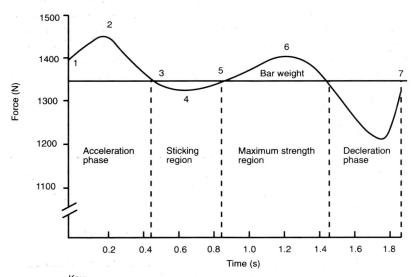

Key:
Forces exerted by the lifter at:
1. Chest
2. Peak acceleration
3. Peak velocity
4. Minimum acceleration
5. Minimum velocity
6. Peak acceleration M.S.R.
7. Maximum displacement

Fig. 9.18 Applied force–time curve during a maximal bench press. Note the differing phases of the movement (courtesy of Wilson *et al.* 1989).

than the load on the bar, as the effective resistance of the weight on the musculoskeletal system is low at this joint position. In this instance, rather than submaximally contracting, the musculature can accelerate the load as fast as possible thereby increasing the applied force above that due to the bar alone.

Compensatory acceleration training involves attempting to move the load as fast as possible throughout the entire movement range. This system has good application when the lift is towards the beginning of the range of motion. However, towards the end of the motion it cannot be used as most weight training exercises require that the bar achieve zero velocity at the end of the range. Consequently the load must be decelerated over the latter part of the movement and hence compensatory acceleration is not possible at this stage of the lift.

Force changes throughout a lift

Compensatory acceleration training outlines a very important factor often overlooked in resistance training. This relates to the fact that the force applied by an individual when lifting a weight is not constant throughout the movement. The force due to the weight of the bar is generally the only force that people consider when lifting weights. However, as outlined above, the force applied has both

a weight and acceleration component. Figure 9.19 outlines the force applied during a typical bench press performed by an experienced power-lifter at maximal effort with a load of 81% of maximum.

As can be seen in Fig. 9.19, the applied force varies substantially from a maximal force of approximately 1780 N (equivalent to ~180 kg force) to a minimum force of approximately 1490 N (equivalent to ~150 kg force). The load on the bar was 165 kg. Thus the forces exerted throughout an exercise are not constant and the acceleration and deceleration of the bar account for substantial alterations in the forces exerted by the individual.

Implications for injury

Such modifications in the applied force have important implications for the occurrence of muscular injuries, particularly during the eccentric (downward) phase of the exercise. If a bar is rapidly lowered, resulting in a high acceleration, the forces required to slow the bar towards the end of the eccentric phase can be considerably greater than the load on the bar. In such instances very high forces are exerted against the musculature when it is in a lengthened position and the potential for muscular injury is great, even when using submaximal loads. Kretzler and Richardson (1989) have reported that tears to the pectoral muscles most often occurred during the

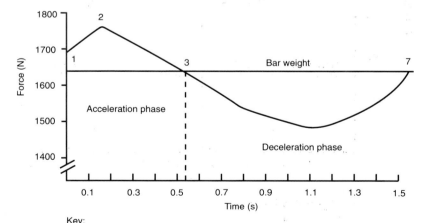

Fig. 9.19 Applied force–time curve during an 81% of maximal bench press. Note the deceleration phase accounts for more than half of the movement (courtesy of Wilson *et al.* 1989).

Key:
Forces exerted by the lifter at:
1. Chest
2. Peak acceleration
3. Peak velocity
7. Maximum displacement

135

performance of the bench press exercise and were reported to take place as additional force was added when the muscle was already at full tension. To reduce the likelihood of the occurrence of muscular injury when training with weights, it is imperative that the weights are lowered in a controlled manner and that minimal acceleration is realized during the eccentric phase. A rapid eccentric phase results in the combination of high forces and a lengthened musculature, which can often lead to muscular injury. Support for a well-controlled eccentric phase was provided by McLaughlin (1985), who reported that elite bench pressers lowered the bar with reduced peak bar accelerations when compared to novice lifters.

Deceleration phase

The applied force–time curve depicted in Fig. 9.19 also outlines another major limitation of weight training, that is, the existence of a deceleration phase. This phase is the part of the lift, towards the end of the movement, where the applied force is below the weight of the bar (Fig. 9.19). It occurs in all weight training exercises, whether using free weights or various weight training machines, as the bar generally must achieve zero velocity at the end of the range of motion. Consequently, towards the end of the movement the bar must slow down (i.e. be decelerated). The length of the deceleration phase is inversely related to the load on the bar. Elliott *et al.* (1989) reported that during the performance of an 81% maximum lift, the deceleration phase accounted for approximately 52% of the concentric movement (Fig. 9.19) and in a maximal lift it accounted for approximately 23% of the movement (Fig. 9.18).

The existence of deceleration phases is one of the most serious limitations of strength training, as they result in submaximal loading on the musculature towards the end of the movement range and are not specific to the performance of most competitive activities. For example, when putting a shot, it is progressively accelerated throughout the entire movement range to achieve maximum velocity at the end of the movement as the shot is released. Thus, relatively high forces are achieved throughout the entire range. However, when per-

forming weight training, the bar is accelerated and achieves its maximum velocity towards the beginning of the movement range and slows down from this point to reach zero velocity at the end of the range. It is interesting to note that plyometric exercises do not require that the body achieve zero velocity at the completion of the exercise and therefore involve the production of high forces throughout the movement range, in a similar fashion to competitive sporting activities. This is an important point which will be discussed further in the section on power training.

EXPLOSIVE STRENGTH TRAINING

The concept of explosive strength training, where relatively light loads are performed at high speed, is currently enjoying popularity among coaches and some sport scientists. This method is seen to make traditionally slow training more dynamic and thus specific to competitive performance. However, such a strategy will result in the occurrence of deceleration phases in more than 50% of the activity and result in athletes under-training the latter half of the movements, because the bar must be decelerated towards the end of the activity so that it may come to rest at the completion of the lift. In essence this method will allow for high forces and accelerations to be experienced for only the first few centimetres of the activity. The remainder of the lift will involve the athlete producing very little force or muscular activity, as the bar simply coasts as it comes to rest at the end of the movement. In reviewing the literature in this area Atha (1981) concluded that '... rapidly accelerating a given load to achieve a fast movement increases the effective loading on a muscle, but only for the period of acceleration. Thereafter, the loading is reduced. Thus far, explosive strength training has not proved as effective as standard isotonic (heavy weight) training in improving strength'.

The effectiveness of explosive strength training may be improved by the use of specific equipment which can serve to reduce the deceleration phase. For example, a popular resistance training exercise for the back musculature is bent-over rowing (Fig. 9.20). As with most standard weight training exercises this movement involves a deceleration phase, as the bar must slow down prior to contacting the chest. However, if it is performed on a bench (Fig. 9.21) the bar can be explosively pulled against the bench and need not be slowed down towards the end of the movement. To facilitate such exercises benches can be designed with a rubber covering which absorbs the impact forces from collisions with the bar.

PNEUMATIC SYSTEMS

There are currently a number of resistance training systems that use compressed air as the form of resistance. Such devices are termed pneumatic systems and are commercially known as Hydrogym or Keiser (Fig. 9.22). One of the major advantages these systems have over traditional weight training is that they involve very small deceleration phases (Fig. 9.23). This is due to the relatively low weight of the system, which tends to limit the development of momentum. Consequently, they allow for the performance of high speed training without the limitation of a relatively large deceleration phase. As such these systems are seen to be advantageous for the development of power for athletic performance and in rehabilitation.

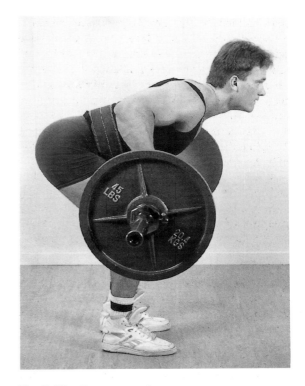

Fig. 9.20 Bent-over rowing.

Variable Resistance Machines

Variable resistance weight machines have an egg-shaped cam (Fig. 9.24) or a lever that varies its length so that the effective resistance of the load can be modified throughout the range of motion. These cams are designed to the human strength curve (see sections on Muscle Mechanics and Neuromuscular Considerations and Fig. 9.8) for various regions of the body, so that they increase the effective resistance of the system during the positions of the lift where individuals tend to be relatively strong, and reduce the effective load in positions that are weak. Modifying the effective load is achieved simply by changing the distance between the load and pivot point, hence altering the torque of the load. Through these modifications in the effective load on the musculature, vari-

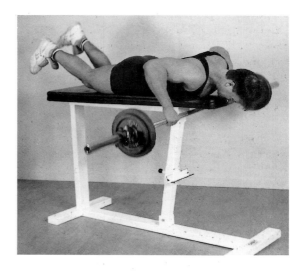

Fig. 9.21 Bench pulls.

able resistance machines allow more of the total range of the movement to be performed maximally. Hence the limitation to free weight performance caused by the sticking region can be reduced by the use of variable or accommodating resistance weight machines.

Despite the advantage that variable resistance devices have over traditional weight training methods, most research has shown that both training methods result in similar increases in muscular strength (Coleman 1977; Pipes 1978).

Heavy Eccentric Training

As previously outlined, a muscle can develop substantially more force during an eccentric muscular action when compared to a concentric or isometric contraction (see section on Force–Velocity Relationship). In fact maximal eccentric force is approximately 1.3 times higher than maximal concentric force (Griffin 1987). This fact is often used to rationalize heavy eccentric training as an effective method of enhancing strength, as the loading placed upon the musculature is seen as an important factor in the development of strength.

Heavy eccentric training is usually performed with loads of 120–130% of the maximum weight that can be concentrically lifted. The loads are lowered slowly, requiring at least 3–4 s for the eccentric phase, and then assistance is received in raising the weights. Such a procedure is relatively simple when performing unilateral exercises, such as a one arm dumb-bell curl, as the non-exercising limb can be used to assist during the concentric phase. However, exercises where both limbs are used, such as the bench press, require one or more assistants.

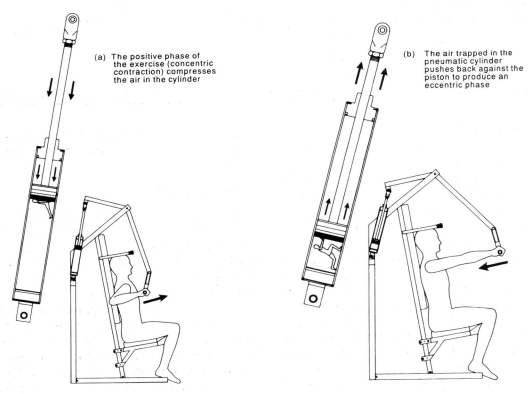

(a) The positive phase of the exercise (concentric contraction) compresses the air in the cylinder

(b) The air trapped in the pneumatic cylinder pushes back against the piston to produce an eccentric phase

Fig. 9.22 A Keiser chest-press system. Note the device uses pressurized air as resistance (from Bloomfield *et al.* 1992).

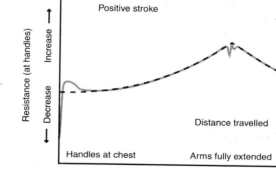

Fig. 9.23 Force–distance curves generated by free weight resistance and the Keiser system. Note that due to the low inertia of the Keiser system the deceleration phase is substantially lower than that produced with free weights (courtesy of Keiser).

POTENTIAL FOR INJURY

Heavy eccentric training is very stressful and should only be used by highly experienced weight trainers. It is essential that the weight be lowered under control and that the bar achieves negligible acceleration. If the supermaximal load is combined with a large acceleration, the force developed will possibly cause an injury. Experienced assistants must be used as spotters, and if the lifter cannot resist the load and the bar begins to accelerate during the eccentric phase, the assistants must be ready to stop the bar's downward movement. Preferably such training should be performed in a power rack, so that the downward motion of the bar is limited by a mechanical stop, such as a steel rod (Fig. 9.61). As a general rule, heavy eccentric training should not be performed in activities that involve a high degree of lower back support such as squats or deadlifts. In these exercises, uneven

assistance from spotters can result in twisting forces on the lower back which may result in serious injury.

USES IN TRAINING

Most elite strength athletes will periodically use heavy eccentric training. This allows them to expose themselves to a level of overload not possible in any other form of training. Further, it enables the use of weights in excess of current maximums and 'getting the feel' of such heavy loads is seen to assist in the psychological battle of performing new maximal lifts. In combining extreme forces with an extending musculature, heavy eccentric training results in the greatest amount of muscle soreness (Talag 1973). Therefore its uses in training tend to be limited to two to four sets performed once per week during a heavy workout.

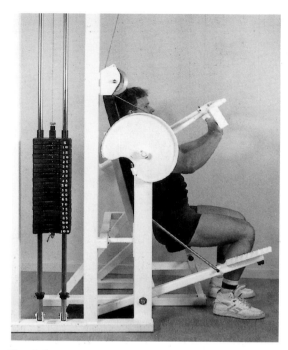

Fig. 9.24 Egg-shaped cam of variable resistance machine.

REDUCING NEURAL INHIBITIONS

In enabling athletes to expose themselves to very high levels of overload, heavy eccentric training is seen to be particularly valuable in reducing inhibitions in the neural system and allowing athletes to access a greater percentage of their true strength potential. Consequently heavy eccentric training is believed to be a good method of reducing the strength deficit (see Neural Adaptations to Resistance Training); however, there is currently little research to support this proposition.

Optimal Training Load

Research has demonstrated that to maximize the development of strength, a load that limits the exercise to between four and eight repetitions should be used (Berger 1963). However, often in the literature the optimal number of repetitions suggested is five to six (Atha 1981). A load of approximately 80–85% is required for the performance of such a set, but in practice it is unusual for individuals to perform repetitions at a single load. For example, after a warm-up an elite strength-trained athlete may perform a pyramid routine where progressively heavier sets are followed by progressively lighter sets. For example, the following sets may be completed:

- 7–8 repetitions × 80% of maximum load
- 5–6 × 85%
- 3–4 × 90%
- 6 × 80%
- 10 × 70%

Furthermore, elite strength athletes will not normally undertake the same load and number of sets on each workout. For example, it is common for elite strength athletes to have a heavy, medium and light day during a training microcycle (often 1 week). An example of a typical training programme used by an elite power-lifter in an attempt to enhance the bench press lift is outlined in Table 9.5.

This model workout can be used by experienced strength athletes attempting to increase their bench press performance. The organization of the workout demonstrates several important factors. First, no two workouts within the week are the same and the routine involves a heavy, light and moderate day. Further, all the muscles which tend to act together are trained on the same day with adequate recovery between exercise sessions and the assistance exercises are regularly varied throughout the week. Such a routine is designed with the principles of specificity, overload, variation and recovery kept in mind.

Research has indicated that compared to any other single combination of load and repetitions, a 5–6 repetition maximum (RM) load results in optimal strength development. However, this does not necessarily imply that a 5–6 RM load is superior to various combinations of load and repetitions performed in a pyramid fashion, because definitive research on this topic is not presently available. Further, the use of a specific load such as 5–6 RM does not allow much scope for variation in a training routine.

Table 9.5 Workout used to improve the bench press performance of an experienced power-lifter

Monday (heavy)
   Bench press 8 sets: 10×40%, 8×60%, 5×80%, 3×90%, 2×95%, 2×95%, 4×90%, 6×85%
   Bench press performed in a power rack with 3 s pause period on the chest between repetitions 4 sets: 8, 6, 5, 8
   Military press 6 sets: 10, 8, 6, 4, 4, 6
   Lying triceps extensions 6 sets: 10, 8, 6, 4, 4, 8

Wednesday (light)
   Bench press 8 sets: 10×40%, 8×60%, 8×80%, 7×80%, 6×80%, 8×70%, 12×60%
   Inclined bench press 5 sets: 8, 6, 5, 5, 8
   Lateral raises 4 sets: 10, 8, 8, 8
   Biceps curls 5 sets: 10, 8, 6, 6, 8

Friday (moderate)
   Bench press 8 sets: 10×40%, 8×60%, 6×80%, 4×90%, 4×90%, 3×90%, 5×85%, 8×75%
   Dips 5 sets : 10, 8, 6, 6, 8
   Press behind neck 6 sets: 10, 8, 6, 4, 4, 6
   Close grip bench press 6 sets: 10, 8, 6, 4, 4, 8

Note: for the bench press exercise, the number of repetitions per set is outlined, as is the approximate load to be used, as a percentage of the current maximum. For the other exercises only the number of repetitions is outlined. The first set of these exercises is a warm-up and should be performed with a light load. For the remaining sets a load should be chosen which limits the set to the number of repetitions which have been specified.

Isometric Training

Isometric literally means 'constant length' and refers to muscular actions that result in no observable change in muscle length. Isometric training involves the performance of a muscular action against a stationary resistance, for example, pushing against a wall. The training normally consists of maximal contractions performed for 2–4 s duration and repeated three to four times each day. Such training routines usually result in reasonably large strength increases for approximately 5 weeks, in previously untrained individuals. However, the strength gains tend to be specific to the joint angles trained. For example, isometric strength training at an elbow joint angle of 150° will increase strength in that position; however, there will be little improvement at an elbow joint angle of 60° (Lindh 1979). Consequently it is often necessary to perform isometric training using a number of positions throughout the range of motion to achieve strength gains throughout that range.

Isometric exercises can be performed with little or no equipment. Often the force can be resisted by another limb, against a partner or exerted against a wall. A large number of isometric exercises can be performed with the use of a barbell and a lifting rack. Pins can be inserted in the rack and the bar pushed against the pins so that a number of exercises can be performed.

As very few sporting activities are isometric in nature the application of isometric training to sport is very limited. However, it can be used in an attempt to maintain strength in instances when no other form of resistance training is available, for example, when travelling. Isometric training can also be useful during rehabilitation from injury when joint mobility is impeded. For example, after an anterior cruciate ligament tear, movement about the knee joint is very limited and painful. In such instances, isometric actions of the quadriceps and hamstring muscle groups can be performed in an attempt to maintain muscular size and strength until the rehabilitation proceeds to more dynamic forms of exercise. In these instances isometric training can also be used for other body parts which are uninjured but which cannot be trained because of lack of mobility.

Future Directions in the Development of Muscular Strength

To a large extent the development of strength is dependent upon exposing the musculature to high levels of overload. Currently there are several machines that are being developed in order to increase strength beyond the levels achieved by more traditional methods.

FUNCTIONAL ISOMETRICS

This is a training technique that has been adopted in a variety of forms over the past 30 years. It involves the performance of a normal isotonic lift, with one or more isometric contractions superimposed during the lift. For example, a squat lift is performed in a rack that has pins which serve to limit the upward movement of the bar. The lifter would perform a normal squat lift starting from the bottom position and raise the bar until it contacted the pins. At this point the lifter would perform a maximal isometric contraction against the pins for several seconds, lower the bar and repeat the lift. The pins are located either at the sticking point of the lift, so that this weak point can be strengthened, or towards the top of the lift. O'Shea and O'Shea (1989) reported that this form of training resulted in significantly greater increases in strength (27%) than those achieved through traditional weight training (11%). Functional isometrics are reported to be used successfully by world class strength athletes such as throwers and lifters (O'Shea *et al.* 1988).

By superimposing a maximal isometric contraction in a normal isotonic lift, greater forces can be achieved by the athlete, as the isometric force is often greater than forces produced during the concentric phase. Therefore, greater overload is experienced and greater training gains are realized. To maximize the benefits of functional isometrics in a squat lift, the pins should be located just before the end of the lift (knee angle ~170°). This will allow the lifter to exert forces in excess of 1.5 times the weight used during a maximum squat in the isometric contraction, as the musculoskeletal system is in a mechanically advantageous force-producing position. Such a technique will not only allow greater forces to be applied but also increases the range over which maximal forces can be exerted, because during traditional weight training the lifter would be in

the deceleration phase of the lift at a knee joint angle of ~170°. Consequently, when performing a traditional maximal squat, towards the end of the movement range an applied force of less than bar weight would normally be produced. However, when performing functional isometrics, an applied force of 1.5 times bar weight can be achieved for several seconds during the end of the movement.

The use of functional isometrics has been mainly limited to the squat movement and has not been well investigated; however, in theory it would seem to represent a simple but effective way of enhancing muscular strength. With relatively small modifications to standard training equipment the idea could be adapted to a whole range of exercises, allowing these activities to be performed with greater levels of force and a reduced deceleration phase.

SAFETY CONSIDERATIONS WHEN PERFORMING FUNCTIONAL ISOMETRICS

Functional isometrics will allow greater forces to be achieved, but a sustained isometric contraction is stressful to the system and will result in extremely high blood pressure during the performance of the exercise. Therefore individuals susceptible to heart attacks and/or strokes should avoid this type of activity. It should only be used by highly experienced individuals who regularly perform maximal isotonic lifts.

FREESPOT

The Freespot is a newly developed weight training system based upon a free weight bar which is in series with a winch motor and a brake, so that the load on the bar can be readily modified (Fig. 9.25). The bar is attached to the motor by cables. The system is termed the 'freespot', as the interaction of the motor and bar is such that when the lifter cannot lift the load on the bar the motor will be engaged and gradually assist the athlete so that the lift can be completed. In this system the motor acts in much the same manner as a spotter but it is more reliable, as the system is controlled by a computer which monitors the velocity of the bar by use of a rotary encoder. When the encoder

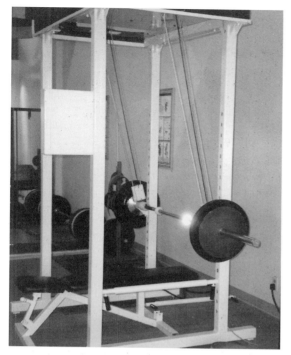

Fig. 9.25 The Freespot system.

senses a velocity of zero, the motor is rapidly engaged to assist the lifter to an extent that just enables the load to be lifted. This allows maximal loads to be lifted with safety and removes the fear element from the performance of heavy weight training, reducing inhibitions and promoting maximal effort.

The other major advantage of this system in terms of strength development is that it can be effectively used to perform heavy eccentric training so that supermaximal weights can be used with safety. For example, a squat lift of 130% of maximum can be used as the training weight. The load can be lowered by the athlete and during the concentric phase the motor is engaged to help complete the lift and this sequence can then continue allowing the performance of several repetitions. If the load is too heavy and the lifter cannot handle the resistance during the eccentric phase, the brake is engaged once a critical threshold velocity is reached. Alternatively, if the bar is released by the lifter, a grip switch is activated

which also engages the brake so that the bar is stopped.

The Freespot is a relatively recent development with only a few machines currently in existence. However, the integration of motors and brakes in resistance training holds great promise for the future development of strength, particularly if it can be achieved in a free weight environment so that the coordination and multi-joint nature of the movement can be preserved.

LIFECIRCUIT

When weights are normally lifted in a set of eight repetitions, a load of approximately 70% of maximum is used. Thus the first few repetitions are performed fairly easily and are submaximal efforts. It is only during the last few repetitions that the musculature fatigues to such an extent that 70% of maximum load represents a maximal effort. Furthermore, the effort is only maximal during the concentric phase, particularly during the time the bar is in the 'sticking region', as eccentric strength is approximately 30% greater than concentric strength. As a result, during the performance of a typical exercise, very little of the motion is actually performed at maximal effort. If developing strength is dependent upon overloading the musculature, there would seem a great deal of scope to increase this loading in excess of that produced by traditional weight training.

The LifeCircuit products have gone part of the way to redressing this free weight limitation. The system is simply a computer-controlled motor which provides resistance to the movement. However, the resistance during the eccentric phase can be made higher than that encountered during the concentric phase, so that the activity can be worked maximally on both the concentric and eccentric phases. The system also allows the resistance to be altered between repetitions within a set. Thus high resistance is experienced over the first few repetitions and as the musculature fatigues the resistance is reduced. As a result the system allows near maximal resistance to be achieved on every repetition during both the eccentric and concentric phases (Fig. 9.26).

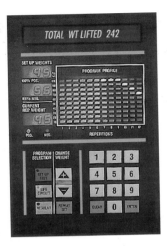

Fig. 9.26 LifeCircuit resistance system. Note the device allows for a heavier load to be used during the eccentric phase as compared to the concentric phase, and provides for progressive fatigue throughout a set.

PNEUMATIC SYSTEMS

The capacity to alter the loading between the eccentric and concentric phases and between differing repetitions within a set is also a feature of some pneumatic systems, such as that produced by Keiser. In fact Keiser goes one step further than LifeCircuit and allows the individual the capacity to alter the resistance within a repetition. The load is modified manually by the user by pressing a button which changes the pressure in the cylinders, thus modifying the resistance. However, such manual modifications may not be particularly accurate during the execution of maximal effort exercises.

USE OF EFFECTIVE SPOTTING

The LifeCircuit and Keiser systems modify the load throughout the exercise so that it maximizes the overload experienced by the lifter. A similar effect can be achieved through the use of good spotting when using free weight methods. The spotter can apply a force increasing the load on the bar during the eccentric phase and apply an assisting force thereby reducing the load while in the 'sticking region' of the concentric phase. Such force application can be modified throughout the performance of a set to allow for the occurrence of progressive fatigue.

POWER TRAINING METHODS

The development of muscular strength has been subject to much research during the past 50 years and a great deal is known about the effect of resistance training on strength. However, research into the development of explosive power is a more recent phenomenon and therefore much less is known regarding the development of power and athletic performance.

Over the past 20 years the use of resistance training has progressed from an activity performed by relatively few strength athletes, to become a permanent feature of the training routines of most sportspersons. In this progression the main objective has shifted from the goal of enhancing muscular strength and size, to the improvement of muscular power and competitive performance. In order to improve performance a number of training options are available to the athlete. These include traditional weight training, where relatively heavy weights are lifted for relatively few repetitions, through to dynamic plyometric training, where the acceleration and deceleration of body weight serve as the training overload.

Although there is a variety of resistance training methods one can use to enhance muscular power, and hence dynamic performance, there appear to be at least three distinct theories as to which method results in optimal performance gains in dynamic sports such as sprints, jumps and throws. These are as follows:

- Traditional strength training
- Plyometric training
- Maximal power training

The purpose of this section is to present effective training methods for each of these forms of power training and to outline the results of recent studies in which the effects of these different training modalities on the development of dynamic athletic performance were compared.

Traditional Strength Training

Traditional heavy strength training involves lifting heavy loads (80–90% of maximum) using few repetitions (4–8 RM; Fig. 9.27). This method is seen to result in optimal increases in strength (Berger 1962) and has also been reported to enhance power and movement speed to a greater extent than training with relatively light loads (Schmidtbleicher & Haralambie 1981; Schmidtbleicher & Buehrle 1987). The rationalization of these findings is based on the size theory of motor unit recruitment which suggests that the large fast twitch (FT) motor units, which are predominantly responsible for the production of powerful movements, will only be recruited if relatively large forces are required. Consequently, heavy loads must be used in training to develop dynamic athletic performance as only heavy load

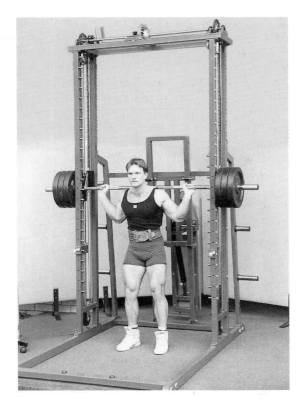

Fig. 9.27   Heavy squat exercise performed in a Smith machine.

training guarantees the recruitment of all motor units, both fast and slow (Schmidtbleicher 1988). Proponents of this theory maintain that power and athletic performance can be best developed by the use of traditional heavy load strength training, provided that the athletes attempt to lift the weights explosively (Behm & Sale 1993). This latter requirement is important in developing the neural pathways that will allow for the enhancement of dynamic athletic performance.

Plyometric Training

Traditional plyometric training uses the acceleration and deceleration of body weight as the overload in dynamic activities such as depth jumps and bounds (Fig. 9.28). This training method improves muscular power, thereby enhancing dynamic competitive performance such as jumping (Bosco *et al.* 1982). Plyometric exercises have been a common resistance training method in many Eastern Bloc countries for at least 25 years (Duda 1988). During the 1960s Yuri Veroshanki, a Russian athletics coach, used plyometric training methods with much success for athletes involved in jumping events. Plyometrics were again in the spotlight during the 1972 Munich Olympics when the Russian, Valery Borzov won the 100 m in a time of 10.0 s and also won the 200 m sprint event, as much of his success was attributed to the use of plyometric training methods. This anecdotal evidence supporting the use of plyometrics has since been confirmed by research demonstrating that this training modality is effective in increasing muscular power and performance (Hakkinen *et al.* 1986; Adams *et al.* 1992).

   Coaches and athletes maintain that plyometric training represents the bridge between strength and power and perceive it as a method of training that will directly enhance competitive performance (Chu 1992). They often see strength training as a means of increasing general strength and plyometrics as a way to apply this strength to improve performance. Such a perception appears well supported in the literature, with many studies reporting that the combination of plyometric and strength training resulted in superior performance

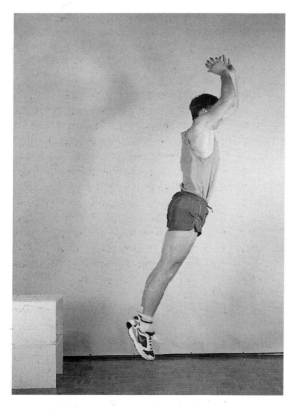

Fig. 9.28 Plyometric exercise: depth jumps.

allows for greater improvements in the maximal rate of force development and thus power, in comparison to traditional weight training methods

- Plyometric exercises do not involve a large deceleration phase during concentric movement, which occurs in traditional strength training, as the body does not have to achieve zero velocity at the end of the exercise (see section on the Deceleration Phase). Thus plyometric exercises involve the production of high forces and accelerations throughout the entire range of motion, specific to most competitive movements

- Plyometric exercises are performed at higher velocities than those achieved using traditional strength training. This increased velocity enhances the specificity of this training modality to competitive performance, improving the transference of training gains to the competitive situation

- Plyometric exercises involve a dynamic stretch–shorten cycle (SSC) movement similar to that adopted in most sporting actions. Research has demonstrated that the performance of plyometric exercises promotes the ability to utilize the SSC by enhancing the use of elastic energy and the stretch reflex (Schmidtbleicher *et al.* 1988)

DISADVANTAGES OF PLYOMETRIC TRAINING

Despite these advantages, this training modality is a relatively recent phenomenon and has a number of limitations associated with its use, which are as follows:

- Due to the dynamic nature of plyometric exercises, high impact forces can occur when landing from activities such as depth jumps or bounds. Impact forces in the order of three to four times body weight are not uncommon when performing high intensity training. These high transient forces placed on the musculoskeletal system can result in the occurrence of musculoskeletal injuries such as anterior compartment pressure syndrome, tibial stress syndrome or even stress fractures. The

gains when compared to plyometric or strength training alone (Adams *et al.* 1992).

ADVANTAGES OF PLYOMETRIC TRAINING

Plyometric training involves a number of advantages over traditional heavy weight training methods. These include the following:

- Plyometric exercise tends to be performed in a much more explosive way than traditional strength training. For example, a depth jump will be performed in 300–500 ms, whereas a heavy squat may take several seconds to perform. Consequently *plyometric training requires the athlete to rapidly develop force, promoting the development of muscular power.* Hakkinen *et al.* (1985a,b) have reported that the dynamic nature of plyometric training occurrence of injury is reduced if the individual has a relatively high level of strength prior to performing this type of training. Furthermore, landing on a compliant surface, such as rubber matting, and using shock absorbing shoes will also assist in reducing the effect of the impact forces

- Plyometric training has traditionally been performed using mainly body mass as the load for lower body activities, or medicine balls of standard masses (3–10 kg) for the upper body. No systematic method has yet been adopted to determine the optimal load for the development of power, with these loads being used simply because of their convenience. For example, there is no scientific reason for using medicine balls weighing 3–10 kg. Research has demonstrated that power is maximized at a load of approximately 30–45% of maximum, which was outlined in the discussion of muscle mechanics and neuromuscular considerations; however, plyometric exercises are not typically performed at this load

- There is a limited number of exercises that can be performed plyometrically. Most plyometric activities are essentially limited to the lower body and dominated by muscular actions involving extension of the thigh and leg. Upper body activities using medicine balls are usually performed with such low loading as to represent inadequate levels of overload on the musculature. Many other activities, such as the recovery of the leg during sprint running, simply cannot currently be carried out in a plyometric fashion

- Plyometric exercises are generally performed with very limited or no feedback, despite the fact that knowledge of the result of the exercise is important in facilitating training motivation. In a recent publication by Chu (1992), only 12 of 89 exercises provided any feedback during the performance of the activity, with a further 12 involving feedback after the completion of the exercise. The type of feedback associated with these exercises included the number of times the athlete could contact an object or the time taken to execute the

exercise. No plyometric exercises involve feedback with relation to the power output of the activity, which is perhaps the most relevant variable. When performing traditional strength training exercises athletes know the load they are lifting or the resistance they need to apply and this serves as a constant source of encouragement. For example, an athlete may perform a new personal best of four repetitions with 150 kg on the bench press and use this to set a personal goal for the next training session, that is a new maximum lift of 165 kg. Although an athlete's performance during plyometric training can be estimated at regular intervals in tests such as the jump and reach, in daily training there is very little feedback or knowledge of the result. With plyometric training, the individual is essentially 'training blind'

- Due to the relatively high velocities achieved when performing plyometric training, the forces produced during these exercises tend to be lower than those achieved during traditional strength training (see section on Force–Velocity Relationship). Consequently this form of training does not develop muscular strength as well as traditional strength training

PLYOMETRIC TRAINING STRATEGIES

Training prerequisites

Strength development is essential prior to the use of high intensity plyometric exercises, such as jumping, hopping and bounding, if positive gains in power are to be expected. Without a good strength base, the legs or arms of the athlete will not be able to withstand the extreme forces generated by plyometrics and without this base the risk of injury is very high (Roundtable NSCA 1986). Further, as outlined previously (see section on Relationship between Strength, Power and Endurance) there is a strong relationship between strength and power so that one cannot have a high degree of power without first being relatively strong. An ability to recruit all of the available force very rapidly is of little consequence if the level of force is low. Thus *the current level of strength of the athlete will always represent the upper limit to his or her power potential.* Consequently, before performing high level plyometric training, at least a year of intensive strength training should be undertaken, and prior to performing high impact activities such as high depth jumps, the athlete should be able to squat at least 1.5 times body weight (Roundtable NSCA 1986).

Training principles

It is important to realize that the same training principles used when developing strength training routines are also relevant when developing plyometric training programmes. Thus the principles of overload, specificity, variation and recovery are just as applicable to plyometric training as they are to strength training. Therefore, when performing plyometric training the load placed on the system should be progressively increased. This is achieved by increasing the height of the drop and/or the addition of extra load through the use of weighted vests. An example of a progressive overload plyometric training routine can be seen in Table 9.6.

Table 9.6 Plyometric training routine for depth jumps

Week	Sets × repetitions	Drop height (cm)
1	3×8	20
2	3×8	20
3	4×8	2×20; 2×30
4	5×8	1×20; 2×30; 2×40
5	6×8	2×20; 2×30; 2×40
6	6×8	2×30; 2×40; 2×50
7	6×8	2×40; 2×50; 2×60
8	6×8	2×50; 2×60; 2×70
9	6×8	2×60; 2×70; 2×80
10	6×8	2×60; 2×70; 2×80

If athletes experience soreness in the tibial region or other skeletal structures of the foot or leg, this is generally caused by increasing the load too soon in the training cycle. In such instances the drop heights should be lowered and/or the weight carried by the athlete decreased.

Plyometric training 'tips'

Optimal drop height Research has not conclusively determined what the optimal drop height is for depth jumps. However, one approach is to use the height that results in the greatest rebound height. This varies for different individuals but is generally between 0.3 and 0.7 m (Asmussen & Bonde-Petersen 1974; Komi & Bosco 1978) and is termed the best drop jump height. This height can be readily determined by having athletes perform drop jumps from various heights and recording the height jumped.

Ground contact time Most coaches and scientists are of the opinion that plyometric exercises must be performed so that ground contact time, or time in contact with a medicine ball, must be *as short as possible.* In fact often the athletes are instructed to imagine they are landing on a hot surface and must rebound very quickly. Such a strategy serves two purposes. First, by reducing contact time, the athlete will be required to rapidly develop force and the power of the activity (work/time) will generally be increased. Second, a dynamic SSC movement performed over a short duration will reduce the likelihood that the athlete will experience a delay between the eccentric and concentric phases, and thereby maximize the use of elastic energy during the plyometric exercise.

Rest and recovery periods To be effective, plyometric training must be carried out explosively and athletes need to be in a fresh state before a training session. Therefore, plyometric training sessions should be performed prior to fatiguing activities such as strength training. Similarly, relatively long rest periods, of approximately 5 min, should be imposed between repeated plyometric activities to enable full recovery of the neuromuscular system to occur. This will ensure that the athlete can continue to perform in a dynamic fashion.

Feedback As previously outlined, plyometric training is often performed with little or no feedback. If the training consists of exercises such as repeated vertical jumps and the athletes have no way of determining the height of the jump, it is difficult to motivate them over a period of months to continue to strive for maximal effort. Every attempt must be made to give the athletes some meaningful feedback. Simply hanging some targets from the ceiling for the athletes to try and reach will give them some idea of how high they are jumping, which will in turn aid motivation.

Chu (1992) recently published a book on plyometrics that includes a very comprehensive list of plyometric exercises for a wide variety of sports. The reader is referred to this text for further information on plyometric training.

Maximal Power Training

Maximal explosive power training involves the performance of dynamic weight training at the load which maximizes mechanical power output (Fig. 9.29). This training strategy involves lifting relatively light loads (~30–45% of maximum) at high speed. Such training results in the production of the highest mechanical power output of the musculature which has been reported to result in the

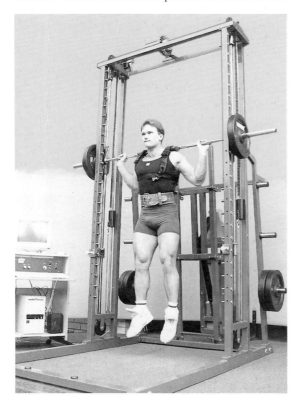

Fig. 9.29 Maximal power exercise: plyometric squats performed at the load which maximizes power output.

greatest training gains in power (Berger 1963; Kaneko *et al.* 1983; Moritani *et al.* 1987). In observing the effects of training at 0, 30, 60 and 100% of maximum, Kaneko *et al.* (1983) reported that 30% of maximum load resulted in the greatest increase in maximal mechanical power output, while the 100% load resulted in the greatest improvements in strength. On the basis of the results obtained by Kaneko *et al.* (1983) and Moritani *et al.* (1987) it was suggested by Moritani and associates that any training method which aimed to improve power should use a training load of 30% of maximum. This claim was strongly supported by research previously conducted by Berger (1963) who reported that the performance of squat jumps at a load of approximately 30% of maximum resulted in greater increases in vertical jump height (2.8 cm) than those achieved in traditional weight training (2.3 cm), isometric training (0.8 cm) or unweighted vertical jumps (−1.0 cm).

MAXIMAL POWER EXERCISES

One extremely important point to realize when considering the application of maximal power training is that the exercises used must not be standard weight training exercises such as bench press or squats, where the bar must achieve zero velocity at the end of the movement range. In such instances maximal power training is relatively ineffective, because of the existence of a particularly large deceleration phase. For example, Fig. 9.30 depicts the forces produced throughout a squat lift performed at 30% of maximum. As can be seen, high forces were exerted at the start of the concentric phase and, due to the momentum developed, the forces exerted throughout the remainder of the lift were very low. Consequently, when performing maximal power training with traditional weight training exercises, the majority of the exercise is spent decelerating the load so that the bar will stop at the end of the movement. This means that high force levels are achieved only through a very small range of the movement and suboptimal training gains result (Schmidtbleicher & Haralambie 1981; Schmidtbleicher & Buehrle 1987). This is also the reason why this form of

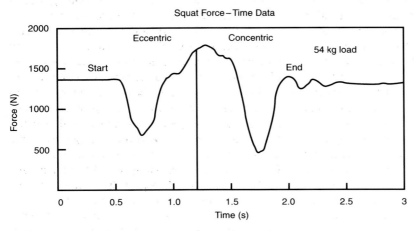

Fig. 9.30 Force–time profile for a traditional squat exercise performed at 30% of maximum (courtesy of Wilson *et al.* 1993).

training is not presently popular with athletes or coaches.

Effective performance of maximal power training

Maximal power training should be performed using activities that allow for the production of high forces and accelerations throughout the entire movement range, such as those that are realized when performing weighted squat jumps. A squat jump movement allows the subjects to leave the ground with the load at the completion of the lift. This eliminates the deceleration phase, as the movement does not come to rest at the completion of the exercise. Large accelerations and forces can then be exerted throughout the entire movement range, as opposed to only a small part of the range. For example, Fig. 9.31 depicts the force–time profile for a weighted squat jump performed by the same subject and at the same load as the traditional squat exercise depicted in Fig. 9.30. Figure 9.31 clearly shows that high forces are exerted throughout the entire range of motion and hence there is no deceleration phase when performing this type of exercise. Similarly, maximal power training can be effectively performed with the use of specialized equipment, as depicted in Fig. 9.21, which reduces the deceleration phase (see Explosive Strength Training).

MAXIMAL POWER TRAINING ROUTINES

Maximal power training is a recent phenomenon and has been subjected to relatively little scientific scrutiny or even field testing. In essence the training modality is a combination of strength training and plyometrics. It allows for greater loading

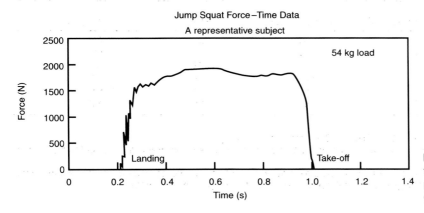

Fig. 9.31 Force–time profile for a squat jump exercise performed at 30% of maximum (courtesy of Wilson *et al.* 1993).

than plyometrics, enabling a higher power output to be achieved, but because of this there may also be an increase in impact forces resulting in a higher incidence of soft tissue injury. The additional load will also result in a muscular action which is performed with a greater contact time and at a reduced velocity when compared to plyometric exercises. Despite these differences, maximal power training and plyometric training are essentially similar so that *maximal power training could be considered a form of plyometric training that is specifically performed at a load which maximizes the power output of the exercise.* Training methods similar to those used for plyometric training should therefore be adopted for maximal power training.

A Comparison between Power Training Methods

A study was performed (Wilson *et al.* 1993) which compared three different methods of training, to determine which one resulted in the greatest increase in running, jumping and cycling. This study involved 64 experienced subjects who were currently undergoing resistance training and had been in training for a period of at least 1 year. Subjects were randomly allocated into four groups which consisted of traditional weight training, plyometric training, maximal power training and a control group.

A summary of the effect of each training modality on each test item from the pre- to post-testing occasions is outlined in Table 9.7. The experimental group who trained with the load that maximized mechanical power achieved the best overall results in enhancing dynamic athletic performance.

The results of the above and other studies (Berger 1963; Kaneko *et al.* 1983; Moritani *et al.* 1987) strongly suggest that to enhance athletic performance, athletes should train using a load that maximizes the mechanical power output of the lift, that is, at approximately 30–45% of maximum. Such a conclusion is logical in view of the fact that a large number of sports are power dominated and thus the nature of the training stimulus should be directed at the enhancement of power output as opposed to the load lifted or the speed at which the movement is executed.

CONCLUSION

Traditional weight training was designed originally to enhance muscular strength and it is seen to be effective in this goal. Since strength is related to power it will also serve to have a diminished effect on power and thus dynamic athletic performance. Plyometric training was designed to directly enhance muscular power and therefore competitive performance; however, no systematic method has been developed to determine the optimal load for plyometric training. In fact plyometric

Table 9.7 Summary of the significant changes observed, pre- to post-training, from each of the training modalities. The percentage changes for results that were statistically significant or that approached statistical significance are presented

Test items	Groups			
	Maximal power (%)	Plyometric (%)	Weight (%)	Control (%)
CMJ	18*	10%*	5*	NS
SJ	15*	NS	7*	NS
Leg extension 300 deg/s	7*	NS	NS	NS
30 m sprint	1.5**	NS	NS	NS
6 s cycle	5*	NS	6*	NS
Maximum strength	NS	NS	16*	NS

Data from Wilson *et al.* 1993.
Statistically significant change *P<0.05, **P<0.1. NS, no significant change.
The CMJ and SJ are vertical jumping tests performed with and without the use of a preparatory counter-movement, respectively.
Note: the performance increases recorded for the maximal power group from the pre- to post-testing occasions in the CMJ and SJ tests were significantly greater than those achieved by the weight training group.

training tends to be performed at body weight only, as this is a convenient load to use. The optimal training strategy to enhance dynamic athletic performance appears to be a hybrid between traditional weight training and plyometric training, that is, to perform plyometric weight training at the load which maximizes mechanical power output. In this way weight training is used to enhance muscular power directly, rather than simply increasing muscular strength.

PRACTICAL APPLICATIONS

The above discussion strongly suggests that performance gains in power-oriented activities are best achieved through the use of plyometric weight training at the load that maximizes mechanical power output (~30–45% of maximum). In order to obtain the full benefits of this type of training, these exercises must be performed in a plyometric fashion so that the subject actually throws or jumps with the resistance. This enables high forces and accelerations to be achieved throughout the entire range of motion. Obviously such movements cannot be performed with free weight exercises, such as the bench press, as the possibility of injury is very high. Recently the Plyometric Power System has been developed to enable the performance of maximal power training exercises with safety and several systems are currently in use throughout Australia and the USA. However, if one does not have access to such specialized equipment, loaded squat jump exercises have been successfully performed for many years (Capen 1950). Medicine ball work is another means through which optimal power training can be performed, but one must use very heavy medicine balls so that the appropriate load can be obtained. However, caution must be used when performing such exercises as the impact forces can be high.

Future Directions in the Development of Explosive Power

THE PLYOMETRIC POWER SYSTEM

The Plyometric Power System has been developed as a testing and training device for the assessment

and development of muscular power. It allows standard weight training activities to be performed in a dynamic, plyometric fashion and was developed to overcome the previously outlined disadvantages of plyometric training, so that more effective use of plyometric training principles could be achieved. The machine is designed to effectively and safely allow a loaded bar to be thrown from the hands repeatedly (Fig. 9.32), while jumping actions such as squat jumps can also be performed with the bar secured to the back by a harness (Fig. 9.29). By incorporating the proven benefits of traditional weight training with the advancement of plyometric techniques, this machine affords the opportunity to powerfully perform typical resistance exercises at high velocities and accelerations. The system is designed so that any jumping, throwing or pushing movement that can be performed with a traditional free weight bar can also be performed dynamically using the Plyometric Power System. Consequently, exercises such as squats, bench presses and military presses can be performed plyometrically, thereby enhancing muscular power.

The Plyometric Power System makes more effective use of plyometric training principles and

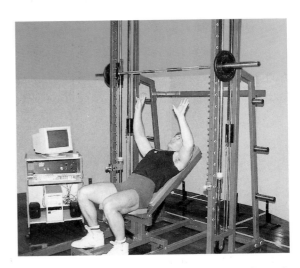

Fig. 9.32 Plyometric inclined bench press performed on the Plyometric Power System.

serves to eliminate the following disadvantages of plyometric exercises:

- The high injury risk associated with the performance of plyometric exercises
- The limited feedback associated with the performance of plyometric exercises
- The inadequate loading associated with the performance of plyometric exercises
- The relatively few exercises that can be performed plyometrically

Reducing injury risks

The system includes safety catches so that the athlete will not be struck by the bar if it is not caught, or if an incorrect landing occurs during jumps. A braking device is also included which can be used to completely or partially reduce the eccentric load if desired. This computer-controlled brake is unidirectional and will only affect the downward movement of the bar. Its function is to reduce the high impact forces often experienced when performing high intensity plyometric activities, such as heavily weighted squat jumps or bench press throws. When the bar reaches the peak of its height the computer will engage the brake to an extent previously specified by the user. This will decelerate the bar prior to ground contact, reducing or even eliminating the impact force (Fig. 9.33). As the athlete lands or catches the bar, the brake is disengaged by the computer and a normal eccentric contraction can be performed. The brake is designed so that the intensity of the braking effect can be infinitely varied. Further, the brake can be set to operate during the entire eccentric phase or only a portion of it.

Enhanced feedback of plyometric performance

A computer (Fig. 9.34) interfaced with the machine provides detailed information on each repetition performed including:

- Height thrown or jumped
- Work done
- Power output
- Velocity
- Contact time
- Fatigue index, which quantifies strength–endurance

All this information is calculated and displayed on the screen instantaneously. The calculation of power output allows the system to be used to determine the load at which an athlete achieves maximal power output. This is done by performing repeated sets of an exercise with loads varying from 20 to 60% of maximum. The power output is recorded on each set and hence the load which

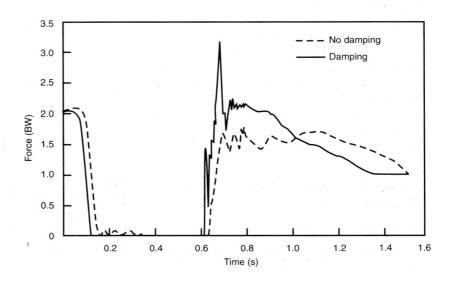

Fig. 9.33 Impact force produced during a loaded squat jump with and without the use of the dampening device of the Plyometric Power System (courtesy of Newton & Wilson 1993).

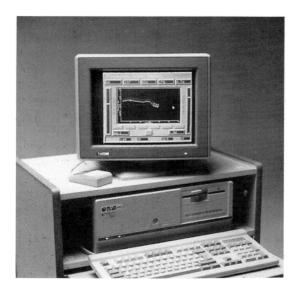

Fig. 9.34 Computer display of the Plyometric Power System (courtesy of Plyopower Technologies).

maximizes mechanical power output can be established and used to perform maximal power training.

Another innovative feature of the computer system is the instantaneous auditory feedback provided to the athlete when a predetermined level of performance has been achieved. Using this facility an athlete or coach can preset a performance level which may be a specified distance, work or power output. For example, a coach may specify that the athlete must perform 10 squat jumps at a load of 50 kg, each to a height of at least 40 cm (or a power output of 1000 W). On every repetition that the athlete reaches or exceeds a height of 40 cm (or 1000 W), the computer gives an instantaneous high tone beep. If the athlete fails to reach the performance criterion a low tone gong is emitted. This function has the effect of motivating the athlete while performing the set to achieve the target level of performance. By using this device the athlete is no longer 'training blind' when performing plyometric exercises.

In essence the Plyometric Power System is a combination of traditional free weight and plyometric training techniques, designed specifically to eliminate the disadvantages of plyometric

training, so that athletes can safely overload their musculature in a more explosive and dynamic fashion than has previously been possible.

The Plyometric Power System is perhaps the first step into future power training. Currently it is limited to movements that are performed in a vertical plane and thus lacks specificity to many sports. However, the technology used in the device could readily be applied to other movement planes and body postures. Just as the barbell revolutionized the development of strength, the Plyometric Power System and related devices may make a similar contribution in the area of power.

STRENGTH–ENDURANCE TRAINING METHODS

Many sports involve the performance of high intensity activities over a prolonged period of time. In such instances the maximum strength or power of the muscle is not the most important factor, but rather it is the ability to maintain a high level of strength and power over a relatively long period of time. Sports where this ability is very important include most swimming events, middle distance running, kayaking, skating, rowing, cycling and skiing. Even in traditional power events, such as the 100 m sprint, the ability to maintain a high level of power over an extended duration is of great importance.

In terms of the development of muscular function, a vast amount of research has been directed at the improvement of strength; substantially less research has examined the enhancement of power; and very little has been done in the area of strength–endurance. At present there are three methods used to improve strength–endurance, which are as follows:

- Traditional heavy weight training
- High repetition training
- Variable load training

Traditional Heavy Weight Training

As previously outlined there is a strong direct relationship between muscular strength and endurance, so that a stronger muscle will have a greater endurance capacity when it is compared to a weaker one. Consequently, one method to increase strength–endurance is to simply enhance strength, using the heavy weight training methods already discussed. The strong relationship between strength and endurance has resulted in some scientists such as Jones (1974) claiming that the physical capacities of strength and endurance are 'exactly the same, and thus should be trained in an identical fashion'.

High Repetition Training

High repetition training involves the performance of relatively high numbers of repetitions using relatively low loads. Between 30 and 50 repetitions per set are performed, using loads of 30–50% of the athlete's maximum, for three or four sets. Alternatively this training involves performing as many repetitions as possible in a specified time period. For example, rowers may perform the bent-over rowing exercise for 6 min using a relatively low load. This time interval is chosen as it is specific to the duration of the 2000 m eight-oar event. However, the use of such low loads provides insufficient overload for the musculature to increase in strength. McDonagh and Davies (1984), in reviewing a number of research findings, suggested that loads of less than 66% of maximum resulted in no increase in maximal strength, even when 150 contractions per day were used as the training stimulus. However, the performance of such high numbers of repetitions results in the production of large quantities of lactic acid and other waste products. Repeated exposure to these high lactate levels enhances the athlete's tolerance to the fatiguing effects of lactic acid, which may increase endurance. In fact the accumulation of lactic acid when performing high repetition training tends to be higher than that which is achievable when performing the actual competitive activity. This type of training also results in specific local muscular adaptations which promote local circulation, enhance metabolism and waste removal, thereby further enhancing endurance.

COMPARISON BETWEEN HEAVY WEIGHT AND HIGH REPETITION METHODS OF STRENGTH–ENDURANCE TRAINING

In comparing the heavy weight and high repetition methods it is apparent that at least two mechanisms of improving strength–endurance are possible. The former is based upon increasing muscle strength and the direct effect this has on strength–endurance. The latter is based on the enhancement of the tolerance of the athlete to the fatiguing effects of waste products, such as lactic acid, through repeated exposure to relatively high concentrations, and other local muscle adaptations. Anderson and Kearney (1982) compared these two training methods and demonstrated that the high repetition and heavy weight training methods resulted in similar improvements in endurance.

Variable Load Training

With two independent mechanisms for the development of strength–endurance, it logically follows that a training system should be designed to incorporate both mechanisms. This system is termed variable load training and represents a combination of the *heavy weight* and *high repetition* training forms. It is designed to expose the athlete to a sufficiently high load to promote the development of strength and also allow the performance of enough repetitions to enhance an athlete's tolerance to lactic acid and other local muscle adaptations. Such a training system is achieved by using a number of progressively reducing loads throughout a set. For example, an athlete may perform the following set with approximately 3–5 s rest between load changes:

- 10 repetitions with ~70% of maximum
- 10 repetitions with ~60% of maximum
- 10 repetitions with ~50% of maximum

Such a method allows exposure to relatively heavy loads (i.e. 70% maximum) to develop strength, as well as the performance of a relatively large number of repetitions (i.e. 30) to enhance endurance. More repetitions and reductions of the load can be achieved depending on the duration of the event.

Variable load training can be used on most strength training exercises and is best practised when a coach or partner is present to rapidly modify the load. Pin-weighted machines are particularly useful for such training, as the modification of the load can occur very rapidly and with little effort. This training method has been used for many years by bodybuilders attempting to simultaneously increase the volume and intensity of their training. *Variable load training would currently appear to represent the best form of training for the development of strength–endurance.*

Future Directions in the Development of Strength–Endurance

Many dynamic sports require high intensity actions over a relatively long period of time. The dynamic nature of these sports, such as swimming, rowing and middle distance running, would suggest that the dominant requirement was power–endurance rather than strength–endurance. Indeed strength may only be important in such instances due to its relationship to power and endurance (see section on the Relationship Between Strength, Power and Endurance). It is interesting to note that much of the research and current training techniques in this area are based upon the performance of traditional weight training methods and thus are centred around strength. Potentially more rewarding may be training systems based upon maximal power training methods, which are modified by increasing the number of repetitions performed to simultaneously promote endurance. Thus exercises such as jump squats, loaded at approximately 20–30% of maximum, performed for sets of 30 repetitions, may represent the future standard for the development of sustained powerful sporting activities.

RESISTANCE TRAINING AND INJURY

The use of resistance training by athletes is seen as a mechanism to directly enhance competitive performance as a result of increases in strength, power and endurance. However, resistance training can also be employed as a means of developing the musculoskeletal structures to such an extent that the incidence of injury from training and competitive performance is reduced. Hence resistance training has an important role to play in injury prevention. A further use of resistance training is in the rehabilitation of injuries, where it can be employed to reduce the recovery time and to develop the musculoskeletal structures so that the likelihood of the recurrence of the injury is reduced.

Injury Prevention

On the basis of vast experience working with athletes and medical practitioners at the United States Military Academy, Peterson (1982) claimed that 'more than half the injuries in sports could easily be prevented through proper strength training'. He claimed that the injury prevention effects of resistance training were the most important consequence of such training. This subjective observation was supported by research conducted by Ekstrand and Gillquist (1983) who reported that soccer players sustaining non-collision knee sprains had reduced quadriceps strength in the injured knee prior to the injury. However, muscle tightness seemed to be more relevant in the incidence of injuries than muscle strength. Bender *et al.* (1964) reported that individuals with strength differences of more than 10% between the quadriceps of the right and left legs were more likely to sustain lower limb injuries when compared to individuals without such strength imbalances.

HOW RESISTANCE TRAINING REDUCES INJURY RISK

Increased size and strength of musculoskeletal structures

Resistance training produces a significant stress on the musculoskeletal structures and, provided that the stress is not excessive, the structures will adapt to this increase in stress. This adaptation will include increases in the size and strength of the muscles as well as the bone, ligaments, tendons and other musculoskeletal structures. It is important to realize that all musculoskeletal structures are living and will adapt in response to training. Many people perceive the skeleton as an inert structure; however, it will adapt to the environmental conditions placed upon it. For example, during the weightlessness experienced in space travel, the reduction in compressive forces results in a significant loss in bone mineral density for the astronauts. Conversely, the high stress that results from heavy resistance training will promote the strength and size of the skeletal structures as well as that of the tendons and ligaments. This increase in size and strength allows the musculoskeletal structures to tolerate the forces that are exerted upon them in various sporting situations, thus reducing the likely occurrence of musculoskeletal injury.

Elimination of muscular imbalances

Many sports involve the use of some muscle groups to a greater or lesser extent, and as a result lead to the development of imbalances in the body. For example, tennis involves the production of large forces on the dominant side of the body that swings the racquet and the upper body often suffers quite profound muscular imbalances. Chandler *et al.* (1992) reported that college tennis players produced significantly more strength and power in the internal rotator muscles in the shoulder region of the dominant arm compared to the non-dominant arm. The tests were conducted in a position specific to the service action and the disparity between the limbs was in the order of a 25% difference. Perhaps of greater significance to the incidence of injury was the fact that the subjects had similar external rotation strength between the differing limbs. Thus these tennis players had enhanced the function of the internal rotator muscles of the arm, which are dominant for the production of force during the service action. However, the external rotators, which are used to decelerate the racquet at the end of the service action, had not increased their capacity as a result of their use in tennis. Chandler *et al.* (1992) suggested that the resulting muscle imbalance was an important factor in

the incidence of muscle injury. These authors stated that:

> By significantly increasing the strength of the dominant shoulder in internal rotation without subsequent strengthening of the external rotators, muscle imbalances may be created in the dominant arm that could possibly affect the tennis player's predisposition to injuries caused by overloading of the shoulder joint. This study suggests that external rotation strengthening exercises should be implemented in tennis conditioning programs to maintain muscle strength balance, and possibly reduce the chance of overload injury.

Similar findings of internal/external rotation muscle imbalances in the shoulder joint have also been reported by Cook *et al.* (1987) in the examination of muscular function of the shoulder joint of college level baseball pitchers.

Hamstring injuries As in the case of the internal/external rotators of the arm, many authors maintain that a balance in strength between the quadriceps and hamstring muscle groups is important in the incidence of hamstring injuries. It is recommended that the hamstrings muscle group should be at least 60% of the maximal strength of the quadriceps muscle group, but among elite athletes engaged in sprinting, it is recommended that the hamstrings should be 75% of the strength of the quadriceps muscle group. If the hamstrings are weaker than this, the likelihood of knee joint or hamstring strains is increased.

Back injuries Perhaps the most problematic muscle imbalances occur in the back. Many sports involve asymmetric muscular actions that involve one side of the body to a greater extent than the other, for example, racquet sports. In such activities the musculature of the back can be developed to a far greater extent on the dominant side compared to the non-dominant side, resulting in unbalanced forces acting about the spine. Such an occurrence is thought to increase the likelihood of injuries to the back.

Resistance training recommendations

Through the use of resistance training, muscle imbalances that are inherent in many sports can be reduced and even eliminated. Those muscle groups which tend to be underdeveloped can be preferentially trained. In the majority of cases the forces exerted during the performance of sporting activities tend to be relatively low in comparison to those achieved during resistance training. Hence comparatively little resistance training is required to be performed to overcome the imbalances created through many thousands of hours of actual sporting activity. If the muscle imbalances involve differences between limbs, then *unilateral (one-limbed) resistance training exercises must be adopted.* For example, if differences exist in arm or leg strength when the athlete is performing bilateral exercises such as squats or bench presses, it is difficult to remove such imbalances, as the dominant limb tends to produce the majority of the force which can serve to accentuate the problem. The performance of unilateral exercises, such as a dumb-bell press or a single limb leg extension or leg press, will enable the weak limb to be adequately trained and the imbalance to be corrected.

Prevention of muscle imbalances

Coaches and athletes should be aware that the performance of many sports will result in relatively specific muscle imbalances and *resistance training should be performed early in an athlete's development to prevent the occurrence of such imbalances,* before they have had an opportunity to develop. Thus baseball pitchers and tennis players should routinely include exercises for the external rotators of the arm, such as illustrated in Fig. 9.35. Athletes involved in sports that require explosive lower body movements should include resistance exercises for the hamstring muscle group; while athletes involved in repetitive high impact sports, such as gymnastics, should include work for the tibialis anterior muscle. This is another instance of where prevention is better than cure and resistance training can be viewed as a very inexpensive form of health insurance.

Injury Rehabilitation

When an athlete is injured the nature of the injury and the reduced workload experienced by the injured muscle group will result in a loss of muscular function. This loss can often lead to muscular imbalances and the atrophy of muscle, bone, ligaments and tendons, which serve to increase the likelihood of recurrence of injury. Ekstrand and Gillquist (1983) reported that 35% of moderate and major injuries observed in soccer were preceded by a minor injury to the same region of the body. Thus it appears that inadequate rehabilitation from injury is an important factor in the recurrence of injuries.

Often athletes and coaches have difficulty in determining when athletes are rehabilitated to the point where they can safely resume participation

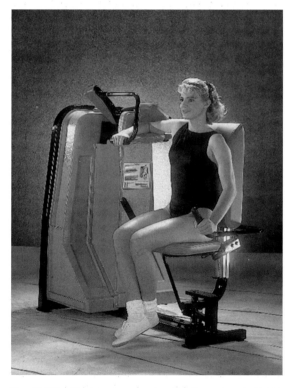

Fig. 9.35 Resistance exercises for the external rotator muscles of the arm.

in sport. Arvidsson *et al.* (1981) and Grimby *et al.* (1980) reported that 5–10 years after knee operations, athletes who had resumed sporting activities still exhibited a persistent 20% loss in muscle strength in the previously injured leg. These athletes were often not aware of the muscle imbalance and perceived themselves to be fully rehabilitated. Ekstrand *et al.* (1983) performed an injury prevention study that involved athletes engaging in a number of practices which were seen to reduce the incidence of muscular injury. These included flexibility training, prophylactic ankle taping and a controlled rehabilitation training schedule that prevented players returning to competition until they had regained 90% of their previous maximum strength. The use of these procedures significantly reduced the incidence of injury, so that there were 75% fewer injuries than there were in the control group.

The actual form of resistance training used in rehabilitation will be dependent on the nature and extent of the injury sustained. The formulation of such training routines is beyond the scope of this chapter; however, it is clear that failure to adequately rehabilitate injuries is very common and remains an important factor in the recurrence of injury.

RESISTANCE TRAINING AND THE USE OF ANABOLIC STEROIDS

The subject of ergogenic aids in sport is very controversial and at times highly emotional. The use of these substances represents cheating and is against the very essence of fair play and cannot be condoned under any circumstances. Nevertheless throughout this section of the chapter an attempt is made to treat the subject scientifically and from a neutral point of view.

There are many forms of ergogenic aids that have been used over the centuries by athletes in an attempt to enhance competitive performance, but the most widely used drugs which are known to increase strength and power are anabolic steroids. These synthetically produced chemicals are closely related in both structure and function to the male sex hormone testo-

sterone. They have two general actions which are as follows:

- An anabolic tissue building effect which stimulates the development of muscle mass
- An androgenic masculizing effect

Incidence of Use

Bodybuilders were reportedly using testosterone in the late 1940s and early 1950s and Soviet and American weightlifters began using these compounds in the 1950s. In 1958 the popular oral anabolic steroid, methandrostenolone, commonly known as Dianabol, was released and the use of anabolic steroids in sport began in the early 1960s. In fact Dr Tom Waddell, a US decathlete, estimated that one-third of the entire US track and field team had used steroids at the 1968 pre-Olympic training camp (Todd 1987). Currently it is difficult to determine the incidence of drug use by various athletes; however, Chinery (1984) stated that 'over 2.5 million athletes worldwide, used anabolic steroids during 1982'.

Performance Enhancement through the Use of Anabolic Steroids

For many years, research data have been available which suggested that anabolic steroids were not effective at increasing muscular function or development (Fahey & Brown 1973; Stromme *et al.* 1974). Such studies were performed using previously untrained athletes for relatively short training periods. These data have been used by various individuals in the medical and scientific communities to claim that anabolic steroids are completely ineffective when used by elite athletes and that the reported anecdotal effects are entirely psychological. However, research performed using experienced strength trained athletes has demonstrated that the use of anabolic steroids, when combined with high intensity strength training, promoted the development of muscular size and strength to a greater extent than the use of training alone (Wright 1980). These data have resulted in the American College of Sports Medicine (1987) concluding that, in some cases, the use of anabolic steroids is effective at increasing muscular strength and lean body mass.

The American College of Sports Medicine (1984) has suggested the following effects of the use of anabolic steroids. These are as follows:

- An anabolic effect whereby the steroids promote nitrogen retention resulting in an increase in muscular size and density. This is seen to result from a combination of increased protein synthesis and a reduction in the catabolic effect of glucocorticoids
- An increase in aggressive behaviour which has the effect of facilitating training, particularly heavy resistance training

It is difficult to assess exactly what advantage the use of anabolic steroids represents in sport. Ward (1973) reported that the use of 10 mg of Dianabol per day for 4 weeks resulted in an increase in bench press strength of 13% in previously trained subjects. The control group, who ingested a placebo, increased strength by approximately 4% over this same period. The dosages used in this study would, however, be considered extremely low and used for a relatively short time period in comparison to those reportedly used by many athletes. However, the use of anabolic ster-

oids by athletes is believed to increase muscular strength by at least 10% above the natural potential of the individual.

Wright (1982) reported the changes in body composition in a world class athlete who reportedly used extreme doses of a variety of anabolic steroids for a 7 month period. The drug regimen began with 7.5 mg of Anavar daily and progressed to 250 mg per day plus 56 mg Winstrol, 125 mg Dianabol and 100 mg of Primobolan Depot daily. These reported doses must be considered extreme and at the peak of the 7 month cycle were equivalent to at least 50 times more than the body's natural production of steroids. The changes in body composition experienced by this athlete are illustrated in Fig. 9.36.

Over the 7 month period of drug use the athlete gained 16.5 kg of lean body mass, an amazing increase given the fact that he was already large and muscular prior to the use of steroids. Unfortunately Wright (1982) did not measure any changes in competitive performance as a result of the use of the drugs. The rate of gain in lean body mass was particularly high over the first 6 weeks of commencement of the drugs but there was a much lower rate of progression after this period, despite large increases in the quantity of the drugs taken (Fig. 9.36). This observation highlights one of the

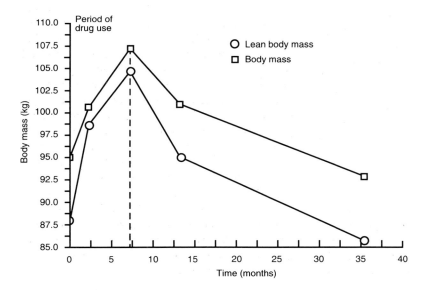

Fig. 9.36 Body composition changes in a world class athlete resulting from intense training and the use of anabolic steroids (adapted from Wright 1982).

important factors in the use of anabolic steroids. When subjected to large quantities of drugs the body will attempt to minimize their effect and return to its normal level of homeostasis. Thus the anabolic effect of these compounds tends to diminish as a function of the time of their use, even if increasing doses are administered. Consequently, long-term continuous use with progressively increasing dosages tends to produce relatively small additional performance gains, at relatively high risk of the development of short- and long-term side effects.

DRUG DOSAGES

Surprisingly, the athlete in this example did not report the occurrence of any short-term side effects. However, Wright (1982) maintained that essentially comparable results could have been achieved with much lower dosages, with a greatly reduced risk of short- and long-term effects. Many authors have reported that some athletes use extremely high doses of anabolic steroids as they feel that 'if a little works well, a lot will work much better'. However, the available evidence does not seem to support such a perception and the additional performance gains tend to diminish as a function of the dose and, particularly, the duration of use. In assessing the quantity of drug dose it is important to realize that the normal daily androgen production rate for males ranges from 5 to 15 mg of testosterone. The reported use by athletes of doses of up to 50 times this value would appear to be completely irrational because the body is unable to utilize such large dosages. Such a strategy is analogous to athletes who ingest 10 large steaks in a day in an effort to increase protein and hence the size of their muscles. There is simply no way the body can assimilate that amount of protein.

LONG-TERM EFFECTS

In an age where some athletes are being banned from competition and subsequently allowed to return several years later, it is interesting to note that upon cessation of the ingestion of drugs, the athlete depicted in Fig. 9.36 returned to his former lean body weight. Thus the effect of the drugs, at least for this individual, appeared to be short-term and resulted in no long-term residual performance effects after the drug had been discontinued for approximately a year. However, further studies are required to determine whether this is a general trend.

Health Effects Relating to the Use of Anabolic Steroids

Many reports on the potential health risks associated with the use of anabolic steroids portray these risks as particularly deleterious, in an attempt to reduce the incidence of their use. In reviewing the health risks associated with the use of anabolic steroids, Wright (1980) maintained that the medical community had tended to overstate the health risks. Wright concluded that: 'If steroid use has been as widespread as many athletes, coaches, medical and sports officials have suggested, there are few explanations as to why serious problems in athletics have not surfaced … Perhaps the health risks of prolonged or high dose use of these drugs by athletes could be compared to oral contraceptive use by women'.

Despite the fact that the health risks associated with the use of anabolic steroids may have, in some cases, been overstated, there are some serious consequences from the use of these substances, particularly when relatively high doses of oral steroids are used over prolonged periods of time. Furthermore, while past generations of steroid users generally appear to have had limited medical problems, more recently the use of these drugs has involved far greater doses and more dangerous compounds than those used previously. Subsequently the severe medical consequences that have been forecast for these individuals using anabolic steroids may yet occur.

The possible side effects from the use of anabolic steroids are listed in Table 9.8; however, a complete description of the mechanism and incidence of these effects is beyond the scope of this chapter. There are several important points

Table 9.8 The possible side effects of the use of anabolic steroids

Psychological changes	Euphoria, mania, depression, psychosis, drug dependence
Metabolic changes	Salt and water retention
Hormonal effects	Gynaecomastia
	Testicular atrophy
	Decreased spermatogenesis
	Changes in libido
	Prostatic hypertrophy
	Decreased follicle stimulating hormone and luteinizing hormone levels
Skin and hair changes	Acne, alopecia
Tendon ruptures	
Blood lipid alterations	Increased triglycerides
	Increased low density lipoprotein cholesterol
	Decreased high density lipoprotein cholesterol
Cardiovascular effects	Hypertension
	Atherogenesis
	Sudden death
Kidney tumours	Wilms' tumour
Liver	Elevated transaminases
	Cholestatic jaundice
	Peliosis hepatis
	Hepatoma
	Carcinoma
Additionally in females	Virilizing effects
	Menstrual disturbances
	Infertility
	Breast atrophy
	Clitoral hypertrophy
	Hirsutism
Additionally in children	Premature epiphyseal closure
	Premature virilization

Adapted from Bloomfield *et al*. 1992.

relating to these side-effects however, that are outlined below:

- As a general rule, oral steroids have more serious side effects compared to injectable steroids, with far greater incidences of liver, kidney, cardiovascular and immune system problems being reported following the use of oral, as compared to injectable steroids
- As with any drug, the side effects differ greatly between individuals. Thus some individuals may experience none at all, even with extreme doses, whereas others may experience serious complications even with minimal use. While the use of these drugs should be avoided and *cannot be condoned under any circumstances*, if individuals persist in using them they

should be examined by a doctor on a regular basis
- The presence and extent of side effects are dose and duration dependent, so that the greater the dose and the longer the individual is exposed to the drug, the more likely it is that serious side effects will occur
- The side effects experienced by women appear to be more permanent than those experienced by men. For example, with steroid use most men will experience testicular atrophy; while clitoral enlargement will occur in most women. Upon cessation of drug use, the testicles will generally return to their normal state, but the clitoris will usually remain enlarged. Similarly, the deepening of the female voice and the growth of body hair is generally

irreversible after anabolic steroids are discontinued

Drug Use and Detection

Testing for anabolic steroids was first introduced in the 1976 Montreal Olympic games, and eight athletes were banned, but given the widespread use by some types of athletes, there has been a surprisingly low number of cases detected. One of the problems that has occurred is that athletes use the drugs during training and come off them prior to the competition. By doing this they have been able to increase their training loads, then cease steroid use before competition, so that the drugs are out of their system when their urine is tested. After the cessation of anabolic steroid use, the effect on performance will still be present for some time. The exact duration of this enhancement has not been quantified, but it is thought to be in the vicinity of several months, depending on the drug used. The time taken from cessation of a drug until it can no longer be detected (clearance time) also varies according to the drug and is shortening considerably as detection procedures improve.

Di Pasquale (1987) reported that with improvements in drug detection, the popular oil-based injectable steroids, known as Deca-Durabolin and Durabolin (nandrolone esters), can be detected for more than a year after the cessation of the drugs. However, he further reported that other drugs, such as the popular oral compound Anavar, could only be detected for 3 weeks after cessation of use, while aqueous testosterone suspension could be used up to 2 weeks prior to a competition without detection. These general clearance times are subject to large individual variation. For example, Francis (1990) reported that in training for the Los Angeles Olympics the accepted clearance time for oral steroids was 21 days. However, one male thrower found he could pass a test 7 days after his last daily dose of 85 mg of oral Dianabol and an American woman discovered she could pass only 3 days after her last dose of Anavar. These clearance times are progressively being increased as research into drug detection continues.

Nevertheless, given this information it is obvious that *to begin to eliminate drug use in sport, year-round testing must be vigorously pursued by independent officials* and that simply testing on the competition day is not going to eliminate the use of these substances.

UNDETECTABLE ANABOLIC STEROIDS

Perhaps the most disturbing aspect of the use of anabolic steroids by athletes is the existence of drugs which cannot be currently detected. Di Pasquale (1987) suggested that the structure of a normal anabolic steroid can be slightly modified so that it retains its anabolic properties but cannot be identified as a banned substance by mass spectrometry, as the modified compounds are not currently on the banned list. He reported that such modifications to steroids could result in thousands of effective, but currently undetectable, anabolic steroids and claimed that some athletes were already using such compounds. Francis (1990) reported that many of his sprinters, including Ben Johnson and Angella Issajenko, had been using the steroid furazabol, which was a slightly modified and undetectable version of the popular steroid stanozolol. Francis stated that: 'For the past three years, some of my sprinters had been using an injectable form of steroid furazabol, which we referred to as Estragol. I knew that it could not be detected, since the IOC's lab equipment hadn't been programmed to identify furazabol's metabolites'. Francis further claimed that the drug had been used on many occasions by his athletes without detection; however, somehow Ben Johnson was taking stanozolol, a detectable steroid, prior to the Seoul Olympics, as opposed to furazabol, and paid the ultimate price in forfeiting his gold medal.

Conclusion

The debate over the use of anabolic steroids in sport either in relation to their health effects, detection or their ability to enhance performance will continue for some time. However, there is no debate about the fact that all sporting bodies throughout the world see the use of such aids as *cheating* and against the very essence of fair play and under *no circumstances* will condone their use. They will therefore continue to pursue a policy of detection, in an effort to see that all athletes compete with one another on equal terms. Such a policy will require that year-round unannounced testing be carried out by independent officials. However, further improvements in drug detection are also required to eliminate the use of presently undetectable steroids. Kammerer (1993) sums up the problem in the following way: 'If athletes know that no one will escape detection for drug abuse and all competitors will face the same uniformly enforced sanctions for the use of drugs, most abuse would cease. Athletes are still afraid of being at a disadvantage by not using certain performance enhancing agents, because they believe that a majority of their competitors, in certain sports, do use performance enhancing agents'.

FACTORS AFFECTING THE DEVELOPMENT OF MUSCULAR FUNCTION

Age

Age has an important influence on the development of muscular function. Muscle mass tends to achieve a peak for males between the ages of 18 and 22. For females this tends to occur between the ages of 16 and 19. The amount of muscle mass will remain relatively stable from this age through to the ages of 30–40, provided activity levels are not reduced. After this period muscle mass tends to decline with further ageing, even if activity levels are maintained. In the loss of muscle mass with ageing, generally the musculature of the lower limbs is lost at a faster rate than that of the upper limbs.

The decrease in muscular function is similar to the changes in muscle mass. Peak strength is usually achieved by the age of 20 for females and between 20 and 30 for males. Strength remains relatively stable until the ages of 35–40 and then gradually decreases with further ageing. For example, Clarke *et al.* (1992) reported the changes in muscular function of differing age groups of subjects who were currently performing weight training and those who were inactive. Between the ages of 20 and 35 the maximum strength of the subjects was similar. However, the strength difference between the trained and inactive subjects was approximately 13%. By age 50 both the inactive and active subjects had greatly decreased lean body mass and muscular function. These researchers concluded that subjects engaged in strength training maintained higher levels of muscular strength and endurance than those who were inactive, but that both functions deteriorate by 50 years of age.

Even though muscular function tends to deteriorate with age, this can be minimized with resistance training. In fact many studies have demonstrated that previously inactive individuals can greatly increase muscular function with training, even into old age. For example, Roman *et al.* (1993) reported that 12 weeks of high intensity weight training resulted in significant increases in muscle size, strength and endurance of subjects with a mean age of 68±2 years. The strength potential at various ages can be seen in the current world power-lifting records for the juniors, open and masters divisions, outlined in Table 9.9. As can be seen, the over-40 world records are very similar to those achieved in the under-23 category. In fact there is only a mean 10% difference between the open and over-40 world records. However, the over-50 world records are, on average, some 27% lower than the open records.

RESISTANCE TRAINING FOR THE OLDER ATHLETE

Similar resistance training routines can be used for older athletes as those adopted by their younger counterparts. However, one must be aware that at the commencement of the training the individual may be at a relatively low level of strength and thus correspondingly low training intensities and workloads need to be used. When commencing a training programme for the older athlete, that is, any individual over 35 years, a thorough medical

Table 9.9 Current men's world power-lifting records for differing weight and age categories (kg)

Body mass (kg)	Under-23	Open	Over-40	Over-50
52	552.5*	587.5	587.5	417.5
56	595	625	595	527.5
60	625	707.5	602	527.5
67.5	685	762.5	727.5	602.5
75	742.5	850	730	685
82.5	875	952.5	830	745
90	872.5	937.5	865	722.5
100	862.5	1032.5	920	752.5
110	880	1000	925	857.5
125	912.5	1005	980	835
>125	937.5	1100	910	875

* Total weight lifted. This total represents a combination of the 1 RM squat, bench press and deadlift exercises performed in a power-lifting competition.

examination should be performed to identify potential hazards. This is particularly important for individuals with relatively high blood pressure or with conditions that can be adversely effected by short-term elevation in blood pressure. It is important to realize that some resistance training exercises, for example, maximal squats, deadlifts and leg presses result in extremely high blood pressure values being achieved during their performance. Similarly, isometric exercises can also result in large blood pressure increases during the performance of an exercise and as a result they should be avoided if subjects have a medical history of high blood pressure or a susceptibility to high blood pressure related illnesses.

Once medical clearance has been received the older athlete can be trained in a similar manner to the younger athlete, with the exception that the recovery periods from the training sessions may need to be slightly longer. Typically 2–3 days of recovery are required between resistance training exercise sessions of the same muscle group and this may need to be increased to 3–4 days for the older athlete to allow for adequate recovery. The adaptations induced by training will be similar to those achieved by the younger athletes; however, the extent of the adaptations will be reduced. Nevertheless there are a number of studies that have demonstrated quite substantial strength increases

from previously inactive elderly subjects who have commenced resistance training.

THE YOUNGER ATHLETE

The intensely competitive nature of many sports has resulted in many child athletes requiring high levels of strength, power and endurance at relatively young ages. Consequently, many coaches want to know whether young children should be exposed to high level resistance training and what potential hazards this may cause.

When a male reaches puberty there is an increase of approximately 20-fold in the production of testosterone and this rapidly accelerates the development of lean body mass. In essence, the individual is on natural steroids and if properly prepared can achieve the best gains of his life in muscular function. Ideally competitors should have been exposed to weight training methods prior to reaching puberty so that they are accustomed to resistance training and the exercise techniques are well mastered. This can generally be achieved with 6–12 months of *low intensity training*.

TRAINING ROUTINES FOR THE YOUNGER ATHLETE

Prior to the advent of puberty, weight training can be employed by children; however, the performance benefits will be somewhat limited, due to the low level of circulating androgens, and the training routine should involve relatively light weights for high numbers of repetitions. For example, sets of 15–20 repetitions are probably best, and the emphasis should be on learning the correct technique. Once the athlete has reached puberty, the loads should be increased to the 8–12 RM range and an effort must be made to increase the intensity of the training so that the full benefit of the increased testosterone production can be realized. However, maximal lifts should be avoided, particularly for exercises that involve the lower back, such as squats, deadlifts and power cleans.

During adolescence the skeleton will be growing rapidly and its resistance to compression and tension forces may be diminished. Large forces exerted upon these bones can result in closure of the epiphysis, which prematurely stops the growth of the long bones. Further, the bones will be less resistant to extreme forces and can easily be damaged. Therefore *maximal lifts, particularly when involving the lower back, should be avoided at all times during and prior to puberty.*

For females, puberty results in an increase in the production of oestrogen, which promotes the deposit of body fat. Consequently, unlike their male counterparts, large increases in muscular function are not observed during puberty. Muscle tissue is still developed by females during this time; however, without the production of large quantities of testosterone the rate of development and overall total potential muscle mass is limited. The difference in the effect of puberty on males and females can be readily seen in many sports. For example, most high level male gymnasts are generally in their twenties and past puberty. The increased testosterone production at puberty has assisted them to achieve the level of muscular function that is associated with the sport at this level. Elite female gymnasts tend to be in their early teens and have not reached puberty. Upon reaching puberty the increase in oestrogen will result in an increase in body fat that adversely effects their power to weight ratio. Consequently many of the manoeuvres become increasingly

difficult to perform and most will retire by the end of puberty.

Gender

Males and females differ in many physiological variables. By the time full maturity is attained the average female is approximately 13 cm shorter, 15 kg lighter in total body mass and 20 kg lighter in lean body mass with considerably more adipose tissue than the average male. The large difference in lean body mass is seen to be predominantly due to a much higher production of the hormone testosterone in males, which is approximately 10 times higher in the blood of normal men than in normal women. The larger amount of lean body mass in males results in large sex differences in muscular function.

The difference in strength between the sexes varies depending on the muscle group tested. For example in the upper body (arms, shoulders and chest), men are considerably stronger than women but the differences are less marked in the lower body. Wilmore (1974) reported that females have approximately 40% of the strength of males in the upper body and approximately 70% in the lower body. However, when the strength differences were expressed per unit of lean body mass, females have approximately 55% of the strength of males in the upper body and are equal to males in the lower body. The latter point highlights a very important fact with respect to the differences in muscular function between the sexes. In essence, *male and female muscle is very similar, with the main difference being that males simply have more of it.*

SEX DIFFERENCES IN RESISTANCE TRAINING

Many studies have shown that although females are generally weaker than males, their ability to respond to resistance training is similar and in some cases superior. Generally these studies have been performed for a limited duration (6–10 weeks) and have involved untrained subjects. In such instances large performance gains are achieved mainly because of neural adaptations (see section on Neural Adaptations to Resistance Training). In the longer term the gains in strength are mostly sustained through muscle hypertrophy and because of the limited production of testosterone, females can increase muscle size and function with training, but not to the same extent as their male counterparts. Consequently *women will not develop massive, bulging muscles through resistance training nor will they develop the same level of strength as men.* The few women who develop relatively large muscles through resistance training tend to have particularly high testosterone levels in comparison to the normal female. The difference in training potential for strength between elite male and female strength athletes can be readily seen by comparing the men's and women's world power-lifting records (Tables 9.9, 9.10). In the seven weight divisions that are common to both the men's and women's competition, the total weight lifted by the women is, on average, only 66.4% of that achieved by the men.

Table 9.10 Current women's world power-lifting records

Body mass (kg)	Total lifted (kg)*
44	325.2
48	390
52	427.5
56	485
60	502.5
67.5	565
75	602.5
82.5	600
90	622.5
>90	622.5

* Total weight lifted. This total represents a combination of the 1 RM squat, bench press and deadlift exercises performed in a power-lifting competition.

THE MENSTRUAL CYCLE

One area of interest to the female athlete and coach is the effect of the phases in the menstrual cycle on performance. Most of the research in this area has tended to indicate that performance is either not affected by the variations in the menstrual cycle or that performance tends to be worse during the actual menstrual phase. However, Davies *et al.* (1991) reported that grip strength was greatest during the menstrual phase. Further, several world records are reported to have been set during the menstrual phase. At present then, no clear general trend in performance exists at various phases in the menstrual cycle. It would appear that the effects are subject to large individual differences and female athletes should determine which phase(s) are best suited for competition. If poor performance phases are identified, the menstrual cycle can be altered to prevent the occurrence of them on competition days, by the use of oral contraception. For example, menstruation can be delayed until after a competition by continuation of the medication's active hormone tablets. Conversely a menstrual cycle can be prematurely initiated by ceasing the medication early.

Disabilities

Over the past decade there has been a large increase in the participation of disabled individuals in sport. Indeed the disabled Olympics is becoming a major sporting event throughout the world. With the great increase in the number and the competitive standard of disabled athletes, many are performing resistance training to enhance their performance. The training principles are the same for all individuals and to a large extent, the resistance training programmes adopted by disabled athletes are similar to other athletes. Slight differences will emerge depending upon the specific disability. For example, wheelchair athletes are not able to stabilize their lower body when performing exercises and therefore upper body exercises such as the bench press are difficult as the fixator and stabilizer muscles are not operative and balance problems tend to occur. Thus it is essential that the athletes are securely stabilized by straps or similar devices when performing these exercises. Alternatively specialized equipment can be used to enhance the stability and safety of the exercises, as depicted in Fig. 9.37.

The modifications to training required by disabled athletes will be dependent upon the disability, and thus programmes should be de-

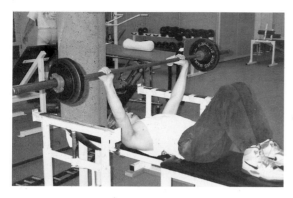

Fig. 9.37 A bench press exercise performed by a disabled athlete. Note the wide design of the bench and the use of safety bars.

signed in collaboration with movement science professionals. Nevertheless several general recommendations can be made:

- Generally it is more convenient and safer for disabled athletes to use exercise machines, as opposed to free weights. This reduces the need to maintain balance, decreases the likelihood of injury and allows for more effort to be directed into the actual lift
- For the many disabled athletes who compete in their wheelchairs, it is generally best to perform resistance training from within their chairs to enhance the specificity of the training, thereby maximizing the transfer of training gains to the competitive performance. This may require some modification to existing resistance training devices so that force can be effectively developed in the competitive action
- Disabled athletes can generally use standard gymnasia for their resistance training, provided that there is sufficient access to the equipment

Aerobic Training

Several researchers have reported that the performance of aerobic training inhibits the development of strength and power. Hickson (1980) compared the changes in strength and aerobic endurance from 10 consecutive weeks of strength training, aerobic endurance training and combined strength/aerobic endurance training. The strength training group increased maximum strength by 44% over the 10 week period, while the combined group only increased strength by 25%. In a similar study Dudley and Djamil (1985) also reported that the combination of endurance training with strength training reduced the gains achieved from strength training by itself. In both of these studies, the combined training group experienced reduced strength gains but endurance was not affected. In fact Hickson *et al.* (1988) demonstrated that heavy resistance training, when combined with aerobic endurance training, can enhance endurance in elite athletes.

Aerobic endurance training has also been reported to adversely affect muscular power. In a recent review paper on this topic, Chromiak and Mulvaney (1990) reported a number of studies which demonstrated that aerobic training in the form of long distance running reduced vertical jump height. Further, after a period of de-training, vertical jump height returned to pre-training values.

INHIBITION MECHANISMS

The reason for the inhibition of strength and power development when aerobic training is performed is not completely understood. One possible cause is that the differing forms of training involve different motor unit recruitment patterns. The endurance training involves the recruitment of the ST fibres, while the heavy resistance training involves FT motor units to a far greater extent. The performance of both strength and endurance training may hinder the organization of efficient motor unit recruitment patterns, such as motor unit synchronization (see section on Neural Adaptations to Strength Training), inhibiting the development of strength and power. Alternatively, the differing forms of training may alter the concentration of hormones such as testosterone. Research has shown that male distance runners have a lower testosterone concentration compared to the average untrained male. A decreased concentration of testosterone would serve to reduce the development of strength and power.

TRAINING RECOMMENDATIONS

Since the performance of aerobic endurance training tends to inhibit the development of strength and power, in sports where these are important factors such training should be kept to a minimum. Often coaches believe that it is important to build up a substantial aerobic base prior to the performance of strength training; however, if the competitive event does not require endurance (e.g. field events) aerobic exercise should be minimized. Even in events such as American football, where powerful bursts of activity are followed by relatively long rest periods, the endurance training performed should not become too intensive or it may compromise the strength and power development of the athletes. If athletes are lacking in strength and power, it may be necessary to reduce the aerobic workload so that they can develop these functions.

Genetic Factors

Strength and power are considered by many to be two of the most trainable physical capacities in sport. For example, it is not unusual for maximal strength to be doubled in response to strength training. A similar increase in movement speed is, however, relatively rare. Nevertheless there are limits to the development of muscular function because of genetic traits which greatly affect the development of these physical capacities. These genetic limitations are outlined below:

- *Fibre type* — as discussed in the section on Muscle Fibre Types, the relative proportion of FT and ST fibres is a very important determinant of the functional capacity of muscle, which is genetically determined. Further, as the hypertrophy resulting from resistance training mostly enhances the size of the FT muscle fibres, a larger proportion of FT fibres may also be important in the development of muscle mass

- *Tendon insertion* — as outlined in the section on Muscle Mechanics the distance between the insertion of the tendon in the bone and the joint greatly affects muscle function. All other factors being equal, the greater this distance, the greater the strength of the individual. Without surgical intervention the location of these insertion points is genetically determined. One of the strongest men in the world, Bill Kazmair, severely damaged his triceps brachii muscle so that it had to be re-inserted into the ulna. The surgeon re-inserted the tendon further away from the elbow joint than its original location and Kazmair reported that this significantly enhanced the strength of the muscle (W. Kazmair, pers. comm. 1990)

- *Body type* — an individual's body type will also have an influence on the development of the physical capacities of strength, power and strength endurance. Individuals with a high degree of mesomorphy will be capable of greater development of muscular size and strength. Hart *et al.* (1991) examined the relationship between body type and bench press performance of 54 subjects following 12 weeks of strength training. After a standardized training period those subjects with a higher degree of mesomorphy were able to lift a greater load than those with a high degree of ectomorphy

- *Lever length* — the length of the bones also represents a genetically imposed limitation in the expression of strength. For example, all other factors being equal, an athlete with relatively long arms will find it more difficult to perform exercises such as the bench press, as the weight must be lifted further, in comparison to an individual with relatively short arms. In recording the anthropometric characteristics associated with the performance of the bench press lift, Hart *et al.* (1991) reported that 'individuals with shorter, more muscular arms at any given body mass performed better in the bench press lift'. Similarly, an athlete with a relatively long femur will find it more difficult to perform a squat lift than an athlete with a shorter femur. These performance limitations of maximal strength need to be recognized by athletes and coaches. However, often such limitations to the performance of strength training exercises may represent advantages in the competitive sport. For example, a rower with relatively long arms may be limited in the weight lifted during the bench press exercise, but this limitation may represent an advantage in rowing, as the increased lever length will enhance the stroke length thus improving rowing performance

Psychological Factors

To recruit all the available motor units and fire them at their maximal rate in a relatively short period of time requires considerable mental effort, determination and often aggression. The nervous system may need to be substantially aroused to produce maximal levels of strength and power. Ikai and Steinhaus (1961) have demonstrated that strength can be increased by actions such as the firing of a gun or aggressive shouting. The use of shouting and other aggressive behaviour is quite common in power-lifting and the throwing events, where each competitor is attempting to maximize muscular performance. The use of such psychological techniques is seen to increase the arousal level of the central nervous system, allowing for the recruitment of more motor units than are normally possible. These techniques enable individuals to come closer to the true strength capacity of their muscles, thus reducing the strength deficit.

Coaches and athletes are reminded that the optimal psychological level of arousal differs between individuals. Elko and Ostrow (1992) compared three mental preparation strategies on the effect of grip strength using novice subjects and reported that the use of imagery resulted in the greatest increase in strength, compared to the use of aggressive arousal techniques. Nevertheless, individual differences need to be considered and an effective individual mental strategy needs to be determined for each athlete. Thus while some athletes will find aggressive behaviour such as shouting to be effective in enhancing strength, others may perform better using visualization techniques.

TRAINING RECOMMENDATIONS

It is important to realize that *resistance training programmes are designed to train the neural system as much as the musculoskeletal structures*. This is particularly the case if athletes are attempting to increase their strength to weight ratio or muscular power. Often athletes undertake strength training exercises in the same way that endurance training is performed, by 'switching off and clocking up the mileage'. Young (1989) has described this phenomenon as the 'going through the motion syndrome' and suggested that to prevent it, athletes should train in competitive groups with coaches and/or training partners encouraging them to push themselves to the limit. Other methods of enhancing training performance include establishing readily definable training goals.

Some athletes whose sport is not purely strength dependent, such as middle distance runners or swimmers, are often resistant to performing strength exercises and lack motivation during their training. For these athletes it is important that the coach explains the benefits of such training, including the strong relationship between strength and endurance and the value of strength training in the prevention of injuries. Further, the resistance training routines adopted should be varied regularly so that athletes do not become bored with the same routine.

STRENGTH AND POWER ASSESSMENT

A variety of measurement strategies have been developed for the assessment of muscular strength and power. These have encompassed the isometric, isotonic and isokinetic modes of contraction with measurement apparatus ranging from the very simple, such as the use of a barbell to perform a 1 RM test, to the very expensive isokinetic dynamometers. In addition, a number of field tests have been used extensively to estimate power developed by the lower limbs.

The many strength and power assessment methodologies are reviewed in Section 3 with evidence provided to lend support to the adoption of selected protocols. Furthermore, Section 3 contains detailed instructions for the accurate collection of strength and power data using the isometric, isotonic and isokinetic modes.

RESISTANCE TRAINING GUIDELINES

Rest Periods

Between repeated sets and exercises during a resistance training routine an athlete will rest. During the rest period the energy stores of adenosine triphosphate (ATP) and creatine phosphate (CP) within the worked muscles will be partially replenished and any accumulated waste products, such as lactic acid, will partially dissipate. If the previous exercise was performed to exhaustion, it will take approximately 3–5 min for the energy stores within the muscle to be completely replenished. The removal of lactic acid is subject to widely varying clearance times, depending on factors such as the amount of lactic acid initially present and whether the rest period was active or inactive. Nevertheless the shorter the rest period the less accumulated lactic acid will be removed, and the greater the number of repetitions performed the higher the accumulation of lactic acid. For example, the use of 10 RM loads performed with a 1 min rest period produces greater levels of lactic acid, when compared to 5 RM loads performed with the same rest period.

STRENGTH AND POWER TRAINING

After the rest period, if the energy systems have not been fully replenished and/or the removal of accumulated waste products has not been completed, then the subsequent work bout will be negatively affected so that a lower level of intensity and volume will result. This occurs because a lack of energy supplies, and/or the presence of waste products, will inhibit the ability of some motor units to fire effectively, thereby reducing the intensity of the overall contraction. Since a high intensity of muscular tension is important for the development of strength and power, it is universally recommended that rest periods of at least 3 min are imposed between repeated maximal work bouts. Put simply, maximal strength or power development will not occur if the musculature is fatigued and thus inhibited in its recruitment of muscle fibres.

Often athletes are under time pressure to perform resistance training and consequently rush through workouts with insufficient rest intervals. It must be remembered that to develop muscular strength the most important factor is the intensity of the muscular contraction, not the total number of sets or repetitions performed. Insufficient rest will result in suboptimal strength gains. If time becomes a major problem, athletes would be much better served by reducing the number of sets or exercises and ensuring that the remainder are performed at maximal intensity. Alternatively, shorter rest intervals can be adopted providing the athlete performs alternating upper body/lower body exercises. For example, a set of bench presses can be carried out, followed by 60 s rest, then a set of calf raises, followed by 60 s rest and then the bench press can be performed again. This rotation is continued until the prescribed number of sets for each exercise is completed. Using this strategy the upper body musculature can recover whilst the lower body is exercising and vice versa. While it would be preferable for the athlete to simply make more time available and adopt a longer rest period, such an approach is sometimes not feasible and the use of the above strategy represents a reasonable compromise between the need for high intensity and short training time.

STRENGTH–ENDURANCE TRAINING

The rest periods adopted when performing strength–endurance training differ depending on the type of training used to develop this muscular function (see section on Strength Endurance Training Methods). If the high repetition training method is adopted, athletes are attempting to increase their tolerance to the accumulation of lactic acid and induce other local muscle adaptations. In this instance relatively short rest periods of 30–60 s are appropriate for they will result in the highest accumulation of lactic acid, facilitating the desired adaptations. Conversely, if the heavy weight or variable load training methods are adopted, one of the objectives of the training is the enhancement of muscular strength. Consequently the exercise must be performed in a fully recovered state so that relatively high training intensities can be realized and therefore relatively long rest periods of 3–5 min will be required.

The Training Year: General Periodization Strategies

The concept of periodization was introduced in the discussion of the training principle of variation and several periodization training strategies were presented. This section outlines how to periodize resistance training throughout a normal competitive year. The structure of the year will depend upon the dominant physical capacity that is to be maximized, that is, strength, power or strength–endurance. Additionally the organization of the year will be dependent upon the nature of the competitive season, that is, whether it involves several major meets spaced throughout a year, as in athletics or swimming, or whether the competitive season involves a prolonged period whereby games are played on a weekly basis, as with most team sports.

PERIODIZATION FOR MAJOR MEETS

Strength

If the sport involves several major competitions spaced throughout a year then a number of periodization strategies are used depending upon the dominant physical capacity involved in the sport. For those sports that predominantly require muscular strength, such as weight- or power-lifting, the athlete will perform a series of successive periodized strength programmes. For example, if an athlete has three major competitions with 12–15 weeks spaced between each, the first competition will be preceded by a 12 week training period where a periodized routine, such as a linear or undulating programme (see section on Periodization, Tables 9.1, 9.2, 9.3), will be adopted. The training cycle should be organized so that a 1–2 week tapering period is imposed prior to the competition. After the first competition, a 1 week rest period should be imposed and the programme will be started again, and this procedure will be repeated throughout the competitive season.

The athlete's goal, as the season progresses, is to use greater loads in each training cycle and competition.

Power

If the dominant physical capacity of the sport is muscular power, for example, with throwers, sprinters or jumpers, then the organization of the training year is somewhat different to the above. The muscular functions of strength and power are closely related and thus a high level of strength is a necessary prerequisite for powerful performance. Consequently the training year will commence with a 2–3 month period of strength training, similar to a strength athlete. As the competition approaches the resistance training programme is progressively modified so that there is an increased content of power and a corresponding reduction in pure strength work. High intensity strength training should be performed throughout the year, but the volume of this training is greatly reduced prior to the competition. For example, during the strength training period two heavy squat sessions may be performed each week. Several months prior to the competition one of the heavy squat workouts should be substituted for a maximal power session of squat jumps. One month prior to the competition, heavy squats should still be performed once per week, but the number of sets and repetitions is reduced and greater quantities of maximal power and plyometric training are performed. Strength work is performed up to 1–2 weeks prior to the competition to maintain strength levels and disinhibit the neural system.

After the competition the resistance training strategy adopted will depend upon the time period to the next major meet. If there is a relatively long period of 4–6 months the athlete may perform a cycle of pure strength work prior to more power-oriented training. If the period is only approximately 2 months, then a combined strength/power routine should be commenced with progressively greater power content and correspondingly lower strength content as the competition approaches.

Strength–endurance

Similar to power, strength–endurance has a close relationship to pure strength, so that a stronger muscle will tend to have greater endurance when compared to a weaker muscle. Therefore strength–endurance athletes, such as middle distance swimmers and runners, require high levels of strength and should perform a 2–3 month strength training cycle at the commencement of their training year. Several months prior to the competition the resistance training routine should be modified so that variable load training is adopted (see section on Strength–Endurance Training Methods). As the competition becomes progressively closer, variable load training should be modified so that a greater volume, at reduced loads, is performed. However, some high intensity work should still be maintained.

PERIODIZATION FOR TEAM SPORTS

Off-season

A typical season for a team sport, such as football or rugby, consists of a 2 month off-season period, a 4 month pre-season period and a 6 month competitive season. The off-season period is often used to rest injuries accumulated during the preceding year and involves athletes participating in 'active rest'. This is where they simply try to keep up a reasonable level of aerobic fitness without performing overly stressful exercise. During this period athletes with specific weak points, for example, muscular imbalances, can undergo remedial resistance training.

Pre-season

The pre-season period is used to enhance the physical capacities of the players so that by the time the competitive season commences they are in peak physical condition. Training performed during the pre-season for team sport athletes should be structured in much the same manner as that specified above for major athletic meets (see section on Periodization for Major Meets). Thus during the pre-season, a power athlete, such as an offensive running back in American football, would perform the same routine as a power athlete, such as a sprinter or jumper (see section on Periodization for Major Meets — Power). Similarly a strength–endurance athlete, for example, a ruck rover in Australian Rules football, would perform a similar pre-season resistance training routine to a middle distance runner (see section on Periodization for Major Meets — Strength–Endurance).

Competition

During the competitive season so much time is spent competing, recovering from the competition and performing specific skill work that there is little time available for resistance training. However, it is important that some resistance training is performed, so as to maintain the physical capacities developed during the pre-season. Generally one intense resistance training session per muscle group per week is required to maintain the developed muscular functions. The maintenance training routine used should be one which stresses the dominant physical capacity involved in the sport. Thus strength–endurance athletes would perform variable load training (see section on Strength–Endurance Training Methods), while power athletes would perform a combination of strength and power work, with progressively more power-oriented work as the season progressed.

Number of Training Sessions

The number of resistance training sessions performed in a week is generally determined by the available time and the relative importance of resistance training to the sport. For example, many elite swimmers will perform 10–12 swimming sessions per week, consequently the time available for resistance training is limited. For the majority of athletes two or three resistance training sessions per week are adequate. Each session should consist of exercises which train the relevant muscle groups involved in the sport, and will be spaced so that at least one day of rest is imposed between workouts.

For athletes involved in sports that are heavily dependent on the physical capacities of strength and power, for example, throwers, lifters and defensive linemen, more resistance training sessions are generally required. These athletes will perform split routines, in which only a portion of the body will be trained in any one session (see section on Split Routines). Generally four to six training sessions are used, with each muscle group trained two to three times per week. Again, at least 48 h recovery is required between exercise sessions of the same muscle group.

Some elite strength athletes, such as weightlifters, perform multiple daily resistance training sessions. By separating the workouts into smaller units, greater intensity can often be achieved. Further, research suggests that hormone levels are maximized during a resistance training session during the first hour of training. After this period hormone levels tend to decrease, even if training is continued. Thus if 2 h of resistance training are required on a given day, it is desirable to split the session into 1 h morning and afternoon sessions, so that the elevation in hormonal levels can be experienced throughout the entire training period. Rogozkin (1976) reported that the use of multiple daily training significantly increased the content and intensity of muscle synthesis compared to a single training session, despite both groups performing the same total amount of work.

Exercise Order

Little research has been performed to examine the effect of the order of exercises upon the training gains achieved. Nevertheless, based upon anecdotal reports and the need to maximize training intensity and hence minimize fatigue, the following training recommendations are suggested:

- Regardless of the training routine adopted, the musculature will tend to fatigue throughout the workout. Thus the exercises initially performed will tend to involve the greatest training intensities. Consequently *the most important exercises should be performed first.* For example, a shot putter should commence the strength training session with the inclined bench press or the squat exercise, rather

than chin-ups or biceps curls, as the former exercises are of more importance to the competitive activity. Alternatively, if an athlete has a specific weakness such as a muscle imbalance, then this muscle group should be exercised first as it represents the most important muscle group to develop. Frequently athletes will perform their favourite or best exercise first, such as the bench press, when often such exercises are not the most important for their competitive performance

- If attempting to develop strength or power, the exercises should be performed in an order that provides the maximum amount of rest between similar exercises. For example, a freestyle sprinter requires a high degree of power in the pectorals, deltoids, latissimus dorsi, quadriceps, triceps brachii and biceps brachii muscle groups. After performing pectoral exercises, the deltoid and triceps muscle groups are often fatigued and therefore exercises for these muscle groups should be spaced as far away as is practicable. Similarly, exercises for the latissimus dorsi and biceps brachii muscles should also be spaced as far apart as possible to minimize the residual fatigue. In Table 9.11 two exercise orders are outlined for a freestyle swimmer, one designed to minimize residual fatigue, while the other is structured to maximize fatigue. The exercise order on the left of Table 9.11 spaces exercises which use similar muscle groups as far away from each other as possible. This serves to reduce the fatigue associated with training similar muscle groups in the same session and allows the subsequent muscle groups to be exercised with greater intensity. The training order outlined on the right of Table 9.11 does not provide for any recovery time between the performance of similarly acting muscle groups and hence the subsequently exercised muscle groups will be fatigued and will experience a reduced training intensity

- If attempting to increase strength–endurance by improving the tolerance to the accumulation of lactic acid, then the exercises should be ordered to maximize the residual fatigue.

Thus exercises that act in similar ways should be performed straight after one another, as shown in the right hand column of Table 9.11

Table 9.11 Differing exercise orders which serve to minimize or maximize residual muscular fatigue

Minimize residual fatigue	Maximize residual fatigue
Latissimus dorsi	Latissimus dorsi
Deltoids	Biceps brachii
Quadriceps	Pectorals
Pectorals	Deltoids
Biceps brachii	Triceps brachii
Triceps brachii	Quadriceps

Warm-up

As with any other strenuous physical activity, it is important to warm the body prior to the performance of resistance training. The warm-up should consist of several minutes of light aerobic exercise, such as riding a stationary bicycle, and be followed by light exercises for the muscle groups to be trained, for example, light dumb-bell presses to warm up the pectoral muscle group. Finally, stretching exercises for the specific muscle groups to be trained should be done and, prior to the use of heavy loads, several light preparatory sets of the exercise should be performed. The warm-up serves to facilitate performance by preparing the neuromuscular system for maximal exertion and also reduces the risk of musculoskeletal injuries. It is important to realize that each new body part trained in a workout may need to be warmed up. For example, if training the chest and the legs, one should not assume the chest training will serve to warm up the legs. After the completion of the chest exercises the legs will need to be warmed prior to commencement of their resistance training.

RESISTANCE TRAINING EXERCISES

This section details 53 resistance training exercises which form a pool from which sport specific res-istance training programmes will be generated in the next section of this chapter.

Strength Training Exercises

Unless otherwise specified the strength training exercises should be executed so that the eccentric phase (generally the downward part) of the lift is performed under control, taking approximately 1.5–2 s to complete, while the concentric portion is executed as rapidly as possible. When using relatively heavy loads all exercises should be performed with at least one spotter standing by in case the lift cannot be completed.

No. 1 Abdominal rotations (Fig. 9.38)

- This exercise is performed using a specialized rotation machine
- The athlete sits within the machine and rotates the trunk to the left and then to the right
- This exercise strengthens the abdominals and is one of the few which involves the trunk

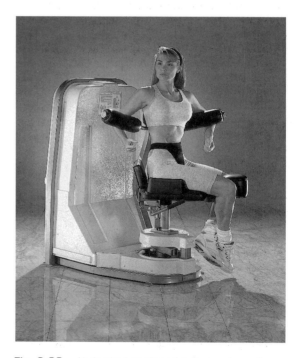

Fig. 9.38 Abdominal rotations (photo courtesy of Cybex).

rotators, that is, the external and internal obliques

No. 2 Ankle curls (Fig. 9.39)

- This exercise is performed using a pulley device which is attached to the foot by a strap
- The exercise involves dorsi-flexing the foot about the ankle
- The exercise commences with the foot plantar flexed so that the toes are pointed forward
- The foot is then curled up so that the toes approach the leg
- This exercise strengthens the tibialis anterior and other muscles of the pre-tibial group

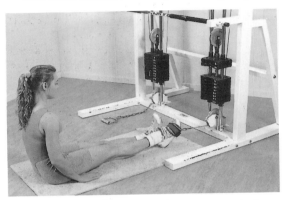

Fig. 9.39 Ankle curls.

No. 3 Trunk extensions (Fig. 9.40)

- This exercise is performed with the athlete lying face down on a trunk extension machine, secured by the ankles
- The exercise commences with the athlete bent over so that the head is almost in contact with the ground. The trunk is raised until it is parallel with the floor. A common mistake is to lift the body above the horizontal position and thus hyperextend the trunk which causes unnecessary stress on the lumbar spine and should be avoided
- The upward and downward movements should both be performed slowly and each take several seconds to complete
- This exercise strengthens the erector spinae muscles of the lower trunk and the gluteal and hamstring muscle groups

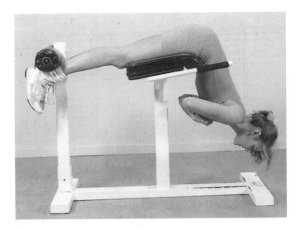

Fig. 9.40 Trunk extensions.

No. 4 Barbell curls (Fig. 9.11)

- This exercise is performed while standing upright with a barbell held in front of the body and the hands spaced about hip width apart
- The bar is gripped so that the palms are facing forwards
- The forearms are initially fully extended at the elbow joint and the bar is raised to shoulder height by flexing at this joint
- The arms should remain in a relatively stable position throughout the lift
- No swinging movements of the trunk should be performed to assist the lift, unless this is a technique adopted to perform heavy eccentric training
- This exercise strengthens the flexors of the forearm, notably biceps brachii, brachialis and brachioradialis

No. 5 Bench press (Fig. 9.41)

- This exercise is performed lying face up on a horizontal bench
- The bar is held at arm's length using a medium width grip, so that the hands are approximately 15 cm wider than the shoulders. The hands firmly grip the bar with the thumbs completely wrapped around it. Do not leave the thumbs underneath the bar, as this increases the likelihood that the bar may leave the hands during the lift, resulting in an accident

- The bar should gently touch the chest at approximately the level of the nipples. No attempt should be made to bounce the bar off the chest
- During the upward movement, the bar is not pushed directly vertical but follows a curved path directed towards the rack, so that at the completion of the lift the bar is positioned directly above the shoulders
- Throughout the lift the athlete's shoulders, head and buttocks should remain in contact with the bench and the feet should be firmly placed on the ground. If, however, the individual has a back condition, the feet should be placed on the bench so that the back is completely flattened
- This exercise strengthens the musculature of the pectorals, deltoids and triceps brachii

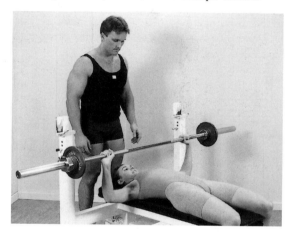

Fig. 9.41 Bench press.

No. 6 Bent-over rowing and bench pulls (Fig. 9.20)

- This exercise is performed standing over a barbell. The legs are slightly flexed about the knees and the trunk bent over so that the back is in a horizontal position
- The lower trunk should be slightly curved inwards with the shoulders pulled back and the buttocks pushed out
- The bar is gripped with both palms facing downwards and the hands approximately 15

cm further apart than shoulder width. The feet are shoulder width apart
- The bar is pulled from the floor to the lower portion of the chest
- The lift is performed while wearing a belt which serves to enhance the support given to the lower trunk and abdominal region. If performed incorrectly this exercise can cause an injury to the vertebral column, particularly when heavy loads are used. Common mistakes include jerking the weight, using a rapid extension of the trunk, and performing the activity with the back curved outwards as opposed to being curved inwards
- This exercise should be avoided if the athlete has a history of lower back injury
- This exercise strengthens the trunk extensor muscles, as the erector spinae group acts as stabilizers and the latissimus dorsi and forearm flexors as prime movers
- This exercise can be performed while lying on a bench (Fig. 9.21) to reduce the contribution of the erector spinae muscle group and enhance the explosiveness of the exercise by reducing the deceleration phase (see Explosive Weight Training). When performed on a bench this exercise is referred to as 'bench pulls'

No. 7 Close grip bench press (Fig. 9.42)

- This exercise is performed lying face up on a bench
- The bar is held at arm's length using a narrow grip, so that the hands are approximately 30 cm apart. The thumbs should be firmly wrapped around the bar
- The bar should gently touch the lower portion of the chest. No attempt should be made to bounce the bar off the chest
- Throughout the lift the athlete's shoulders, head and buttocks should remain in contact with the bench and the feet should be firmly placed upon the ground. If the athlete has an injured back the feet should be placed up on the bench so that the lumbar spine is flattened
- This exercise strengthens the musculature of the triceps brachii, pectorals and deltoids. When

compared to the bench press (No. 5), this exercise increases the contribution from the triceps brachii and reduces the contribution from the pectoral group

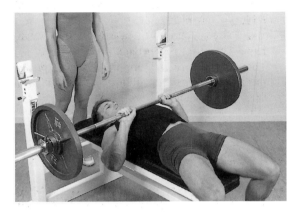

Fig. 9.42   Close grip bench press.

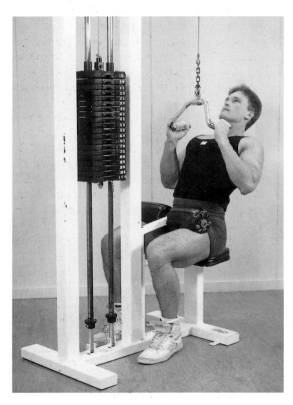

Fig. 9.43   Close grip pull-downs.

No. 8 Close grip pull-downs (Fig. 9.43)

- The exercise is performed seated upright on a lat pull-down machine using a close grip bar so that the hands are spaced approximately 15 cm apart
- The exercise commences with arms outstretched and finishes as the hands are brought down to the upper chest region
- This exercise strengthens the latissimus dorsi and forearm flexor musculature

No. 9 Deadlifts (Fig. 9.44)

- The lift commences with the athlete crouched over the bar, with the feet spaced slightly closer than shoulder width and the bar positioned very close to the individual. The bar is gripped with one palm facing downwards and the other facing upwards and the hands spaced approximately shoulder width apart. This type of grip greatly increases the load that can be held
- It is important that prior to the commencement of the lift, the athlete is predominantly flexed about the knee and that the trunk is slightly flexed forward, but relatively straight. In fact the lower trunk should be slightly curved inwards so that the shoulders are pulled back, the head looking up and the buttocks pushed out
- The bar is lifted explosively to waist height in one coordinated movement of the legs, thighs and trunk. The arms should be straight throughout the lift and not contribute to the upward movement of the bar. The arm musculature is simply too weak to lift the loads encountered during deadlifts and their attempted contribution can result in tears to the biceps brachii and brachialis muscles
- Throughout the lift the bar should be kept close to the body. In fact the bar should be in contact with the lower limbs throughout the entire movement and should be lifted upwards and backwards as the athlete leans back at the completion of the lift. Baby powder can be applied to the athlete's legs in order to reduce the friction of the bar

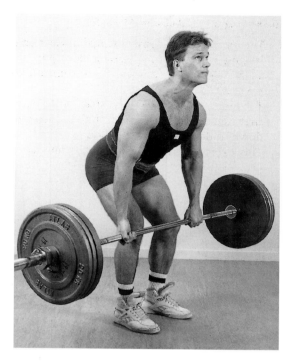

Fig. 9.44 Deadlifts.

- Heavy deadlifts are a test of grip strength as much as thigh and trunk strength and in order to enhance the effectiveness of the grip it is often necessary for the athlete to apply chalk rosin (magnesium carbonate) to the hands
- The bar should be lowered to the floor in a reasonably controlled manner. Again during the eccentric phase the movement occurs mainly due to the flexion of the legs and thighs. The trunk will be slightly flexed at the hips but must remain straight
- The lift is performed with a belt, which serves to increase the support given to the lower trunk and abdominal region. The use of a belt can reduce the shearing force on the vertebral column by increasing the intra-abdominal pressure. If it is performed incorrectly, this exercise can cause major injury to the vertebral column, particularly when heavy loads are used. Common mistakes include insufficient use of the legs and consequently, excessive flexion of the trunk. Thus the movement

almost becomes a stiff-legged deadlift (No. 32). Further, athletes sometimes lift the bar with the shoulders in a forward position and the head down, which results in a humped appearance in the upper back, increasing the likelihood of injury in this region
- This exercise should be avoided if the athlete has a history of lower back problems
- This exercise strengthens the erector spinae, quadriceps, hamstring, gluteal, upper trunk and forearm musculature

No. 10 Dips (Fig. 9.45)

- This exercise is performed using a parallel dip bar
- The movement is commenced at arm's length with the hands spaced slightly wider than shoulder width. A narrower grip will increase the contribution from the triceps brachii muscle, while a wider grip will increase the contribution from the pectoral group
- The body should be lowered in a vertical plane and reach the bottom position when the hands are at approximately the same level as the chest. A lower position is desirable if the athlete has sufficient flexibility
- The bottom position should be maintained for 1 s to dissipate some of the stored elastic energy and hence increase the contribution of the pectoral muscles to the initial portion of the movement
- Additional weights can be applied by use of a strap device, which allows loads to be placed between the legs
- This exercise strengthens the pectoral, triceps brachii and deltoid musculature

No. 11 External rotator raises (Fig. 9.35)

- This exercise is performed using a specialized strength training machine
- The forearms are rotated about the elbow until they reach a vertical position. They are then lowered to the start position
- This exercise strengthens the external rotators of the arm

179

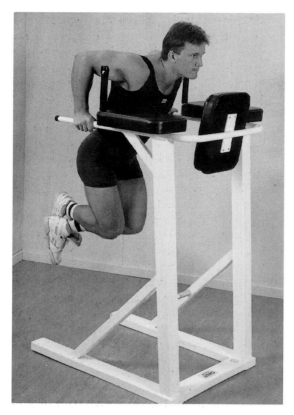

Fig. 9.45 Dips.

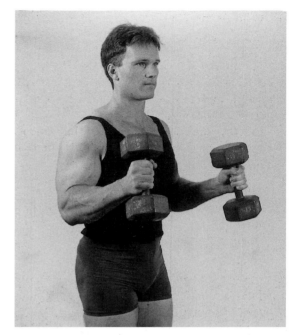

Fig. 9.46 Hammer curls.

No. 12 Front pull-downs (one-and two-handed; Fig. 9.15)

- The athlete stands in front of a lat pull-down machine. The bar is gripped palms down with a grip width of approximately 20 cm
- The forearms are slightly flexed and the elbows point out to the side throughout the movement. A common mistake is to increase the flexion of the forearm as the movement progresses and consequently involve the triceps brachii muscles in the activity
- The movement commences from above the athlete's head and ends as the bar comes into contact with the hips. The forearms should remain slightly flexed throughout
- This exercise can also be performed in an alternate, unilateral manner if two independent pulley systems can be used. Such an exercise is more specific to sports that involve unilateral, alternate arm actions such as kayaking and front crawl swimming. Further, this exercise can be performed in essentially the same manner, with the exception that the athlete faces away from the machine and the bar is brought from head height to the buttocks in an arm action similar to swimming backstroke
- Muscles which are strengthened in this exercise are the latissimus dorsi and teres major

No. 13 Hammer curls (Fig. 9.46)

- This exercise is performed in the same position as barbell curls (No. 4), except that it uses dumb-bells which are held so that the palms of the hands face each other throughout the lift
- The muscle groups which are strengthened are the forearm flexors as prime movers and forearm extensors as stabilizers

No. 14 Head curls (Fig. 9.47)

- This exercise is performed using a specialized weight training machine
- The exercise commences with the head in a flexed position with the chin close to the chest. The head is then moved backwards into an extended position
- Both the concentric and eccentric movements are performed slowly under control with each phase requiring approximately 2–3 s
- Care should be taken to ensure that the head is not hyperextended
- The musculature about the neck is strengthened in this exercise, particularly the trapezius muscle

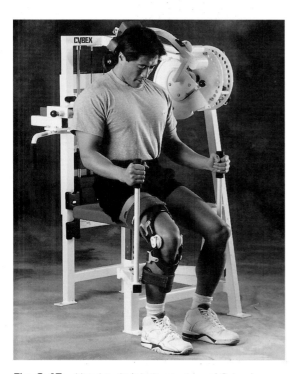

Fig. 9.47 Head curls (photo courtesy of Cybex).

No. 15 High pulls (Fig. 9.48)

- This exercise is a version of the popular power clean movement, modified to make its execution technically easier to perform. The lift commences with the athlete crouched over the bar, with the feet spaced slightly closer than shoulder width and the bar positioned very close to the athlete. The bar is gripped by the athlete with the palms facing downward and the hands spaced approximately shoulder width apart
- It is important that at the commencement of the lift, the athlete primarily flexes the legs and that the trunk is slightly flexed forward, but relatively straight. In fact the lower trunk should be slightly curved inwards so that the shoulders are pulled back, the head looking up and the buttocks pushed out
- The bar is explosively lifted to shoulder height in one coordinated movement of the legs, thighs, arms and trunk. The contribution of the arms to the lift should be relatively small, with the thigh and trunk musculature providing the necessary momentum to carry the bar to shoulder height
- Throughout the lift the bar should be kept close to the body with a slight tendency to move towards the athlete's body as the lift progresses
- If the lift is performed over a weightlifting platform then the bar can simply be dropped if the load is heavy. If not then the bar should be lowered to the floor in a reasonably controlled manner
- The exercise is very popular as it is performed in a dynamic fashion, whereby the dominant portions of the movement (i.e. leg and thigh extension) are not limited by the existence of a deceleration phase
- The lift is performed with a belt which serves to increase the support given to the lower trunk and abdominal regions. If performed incorrectly, this exercise can cause major injury to the vertebral column, therefore particular care needs to be taken during its execution. Further, it should be avoided by individuals with a history of lower back problems
- This exercise strengthens the erector spinae, quadriceps, hamstrings, gluteal, upper and lower trunk musculature

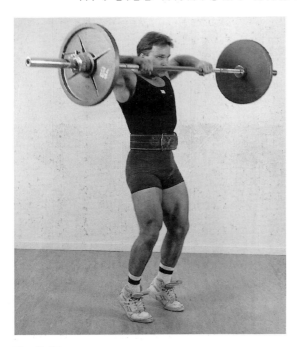

Fig. 9.48 High pulls.

No. 16 Inclined bench press (Fig. 9.49)

- This exercise is performed lying face up on a bench inclined at an angle of approximately 45°
- The bar is held at arm's length using a medium width grip, so that the hands are approximately 10 cm wider than shoulder width
- The bar should gently touch the upper chest between the level of the nipples and the clavicle. No attempt should be made to bounce the bar off the chest
- This exercise strengthens the pectoral, deltoid and triceps brachii musculature. In comparison to the bench press (No. 5), the inclined nature of the exercise increases the contribution of the deltoids and upper pectoralis major muscle fibres and decreases the contribution of the lower pectoralis muscle fibres

No. 17 Inclined sit-ups (Fig. 9.50)

- This exercise is performed on an inclined sit-up board and commences with the athlete lying face up on the board, with the feet strapped in at the top and hands held behind the neck

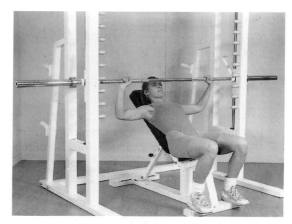

Fig. 9.49 Inclined bench press.

- The legs and thighs are flexed throughout the movement
- The athlete raises the body until the elbow touches the knee. Towards the top of the movement the body should be rotated, so that the right elbow touches the left knee or the left elbow touches the right knee
- The body is then slowly lowered until the head touches the board
- This exercise strengthens the abdominal and thigh flexor muscle groups

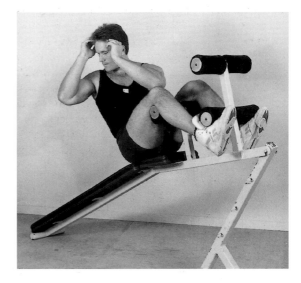

Fig. 9.50 Inclined sit-ups.

No. 18 Leg curls (Fig. 9.16)

- This exercise is performed lying face down on a leg curl machine. Where possible, leg curls should be performed on an inclined leg curl machine, as opposed to a flat bench machine because the inclined bench raises the height of the buttocks and stretches the hamstrings, placing them in a more mechanically advantageous position to produce force. Further, these benches reduce the tendency to accentuate the lumbar spine when performing the exercise, thereby reducing the stress on the lower trunk

- The exercise commences with the legs extended and ends with the legs flexed, so that the heels touch the buttocks

- This is an isolated single joint exercise that strengthens the flexors of the leg about the knee joint, that is, the hamstring group and gastrocnemius. Such exercises may lack relevance to multi-joint sports actions, however they provide the opportunity to build up a specific muscle group. This is of particular benefit when a weak muscle or muscle group needs to be preferentially trained, or during rehabilitation of injured or atrophied muscles

No. 19 Leg press (Fig. 9.51)

- This exercise is performed using a leg press machine and such machines vary considerably in the angle of inclination of the lower limbs

- Similar to the squat exercise (No. 29), the leg press mainly involves the musculature which extends the thigh and leg. However, this exercise involves a smaller contribution of the lower trunk musculature, is technically easier to perform and does not require the load to be stabilized on the upper trunk. For these reasons the leg press is a popular exercise used by athletes in lower body dominated sports

- The concentric phase of the exercise commences with the legs flexed, at approximately 120° and is completed as the legs achieve full extension

- Throughout the movement the hands should firmly grasp the machine to improve the stability of the body

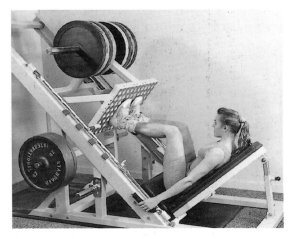

Fig. 9.51 Leg press.

No. 20 Lying leg raises (Fig. 9.52)

- This exercise is performed on a horizontal leg curl/extension machine. The athlete lies on the machine face upwards with the body extended and the feet placed under the top lever of the machine

- The activity commences with the legs extended and ends as the knees are raised to the level of the waist

- The concentric and eccentric phases of the lift should be performed under control

- Throughout the activity the hands must firmly secure the body to the bench

- Some athletes may find this exercise stressful on the lower back and may require a towel or other bracing device to be placed under the back to improve its support

- This exercise strengthens the abdominal and thigh flexor musculature

No. 21 Lying triceps extensions (Fig. 9.53)

- This exercise is performed lying face upwards on a horizontal bench

- The bar is held at arm's length with the hands approximately 30 cm apart. This exercise is often performed with an easy curl bar to reduce the stress placed upon the wrist joints

- The bar is lowered slowly to touch the forehead (forearm flexion) and then returned to

183

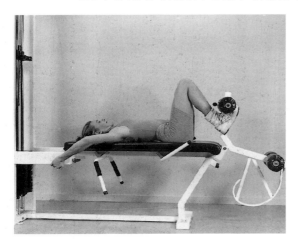

Fig. 9.52 Lying leg raises.

arm's length (forearm extension) as explosively as possible
- Throughout the exercise the arm should not move and the elbows should remain pointing upwards
- This exercise can be stressful on the elbow joints and if it becomes painful, the triceps kickback exercise (No. 38) should be performed instead
- The main muscle group involved in this exercise is the triceps brachii

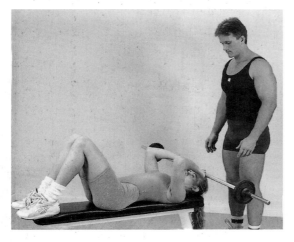

Fig. 9.53 Lying triceps extensions.

No. 22 Pull-overs (Fig. 9.54)
- This exercise is performed on an upright pull-over machine
- It commences with the athlete seated upright in the machine with both arms flexed in a position overhead
- The arms are extended so that they move in front of the body to the level of the waist
- The main musculature involved in this exercise includes pectoralis major, latissimus dorsi and teres major

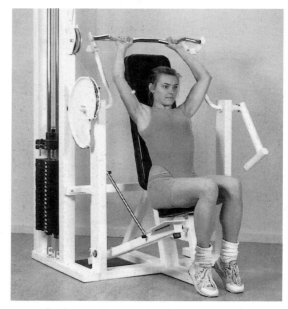

Fig. 9.54 Pull-overs.

No. 23 Reverse curls (Fig. 9.55)
- This exercise is essentially the same as the barbell curl (No. 4) with the exception that the bar is gripped with the palms facing downwards
- This exercise strengthens mainly the brachialis muscle rather than the biceps brachii. The forearm musculature acts in a stabilizing role

No. 24 Reverse pec dec (Fig. 9.56)
- This exercise is performed using a specialized strength training machine

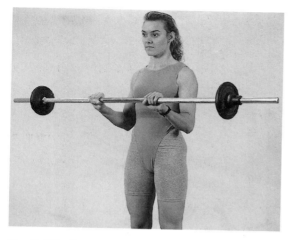

Fig. 9.55 Reverse curls.

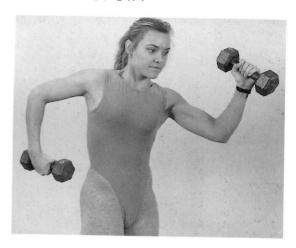

Fig. 9.57 Running dumb-bells.

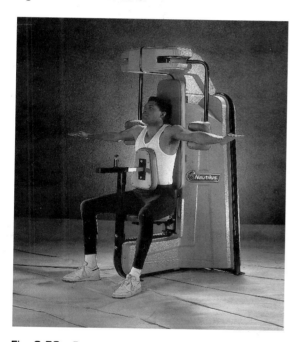

Fig. 9.56 Reverse pec dec.

- The exercise commences with the arms extended forward at shoulder width against the pads of the machine. They are then pushed backwards, moving through a range of 90°
- This is a highly specialized exercise which strengthens the latissimus dorsi and the teres major muscles

No. 25 Running dumb-bells (Fig. 9.57)

- This exercise is performed using dumb-bells with the athlete standing upright
- The forearms are flexed at about 90° at the elbows and the arms move backwards and forwards so that they simulate the arm action as used in running

No. 26 Seated rowing (Fig. 9.58)

- This exercise is performed using a seated rowing machine with the hands positioned approximately 15 cm apart on the bar
- The exercise commences with the hands at the level of the feet. The bar is then moved, predominantly by flexion of the forearms and, to a lesser extent, by extension of the trunk, until the hands reach the lower chest region
- During the exercise the lower limbs should be extended with a small degree of leg flexion. The trunk, though initially flexed, should be straight. In fact the lower trunk should be slightly curved inwards
- A belt should be worn during this exercise to support the lower trunk and abdominal regions
- This exercise strengthens the rhomboids, trapezius and erector spinae muscles of the trunk as well as the extensors of the arm (latissimus dorsi and teres major), and forearm flexors (biceps brachii, brachialis and brachioradialis)

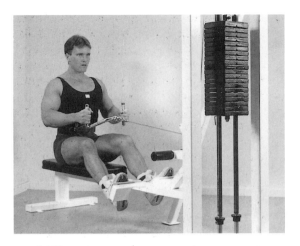

Fig. 9.58 Seated rowing.

No. 27 Shrugs (Fig. 9.59)

- This exercise is performed standing upright with dumb-bells placed in each hand
- The exercise involves elevating the shoulders mainly by contracting the trapezius muscles
- The forearms should be extended throughout the exercise and not contribute to the lift

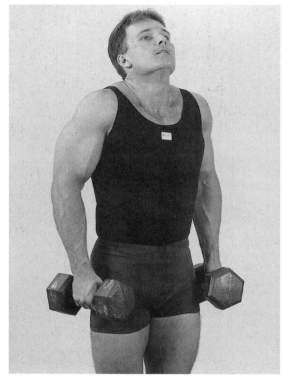

Fig. 9.59 Shrugs.

No. 28 Side bends (Fig. 9.60)

- This exercise is performed while standing erect with a dumb-bell in one hand
- The exercise involves lateral flexion of the trunk so that the athlete bends to the side on which the dumb-bell is located and returns to the upright position. At the maximum position of lateral flexion the dumb-bell should be located approximately at the level of the knee
- When the exercise has been completed on one side, the dumb-bell is switched to the other hand and the activity repeated
- Both the eccentric and concentric phases of this activity should be performed slowly, requiring approximately 3 s to complete each phase
- This exercise strengthens the external and internal obliques, quadratus lumborum and the erector spinae muscles

No. 29 Squats (Fig. 9.61)

- This exercise is performed while standing erect with a bar placed on the upper trunk. The bar should be located on the trapezius muscle and not on the cervical spine. If the athlete feels that the location of the bar is uncomfortable, a rubber mat or a towel should be placed between the bar and the trunk. The bar should be held against the body firmly by the hands. For safety reasons the squat exercise should be performed in a power rack which has bottom safety stops, so that the bar can be rested upon these stops if the lift cannot be completed
- The feet should be positioned slightly further apart than shoulder width, with the toes facing forward
- The movement commences from an upright posture and the athlete lowers the body, mainly by flexing the thighs and, to a lesser extent the legs, until a knee angle of approximately 120°

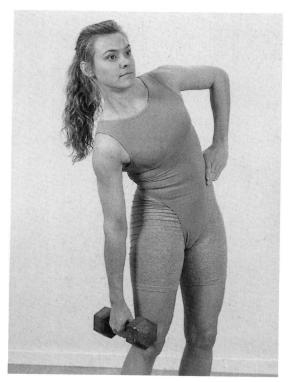

Fig. 9.60 Side bends.

is achieved. At this point the bar is raised by extending the thighs to achieve an upright posture

- Throughout the lift the shoulders are pulled back, the elbows rotated to a forward position, the head held up and the trunk, though angled slightly forward, should be relatively straight. In fact the lower trunk should be curved slightly inwards
- Squats are very popular among athletes; however, they are often performed incorrectly. The most common problem involves leaning too far forward during the exercise, which greatly increases the stress placed on the lower back. Athletes must keep the trunk very rigid and basically upright throughout the lift. It is vitally important that the upper back remain rigid and athletes should be encouraged to look upwards, keep the shoulders back and rotate the elbows into a forward position

- The technique in the squat can be readily assessed by watching the individual from the side. The weight should be located almost directly above the hips and ankles throughout the lift. If athletes have a tendency to fall forward during the lift then the exercise should be performed on a Smith machine (Fig. 9.27) so that the bar motion remains in a vertical plane
- Squats can sometimes be difficult for many athletes in lower-body dominated sports, as their lower bodies are developed more than their upper bodies, and thus the limitation to performance is generally the ability of the upper body to stabilize the load on the back. This problem can be reduced by the use of a Smith machine (Fig. 9.27) or by performing the leg press exercise (No. 19) instead
- The squat exercise strengthens the quadriceps, hamstrings and gluteal muscle groups as well as the erector spinae muscles

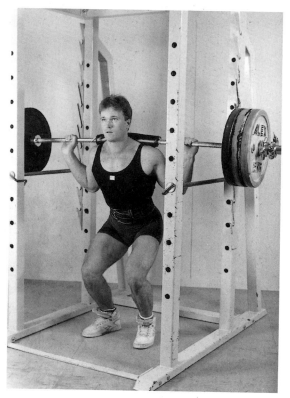

Fig. 9.61 Squat exercise performed in a power rack.

No. 30 Standing calf raises (Fig. 9.62)

- This exercise is performed in an upright position using a standing calf raise machine. The balls of the feet are placed on the bottom of the machine and the exercise is achieved by alternately plantar- and dorsi-flexing the feet about the ankle joint

- The exercise commences with the feet plantar-flexed so that the heels are slightly above the ground. The athlete then raises the body by contracting the calf musculature until a maximal height is achieved

- The lower limbs should be kept straight throughout the exercise

- It is not uncommon for this exercise to be performed with a great deal of weight, even by athletes who have not previously performed weight training. The calf musculature receives a large quantity of work during the many sporting activities that involve running and similar skills and are generally quite strong prior to the commencement of resistance training. Consequently, relatively heavy loads are required to further enhance the strength of this muscle group

- This exercise strengthens the gastrocnemius and soleus muscles

No. 31 Standing push press (back and front; Fig. 9.63)

- This exercise is usually performed standing erect with the bar held in front of the athlete at the level of the neck. However, more recently the exercise is being performed from a position with the bar located on the top of the athlete's back, behind the head. The latter position is considered safer, as it prevents the bar contacting the athlete's chin on its upward movement. Further, it reduces the curvature in the spine when the bar is lifted overhead, as compared to the 'in front of the neck' technique. The 'behind the head' push press should be performed in front of a mirror so that the location of the bar can be accurately monitored

- If the 'behind the neck' position is used, the feet should be placed slightly closer than shoulder width apart. If the 'in front of the neck' position is used, the same feet position should be adopted, with the exception that one foot

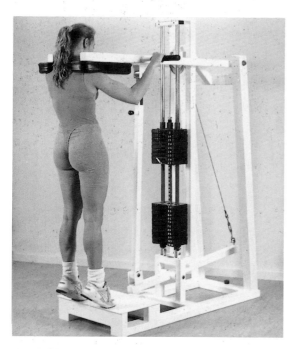

Fig. 9.62 Standing calf raises.

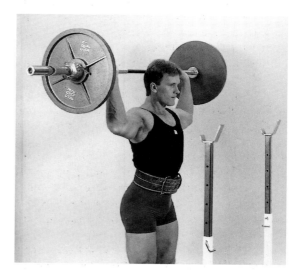

Fig. 9.63 Standing push press.

should be placed about 20 cm in front of the other. This will serve to limit the stress exerted on the lower trunk during the lift

- The movement commences with a dynamic short range flexion and extension of the thighs and legs. This is rapidly followed by a powerful contraction of the upper body musculature which serves to rapidly push the bar to an overhead position in which the arms are completely extended

- A belt should be worn throughout this movement to support the lumbar and abdominal regions

- This exercise strengthens the deltoid, triceps brachii and trapezius musculature as well as the quadriceps group

No. 32 Stiff-legged deadlifts (Fig. 9.64)

- This exercise is performed with a barbell held while standing erect on a bench or box. The box is required to allow the athlete to achieve a full stretch position, with the bar touching the feet, without the weights touching the ground

- The bar is gripped with the palms down. However, for heavy lifts an alternate grip, as used in deadlifts (No. 9), may be necessary

- The exercise is commenced from an upright position with the barbell lowered, mainly by flexion of the trunk about the hip, until the bar touches the athlete's feet. The bar is then raised until the upright starting position is achieved

- Throughout the movement the knees should be slightly flexed to remove the pressure on the knee joint and the back should be kept straight at all times

- Both the eccentric and concentric phases of the lift should be performed under control. This exercise, if performed in an explosive or jerky manner, could result in an injury to the lower trunk, so great care should be taken while executing it

- The lift should be performed with a belt to enhance the support of the lumbar and abdominal regions; however, if the athlete has a

history of lower back problems this exercise should be avoided

- The main muscle groups strengthened by this exercise are the extensor muscles of the thigh (hamstring and gluteal groups) and trunk (erector spinae group)

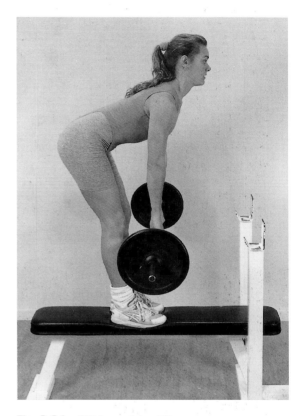

Fig. 9.64 Stiff-legged deadlifts.

No. 33 Swim bench pulls (Fig. 9.65)

- This exercise is performed on a swim bench machine which allows for the simulation of the upper body arm actions used in swimming against various levels of resistance

- The arm action used by the swimmer in simulating front crawl, butterfly or breast-stroke actions, should be similar in cadence and technique to that used by the swimmer in competition

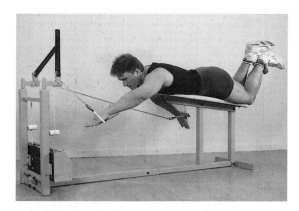

Fig. 9.65   Swim bench pulls.

No. 34 Thigh abduction (Fig. 9.66)

- This exercise is performed in a thigh abduction machine. Commencing with the limbs together, the thighs are then abducted to achieve a position as wide as possible without experiencing discomfort
- As the name suggests, this exercise strengthens the abductors of the thigh, that is, the gluteus medius and minimus muscles

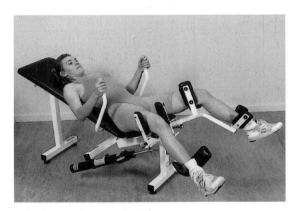

Fig. 9.66   Thigh abduction.

No. 35 Thigh adduction (Fig. 9.67)

- This exercise is performed in a thigh adduction machine. The movement commences with the limbs spread as wide apart as possible without incurring discomfort. The thighs are then adducted, that is, brought together

- Both the eccentric and concentric portions of the movement should be performed slowly and under control
- As the name suggests, this exercise strengthens the thigh adductor group, that is, the pectineus, the gracilis and the adductors magnus, longus and brevis

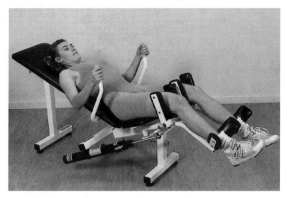

Fig. 9.67   Thigh adduction.

No. 36 Thigh extensions (Fig. 9.17)

- This exercise is performed in an upright position one limb at a time, using a total hip machine. The movement commences with the thigh flexed in a horizontal position
- The thigh is then pulled down until it is directly beneath the body and the movement is subsequently repeated
- This exercise attempts to simulate the leg recovery action in sprinting, when the leg is brought downwards just prior to heel strike
- This exercise strengthens the extensors of the thigh about the hip joint, the hamstring group, the adductor magnus and gluteus maximus

No. 37 Thigh flexions (Fig. 9.68)

- This exercise is performed in an upright position one limb at a time, using a total hip machine
- Basically the exercise attempts to simulate the initial recovery of the leg during sprinting. The thigh is rapidly flexed until it reaches the horizontal position

- This exercise strengthens the thigh flexor musculature including the iliopsoas group and the rectus femoris muscle

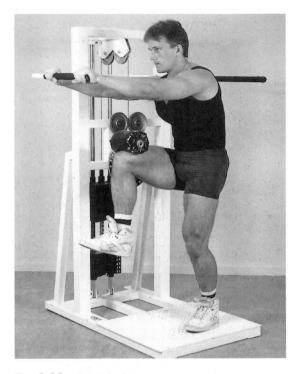

Fig. 9.68   Thigh flexions.

No. 38 Triceps kickbacks (Fig. 9.69)

- This exercise is performed using a cable weight system which has two independent loads
- The athlete is positioned facing the machine in a bent over posture. The exercise commences with the hands close to the shoulders and involves extension of the forearm
- The exercise attempts to simulate the final portion of the arm action of a front crawl or butterfly swimmer. Front crawl swimmers should perform the exercise in an alternate fashion, while butterfly swimmers should perform the arm action simultaneously
- The arms should be held close to the body throughout the exercise
- The exercise mainly strengthens the triceps brachii muscle

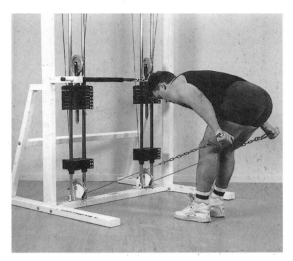

Fig. 9.69   Triceps kickbacks.

No. 39 Upright rows (Fig. 9.70)

- This exercise is performed while standing erect with a barbell held at arm's length, at the level of the hips
- The hands grip the bar palms down and are positioned approximately 10 cm apart
- The bar is raised upwards until it reaches the level of the neck
- The elbows are kept high throughout the movement and the bar follows a path very close to the body
- The exercise strengthens the deltoid and trapezius muscles

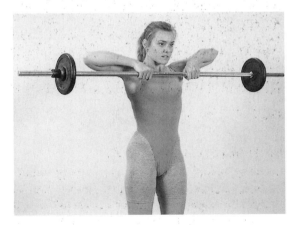

Fig. 9.70   Upright rows.

No. 40 Wide grip chins (Fig. 9.71)

- This exercise is performed using a chin-up bar. The bar is gripped palm down with the hands spaced approximately 15 cm further apart than shoulder width
- The movement commences with the arms fully extended and ends with the chin raised to bar height. The exercise can be performed either with the body raised so that the bar is in front, or behind the head
- The upward movement should not involve much body sway
- The dominant muscle groups involved in this exercise are the latissimus dorsi, the teres major and the forearm flexors (biceps brachii, brachialis and brachioradialis)

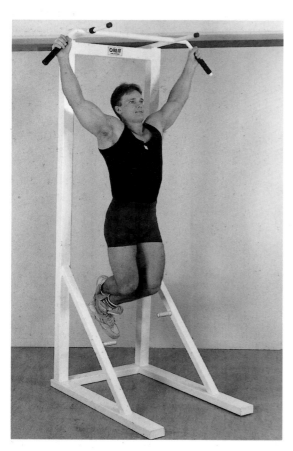

Fig. 9.71 Wide grip chins.

No. 41 Wrist curls (Fig. 9.72)

- This exercise can be performed with a barbell or a dumb-bell. The athlete sits on the end of a bench with the hands positioned palm up and overhanging the knees
- The load is held within the hands and rotated upwards and downwards by flexion and extension movements of the hand about the wrist joint. Upon rotation the load should move to the fingers during the descent and back to the palms during the upward movement
- This exercise mainly strengthens the hand and finger flexor muscles located in the forearm

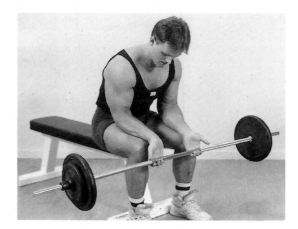

Fig. 9.72 Wrist curls.

Power Training Exercises

MAXIMAL POWER EXERCISES

Unless otherwise specified these exercises should be performed on the Plyometric Power System (PPS) using a load that maximizes the power output of the exercise. This is determined by modifying the load used on several trials and recording the power output on the computer system. The load that maximizes power output should be used in training. If the impact force is high when performing the maximal power exercises then the brake device of the PPS should be engaged to reduce the peak force. The athlete should be given auditory feedback by the computer system when performing the exercises through the use of the threshold function of the computer. When performing maximal power exercises the bottom safety stops of the PPS should be set so that if the bar is incorrectly caught, or if an incorrect landing is performed, the bar will contact the safety stops prior to striking the athlete's body. *All maximal power and plyometric exercises should be performed as explosively as possible, with minimum contact time.*

If the athlete does not have access to a PPS, a low friction Smith machine may be used. However, several spotters must be employed to support the bar in case it is incorrectly caught by the lifter, as this type of machine does not have bottom stops to act as safety catches. Further, a Smith machine will not provide feedback, knowledge of optimal load, nor will it involve a braking device. The performance of maximal power exercises on a Smith machine is not as effective nor is it as safe as using a PPS, nevertheless it is currently the next best option.

No. 42 Plyometric bench press (PPS; Fig. 9.73)

- This exercise is essentially the same as the bench press described earlier in the chapter (No. 5), with the exception that the bar is thrown at the completion of the lift. The bar is subsequently caught and rapidly rethrown. This has the effect of making the exercise mainly power oriented, as opposed to purely a strength exercise

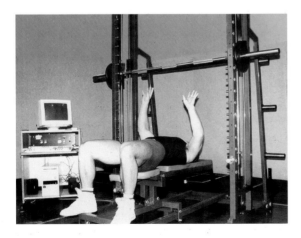

Fig. 9.73 Plyometric bench press.

No. 43 Plyometric inclined bench press (PPS; Fig. 9.32)

- The exercise is essentially the same as the inclined bench press (No. 16), with the exception that the bar is thrown at the completion of the lift. The bar is subsequently caught and rapidly rethrown. As with the plyometric bench press, this makes the exercise mainly power oriented
- The exercise can be performed with one or two hands. For one-handed sports or events, such as the shot put, one-handed training would be most appropriate. When using one hand it should be placed approximately at the centre of the bar

No. 44 Plyometric leg extensions (Fig. 9.74)

- This exercise is performed on a well-padded leg extension machine and involves leg extension and flexion while seated. The lever of the machine is kicked off the feet at the completion of the extension phase and then recaught by the feet and rapidly kicked off again
- The movement range is between the knee angles of 120° and full extension
- The impact force associated with catching the lever is reduced if the athlete gradually slows the lever over the eccentric portion of the exercise. Well-padded footwear should be worn to reduce the effect of the impact upon the feet
- Throughout the exercise athletes should firmly brace themselves by holding on to the handles of the machine
- Unlike the other maximal power exercises this movement is not performed on the PPS and consequently no feedback, knowledge of optimal load, nor use of a braking device is available. Nevertheless it is a dynamic exercise that simulates a kicking action and is useful for many sports

No. 45 Plyometric lying triceps extensions (PPS; Fig. 9.75)

- The exercise is essentially the same as the lying triceps extension (No. 21), with the exception that the bar is thrown at the completion of the lift. The bar is subsequently caught and rapidly rethrown

- A further difference between this exercise and its strength training equivalent is that the bar should be lowered to a position behind the head, as opposed to the forehead. Due to the dynamic nature of the exercise it is simply too dangerous to rapidly lower the weight to the forehead

- The body should be positioned so that the bar passes overhead and contacts the bench if not caught by the athlete

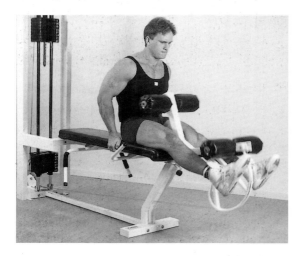

Fig. 9.74 Plyometric leg extensions.

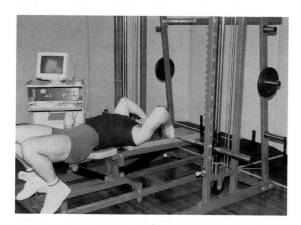

Fig. 9.75 Plyometric lying triceps extensions.

No. 46 Plyometric split squats (PPS; Fig. 9.76)

- The athlete commences in an upright position with the bar strapped to the upper back using a harness. The movement is initiated in the same manner as plyometric squats (No. 47); however, the athlete lands with the legs in a split position with one foot landing approximately 1 m in front of the other. The position of the feet on landing alternates on each jump

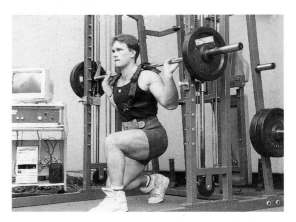

Fig. 9.76 Plyometric split squats.

No. 47 Plyometric squats (PPS; Fig. 9.29)

- The athlete commences in an upright position with the bar strapped to the upper trunk using a harness
- The exercise is essentially the same as the squat (No. 29), with the exception that the athlete jumps at the completion of the lift. The athlete subsequently lands and rapidly takes off, which has the effect of making the exercise more power-oriented
- To limit contact time the minimum knee angle attained should be approximately 140°
- If the athlete has sufficient strength the exercise may be performed alternately, one leg at a time. Such a unilateral action is in most cases more specific to competitive sports

No. 48 Plyometric standing push press (PPS; Fig. 9.77)

- The exercise is essentially the same as the 'in front of the neck' standing push press (No. 31),

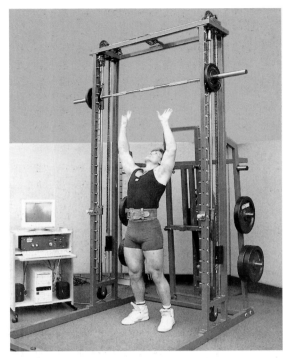

Fig. 9.77 Plyometric standing push press.

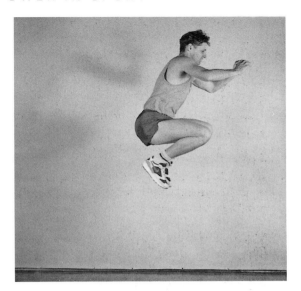

Fig. 9.78 Bounding.

with the exception that the bar is thrown at the completion of the lift. The bar is subsequently caught and rapidly rethrown

PLYOMETRIC EXERCISES

No. 49 Bounding (Fig. 9.78)

- This exercise should be performed on a flat compliant surface, such as an athletic running track or grass. The athlete performs a series of repeated forward jumps, landing and taking off from two legs, attempting to maximize jump height and horizontal distance simultaneously
- The exercise should be executed explosively with minimum contact time. The athlete should imagine landing on a hot surface and attempting to leave the ground as quickly as possible
- A knee angle of approximately 140–150° should be achieved at the bottom position of the bound

No. 50 Chest throws (Fig. 9.79)

- This exercise is performed in pairs with a medicine ball. One athlete lies down with arms outstretched while the other stands directly above and simply drops the medicine ball
- The medicine ball is caught above the level of the chest and rethrown at maximal speed and the activity repeated. The exercise should be performed explosively with contact time kept to a minimum
- Additional overload can be achieved by dropping heavier balls or the same ball from greater heights

No. 51 Depth jumps (Fig. 9.28)

- This exercise is performed by stepping off a box, landing on the ground and rapidly jumping vertically for maximum height
- The box should be at the height that results in maximum rebound jump height. This will vary between individuals, but should be between 30 and 70 cm
- The exercise must be executed explosively with minimum contact time. The athletes should imagine they are landing on a hot surface and attempt to leave the ground as quickly as possible

- The athlete should land on a compliant surface, such as a padded gymnasium floor, athletic track or grass. Additionally, impact-absorbing shoes should be worn
- A knee angle of approximately 140–150° should be achieved at the bottom position of the landing
- Additional loads can be used in this exercise and should be applied in the form of a weight vest. If the additional load is added by using a barbell, a harness device should be worn to firmly secure the load to the trunk. Without the use of a harness the load may leave the trunk during the jump resulting in a potentially injurious collision when it contacts the upper trunk upon landing
- The athlete should receive feedback as to the height of the jump. Performance feedback can be achieved in many forms, for example, the athlete can jump for a target such as a basketball hoop

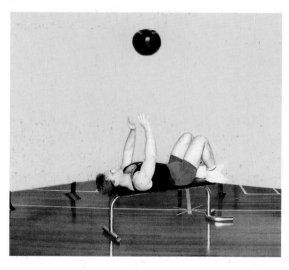

Fig. 9.79 Chest throws.

No. 52 Overhead throws (Fig. 9.80)

- This exercise is performed in pairs (with one person acting as a catcher) with a medicine ball in an identical manner to the chest throw exercise, described previously (No. 50), except that the athlete lies on the end of a bench and the ball is dropped to a level just above the head
- As the ball is caught the forearms are flexed about the elbow (eccentric contraction of triceps brachii), the ball brought below the level of the head and rapidly thrown with a powerful contraction of the triceps brachii (concentric contraction)
- Additional overload can be achieved by dropping heavier balls or the same ball from a greater height

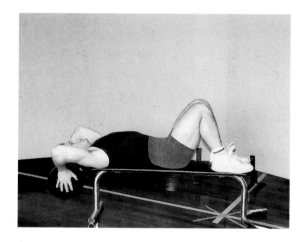

Fig. 9.80 Overhead throws.

No. 53 Plyometric push-ups (Fig. 9.81)

- This exercise is performed in a push-up position with the hands shoulder width apart and the feet resting on a box so that they are just above the height of the shoulder
- The athlete performs a push-up, throwing the body in the air as high as possible. Upon landing the push-up action is rapidly repeated
- The push-up action should be dynamically performed so that the time in contact with the ground is minimized
- The movement should be performed so that the bottom position occurs with an elbow angle of approximately 90°

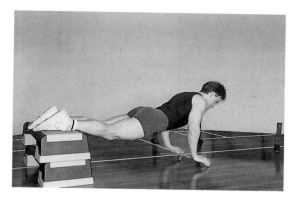

Fig. 9.81 Plyometric push-ups.

RESISTANCE TRAINING PROGRAMMES FOR SPECIFIC SPORTS

This chapter is essentially designed to enable the reader to develop sport-specific resistance training programmes. These programmes need to take into account the training principles of overload, specificity, variation and recovery, as well as the specific requirements of the sport, the individual characteristics of the athlete and the time of the competitive year. Consequently *there is no magical routine that can be used by all athletes at all times.* However, there are exercises that are more suited to some sports than others and this section is designed to identify them. Sport-specific exercises are suggested and model resistance training routines are outlined. *It must be emphasized, however, that these routines are not going to be optimal for all individuals at all times and the information should be used only as a starting point for the coach or athlete, who can then modify it depending on the specific requirements of he sport, phase of the year and individual characteristics of the athlete.* It is assumed that prior to the commencement of the specific exercises outlined in this section, athletes will have experienced at least 6 months of general strength training. An example of such a basic introductory strength training routine is outlined in Table 9.12.

Racquet Sports (Tennis, Badminton, Squash, Racquetball)

Racquet sports are ballistic in nature, requiring powerful and dynamic upper and lower body movements. The resistance training exercises most suited to these sports include: plyometric squats (exercise no. 47); plyometric split squats (46); plyometric lying triceps extensions (45); plyometric bench press (42); overhead throws (52); wrist curls (41); hammer curls (13); external rotator raises (11); high pulls (15); trunk extensions (3); abdominal rotations (1); thigh adduction (35); thigh abduction (34); leg curls (18); thigh extensions (36); standing calf raises (30); upright rows (39); pull-overs (22); and ankle curls (2). Furthermore, specific arm actions can be simulated by using a cable pulley system (Fig. 9.82). An example of a pre-season resistance training routine for racquet sports is outlined in Table 9.13. Due to the unilateral nature of racquet sports it is advisable that where possible resistance training should be performed independently on both sides (i.e. using dumb-bells), to eliminate muscular imbalances.

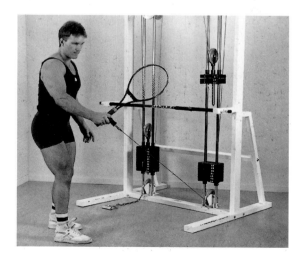

Fig. 9.82 The use of pulley weights to simulate the arm action in racquet sports.

Table 9.12 General introductory strength training routine

Monday	Wednesday	Friday
Bench press	High pulls	Deadlifts
Standing push press	Inclined bench press	Leg curls
Lying triceps extensions	Close grip bench press	Standing calf raises
Squats	Upright rows	Inclined sit-ups
Bent-over rowing	Trunk extensions	Bench press
Inclined sit-ups	Hammer curls	Standing push press
Barbell curls	Abdominal rotations	Lying triceps extensions
Leg curls	Leg press	Wide grip chins
Standing calf raises	Stiff-legged deadlifts	Barbell curls

After a 1 month gradual introductory phase, 3 or 4 sets of 8–12 repetitions should be performed for each exercise.

Aquatic Sports

All the aquatic sports are dominated by the need for high levels of power and strength–endurance. The relative importance of these functions is dependent upon the specific duration of the event.

SWIMMING

Exercises most suited to swimming include: swim bench pulls (exercise no. 33); front or back pulldowns (12); triceps kickbacks (38); close grip pulldowns (7); pull-overs (22); reverse pec dec (backstrokers only; 24); plyometric leg extensions (44); leg press (19); plyometric squats (47); wide grip chin-ups (40); plyometric inclined bench press (43); plyometric bench press (42); bench press (5); bench pulls (6); depth jumps (51); lying leg raises (20); dips (10); trunk extensions (3); external rotator raises (11); wrist curls (41); and thigh extensions (36). An example of a pre-season training routine for a front crawl or butterfly swimmer is outlined in Table 9.14.

WATERPOLO

The sport of waterpolo requires a high level of swimming performance, thus the exercises required for this sport are essentially similar to those outlined for swimming. In addition, waterpolo players require exercises that enhance the overhead throwing action, such as plyometric lying triceps extensions (exercise no. 45) and overhead throws (52), and lower body exercises that enhance the ability of the players to rise out of the water, such as plyometric split squats (46), thigh adduction (35) and thigh abduction (34).

Table 9.13 A pre-season resistance training routine for racquet sport athletes

Monday	Wednesday	Friday
Plyometric squats	Forehand stroke	Plyometric squats
Plyometric lying triceps extensions	Plyometric bench press	Backhand stroke
	Plyometric split squats	Plyometric lying triceps extensions
High pulls	Overhead throws	
Thigh adduction	Thigh abduction	High pulls
Thigh extensions	Pull-overs	Thigh adduction
Standing calf raises	Inclined sit-ups	Thigh extensions
Abdominal rotations	Trunk extensions	Abdominal rotations
External rotator raises	Hammer curls	Standing calf raises
Wrist curls		Ankle curls
Stiff-legged deadlifts		Upright rows

Table 9.14 Pre-season resistance training routine for a front crawl swimmer

Monday	Wednesday	Friday
Swim bench (slow speed)	Swim bench (moderate	Swim bench (fast speed)
Plyometric leg extensions	speed)	Plyometric leg extensions
Plyometric inclined bench	Depth jumps	Plyometric bench press
press	Close grip pull-downs	Front pulls
Plyometric squats	Leg press	Lying leg raises
Front pull-downs	Bench press	Triceps kickbacks
Lying leg raises	Bench pulls	Bench pulls
Triceps kickbacks	Pull-overs	External rotator raises
Chins	Wrist curls	Trunk extensions
Thigh extensions		

ROWING

The resistance training exercises most suited to rowing include: seated rows (exercise no. 26); high pulls (15); plyometric squats (concentric movement only; 47); deadlifts (9); barbell curls (4); wrist curls (41); hammer curls (13); stiff-legged deadlifts (32); leg press (19); and upright rows (39). Rowers should also perform bench press (5), leg curls (18) and inclined sit-ups (17) to help balance the development of their musculature.

CANOEING

Canoeing and particularly kayaking require similar muscular actions to rowing with the exception that the lower body actions are different and the upper body action is unilateral. Consequently, exercises such as leg press (exercise no. 19), leg curls (18) and plyometric squats (47) are of lesser importance, and additional exercises such as abdominal rotations (1), bench pulls (6) and inclined bench press (16) should be performed instead. Furthermore, the arm action of a kayaker can be simulated by the performance of a front pull-down exercise (12) with a pulley system that allows each arm to be exercised alternately.

Gymnastic and Power Sports

GYMNASTICS

Gymnastics is a sport that demands a high degree of muscular power and strength throughout the entire body. Due to the wide variety of move-ments performed in the gymnastic events, the majority of the strength and power exercises described in this chapter are suitable for these athletes. Those which are most suited include: plyometric squats (exercise no. 47); plyometric split squats (46); plyometric bench press (42); plyometric standing push press (48); plyometric push-ups (53); depth jumps (51); bounding (49); high pulls (15); wrist curls (41); hammer curls (13); reverse curls (23); barbell curls (4); dips (10); thigh extensions (36); thigh abduction (34); thigh adduction (35); abdominal rotations (1); lying leg raises (20); wide grip chins (40); deadlifts (9); inclined bench press (16); ankle curls (2); and standing calf raises (30). In fact the importance of strength and power to gymnastics requires that an upper body/lower body split routine be adopted whereby four resistance training sessions are performed per week during the pre-season. An example of a pre-season resistance training routine for gymnastics is outlined in Table 9.15.

DIVING

The sport of diving requires explosive power in the lower limbs to achieve vertical height. The higher the vertical jump, the longer the time in the air, and the greater the number of manoeuvres which can be performed. Consequently, exercises such as plyometric squats (one and two leg take-offs; exercise no. 47), plyometric split squats (46), depth jumps (51) and squats (29) are recommended. Divers also require forearm strength so that the hands can maintain a firm

Table 9.15 Pre-season resistance training routine for a gymnast

Monday	Tuesday	Thursday	Saturday
Plyometric bench press	Plyometric squats	Plyometric standing push press	Plyometric split squats
Plyometric standing push press	Bounding	Plyometric bench press	Depth jumps
Dips	High pulls	Inclined bench press	Deadlifts
Wide grip chins	Thigh extensions	Dips	Wide grip chins
Plyometric push-ups	Thigh abduction	Barbell curls	Thigh adduction
Barbell curls	Ankle curls	Hammer curls	Thigh extensions
Hammer curls	Calf raises	Wrist curls	Calf raises
Wrist curls	Abdominal rotations	Lying leg raises	Abdominal rotations

position on entry to the water. Exercises such as wrist curls (41), reverse curls (23) and hammer curls (13) are therefore important. Additionally, platform divers should perform standing push press (31), stiff-legged deadlifts (32) and lying leg raises (20) so that inverted positions can be easily achieved and maintained on the platform.

WEIGHTLIFTING

The sport of weightlifting has an obvious requirement for strength and power. Exercises that are used include the actual competitive lifts, that is, the snatch and clean and jerk, and smaller components of these lifts including high pulls (exercise no. 15), standing push press (31) and squats (29). To be more specific to the competitive lifts, the squat exercise is often performed with the bar held upon the shoulders in front of the neck (i.e. front squats), and through a greater depth than normal squats. Additional exercises that will assist the weightlifter include: plyometric squats (47); plyometric standing push press (48); deadlifts (9); trunk extensions (3); reverse curls (23); wrist curls (41); bent-over rowing (6); inclined sit-ups (17); and shrugs (27).

Track, Field and Cycling

RUNNING

Running requires a high degree of power and strength–endurance; however, the relative amount of each of these capacities is dependent upon the duration of the event. The exercises most benefi-

cial to runners include: plyometric squats (one- and two-legged; exercise no. 47); plyometric split squats (46); standing calf raises (30); bounding (49); thigh extensions (36); thigh flexions (37); running dumb-bells (25); lying leg raises (20); stiff-legged deadlifts (32); seated rows (26); plyometric bench press (42); ankle curls (2); leg curls (18); leg press (19); thigh abduction (34); thigh adduction (35); inclined sit-ups (17); trunk extensions (3); and close grip pull-downs (8). An example of a resistance training routine used by a runner is outlined in Table 9.16.

FIELD SPORTS (JUMPS)

Jumping events such as long, high and triple jump require a great deal of lower body power. Consequently the exercises most suited to jumping events include: plyometric squats (particularly single-legged jumps; exercise no. 47); plyometric split squats (46); plyometric leg extensions (high jump only; 44); depth jumps (51); bounding (49); thigh flexions (37); lying leg raises (20); thigh extensions (36); standing calf raises (30); ankle curls (2); stiff-legged deadlifts (32); and leg press (19). Performance in triple and particularly long jump is dependent upon achieving a fast run-up speed; consequently the exercises outlined for runners are also applicable to these athletes. Furthermore, long and triple jumpers must absorb very high forces through their lower bodies and therefore should develop a particularly strong musculo-skeletal system to avoid injury. These athletes must also develop the capacity to tolerate high

Table 9.16 In-season resistance training routine for a runner

Monday	Wednesday	Friday
Plyometric squats	Plyometric split squats	Plyometric squats
Thigh extensions	Leg curls	Thigh extensions
Bounding	Lying leg raises	Bounding
Thigh abduction	Leg press	Thigh adduction
Plyometric bench press	Running dumb-bells	Plyometric bench press
Standing leg raises	Calf raises	Standing leg raises
Calf raises	Stiff-legged deadlifts	Stiff-legged deadlifts
Running dumb-bells	Ankle curls	Inclined sit-ups
Back extensions	Seated rowing	Close grip pull-downs

loads so that they do not adversely affect their competitive performance. Therefore, long and triple jumpers should periodically expose themselves to relatively high eccentric loading during training by not engaging the braking device of the PPS during plyometric squats (47) or plyometric split squats (46) and by also performing depth jumps (51) from relatively high drop heights (i.e. up to 1 m). Due to the extreme forces experienced, high eccentric load training should only be performed for a few sets every couple of weeks at a maximum.

FIELD SPORTS (THROWS)

The throwing events require a great deal of strength and power. In fact the large requirement for strength and power in these events often necessitates the need for four or five resistance training sessions per week using an upper body/lower body split routine. The exercises most applicable to the throwing events include: plyometric inclined bench press (one- and two-handed, shot put only; exercise no. 43); plyometric inclined bench press (discus only, performed with a wide grip; 43); plyometric lying triceps extensions (45) and overhead throws (javelin and shot put only; 52); plyometric standing push press (48); plyometric squats (47); plyometric split squats (46); depth jumps (jumping backwards for shot; 51); bounding (49); high pulls (15); inclined bench press (16); pull-overs (javelin only; 22); squats (29); standing calf raises (30); bench pulls (6); abdominal rotations (1); wrist curls (41); hammer curls (13); thigh adduction (35); thigh abduction (34); and external rotator raises (11).

CYCLING

Cycling requires a high degree of power and strength–endurance. The relative degree of each physical capacity is dependent upon the duration of the event. Cycling requires exercises which promote explosive lower body power. In addition, upper body strength is also required to provide a stable platform from which lower body power can be exerted effectively. The exercises most beneficial to cyclists include: plyometric squats (concentric phase only; exercise no. 47); depth jumps (51); thigh extensions (36); thigh flexions (37); squats (29); leg press (19); lying leg raises (20); standing calf raises (30); stiff-legged deadlifts (32); wrist curls (41); hammer curls (13); seated rowing (26); wide grip chins (40); barbell curls (4); and trunk extensions (3).

Mobile Field Sports (Field Hockey, Soccer, Lacrosse)

An integral factor in all mobile field sports is the ability to run fast. Thus the exercises previously outlined for runners are also applicable to these athletes. In addition, these athletes should perform plyometric leg extensions (soccer only; exercise no. 44); plyometric lying triceps extensions (45) and overhead throws (soccer and lacrosse only; 52); abdominal rotations (1); wrist curls (41) and hammer curls (hockey, lacrosse and soccer goalkeeper only; 13); head curls (soccer only; 14); plyometric bench press (42); and upright rows (39). An example of a pre-season resistance training routine for a soccer player is outlined in Table 9.17.

Table 9.17 A pre-season resistance training routine for a soccer player

Monday	Wednesday	Friday
Plyometric squats	Plyometric leg extensions	Plyometric split squats
Overhead throws	Leg curls	Plyometric leg extensions
Bounding	Lying leg raises	Thigh extensions
Thigh adduction	Leg press	Thigh adduction
Plyometric bench press	Plyometric lying triceps	Bounding
Thigh extensions	extensions	Standing leg raises
Stiff-legged deadlifts	Calf raises	Calf raises
Running dumb-bells	Stiff-legged deadlifts	Abdominal rotations
Head curls	Ankle curls	Shrugs
	Thigh abduction	

Contact Field Sports (Rugby, Australian Football, American Football)

The contact field sports require a high degree of muscular size, strength and power. In each of these sports some players additionally require a relatively high degree of strength–endurance. The high degree of strength and power required in these sports generally necessitates that in the pre-season four resistance training sessions are performed per week, using an upper body/lower body split routine. The exercises most suited to contact field sports include: plyometric squats (exercise no. 47); plyometric split squats (46); plyometric bench press (42); plyometric standing push press (48); plyometric lying triceps extensions (American football only; 45); plyometric leg extensions (44); bounding (49); bench press (5); standing push press (31); barbell curls (4);

hammer curls (13); wrist curls (41); bench pulls (6); high pulls (15); deadlifts (9); shrugs (27); lying leg raises (20); abdominal rotations (1); squats (29); thigh adduction (35); thigh abduction (34); stiff-legged deadlifts (32); thigh extensions (36); standing calf raises (30); shrugs (27); and head curls (14). As with the other routines outlined above, the specific training programme will depend upon the position played within the sport, the individual characteristics of the athlete and the particular phase of the competitive year. With these limitations in mind a general example of a pre-season resistance training routine for contact field sports is outlined in Table 9.18.

Set Field Sports

Athletes involved in set field sports have not traditionally participated in resistance training to a large

Table 9.18 A pre-season resistance training routine for contact field sports (rugby codes, Australian football, American football)

Monday	Tuesday	Thursday	Friday
Plyometric squats	Plyometric bench press	Plyometric split squats	Plyometric inclined bench
Plyometric leg extensions	Plyometric standing	Plyometric leg extensions	press
High pulls	push press	Bounding	Bench press
Thigh extensions	Abdominal rotations	Thigh extensions	Lying leg raises
Calf raises	Head curls	Calf raises	Standing push press
Leg press	Inclined bench press	Deadlifts	Lying triceps extensions
Bench pulls	Close grip bench press	Thigh adduction	Barbell curls
Stiff-legged deadlifts	Barbell curls	Shrugs	Hammer curls
Thigh abduction	Hammer curls		Wrist curls
	Wrist curls		

extent. These sports have a particularly high skill base and thus the physical capacities of strength, power and endurance are seen to be of low priority. Nevertheless the running and throwing ability of athletes in baseball and cricket can be enhanced by resistance training, as can hitting power in all sports. Further resistance training can also be used to remove muscular imbalances in these sports and thus help reduce the incidence of injury.

BASEBALL AND CRICKET

Resistance training exercises most suited to baseball and cricket include: plyometric squats (exercise no. 47); plyometric split squats (46); bounding (49); plyometric bench press (42); plyometric lying triceps extensions (45); thigh extensions (36); wrist curls (41); external rotator raises (11); bench pulls (6); stiff-legged deadlifts (32); abdominal rotations (1); upright rows (39); pull-overs (22); standing calf raises (30); side bends (28); ankle curls (fast bowlers especially; 2); thigh adduction (35); and thigh abduction (34). An example of a resistance training routine for cricket and baseball players is outlined in Table 9.19.

GOLF

Resistance training exercises most suited to golfers include: wrist curls (exercise no. 41); bent-over rows (6); plyometric bench press (42); dips (10); front pull-downs (12); pull-overs (22); wide grip chins (40); chest throws (50); hammer curls (13); abdominal rotations (1); trunk extensions (3); stiff-legged deadlifts (32); upright rows (39); side bends (28); lying triceps extensions (21); reverse curls (23); seated rows (26); bench press (5); and external rotator raises (11).

Court Sports (Basketball, Netball, Volleyball)

The sports of basketball, netball and volleyball require a high degree of muscular power, particularly in the lower body. Resistance training exercises most suited to these sports include: plyometric squats (exercise no. 47); plyometric split squats (46); depth jumps (51); bounding (49); plyometric bench press (42); plyometric lying triceps extensions (45); overhead throws (52); chest throws (50) and bench press (basketball and netball only; 5); ankle curls (2); standing calf raises (30); thigh adduction (35); thigh abduction (34); stiff-legged deadlifts (32); thigh extensions (36); leg press (19); standing push press (basketball and netball only; 31); wrist curls (41); abdominal rotations (1); hammer curls (13); lying leg raises (20); and close grip pull-downs (basketball only; 8). A pre-season resistance training routine for basketball players is outlined in Table 9.20.

Martial Arts

WRESTLING AND JUDO

Wrestling and judo require a great deal of muscular strength and power throughout the entire body. Exercises most suited to these sports include: wrist

Table 9.19 Resistance training routine for cricket and baseball players

Monday	Thursday
Plyometric squats	Plyometric split squats
Plyometric bench press	Bounding
Plyometric lying triceps extensions	Overhead throws
Thigh extensions	Thigh extensions
Abdominal rotations	Abdominal rotations
Wrist curls	Stiff-legged deadlifts
Bench pulls	Wrist curls
External rotator raises	Calf raises
Pull-overs	Ankle curls
Thigh adduction	Thigh abduction

Table 9.20 A pre-season resistance training routine for basketball players

Monday	Wednesday	Friday
Plyometric squats	Plyometric split squats	Plyometric squats
Plyometric bench press	Overhead throws	Plyometric inclined bench
Bounding	Depth jumps	press
Plyometric lying triceps	Bench press	Thigh extensions
extensions	Thigh extensions	Plyometric lying triceps
Close grip pull-downs	Leg press	extensions
Stiff-legged deadlifts	Reverse curls	Standing push press
Abdominal rotations	Calf raises	Ankle curls
Wrist curls	Thigh adduction	Close grip pull-downs
Thigh abduction		Lying leg raises
		Calf raises

curls (exercise no. 41); reverse curls (23); hammer curls (13); seated rowing (26); barbell curls (4); shrugs (27); high pulls (15); deadlifts (9); bench press (5); close grip pull-downs (7); plyometric standing push press (48); dips (10); head curls (14); reverse curls (23); plyometric bench press (42); plyometric squats (47); stiff-legged deadlifts (32); lying leg raises (20); leg press (19); abdominal rotations (1); side bends (28); standing calf raises (30); and bench pulls (6). A resistance training routine for these athletes is outlined in Table 9.21.

PUNCHING AND KICKING SPORTS

Sports involving kicking and punching require a high degree of speed and power. Exercises most suited to these sports include: plyometric bench press (concentric phase only; exercise no. 42); plyometric standing push press (concentric phase only; 48); plyometric squats (47); plyometric split squats (46); plyometric leg extensions (kicking sports only; 44); plyometric push-ups (53); depth jumps (51); bounding (49); chest throws (50); abdominal rotations (1); inclined sit-ups (17); lying leg raises (20); thigh flexion (kicking sports only; 37); high pulls (15); seated rowing (26); shrugs (27); head curls (14); thigh adduction (35); thigh abduction (34); stiff-legged deadlifts (32); bench press (5); and standing calf raises (30).

CONCLUSION

Resistance training has resulted in vast improvements in performance in a wide variety of sports over the past 20 years. This chapter has outlined the use of strength and power training in sport from a performance enhancement perspective. Current training practices and principles have been outlined and potential future directions have been

Table 9.21 A resistance training routine for athletes involved in the sports of wrestling and judo

Monday	Tuesday	Thursday	Saturday
Plyometric standing push	High pulls	Plyometric bench press	Plyometric squats
press	Plyometric split squats	Close grip pull-downs	Seated rowing
Abdominal rotations	Seated rowing	Standing push press	Abdominal rotations
Bench press	Shrugs	Reverse curls	Deadlifts
Dips	Standing calf raises	Hammer curls	Thigh extensions
Barbell curls	Leg press	Barbell curls	Head curls
Hammer curls	Stiff-legged deadlifts	Wrist curls	Lying leg raises
Wrist curls	Side bends	Bench pulls	Side bends

proposed. In developing effective resistance training routines, a thorough understanding of the training principles of overload, specificity, variation and recovery are required. Similarly an understanding of the advantages and limitations of current training methods and equipment is also important. While the use of strength training has been fundamental to performance improvement in many sports over the past 20 years, the steady progression from pure strength towards explosive power exercises, will bring far greater performance improvements in the near future.

REFERENCES

Ackland T. & Bloomfield J. (1992) Functional anatomy. In Bloomfield J., Fricker P. & Fitch K. (eds) *Textbook of Science and Medicine in Sport*, pp. 13, 15, 42. Blackwell Scientific Publications, Melbourne.

Adams K., O'Shea J., O'Shea K. & Climstein M. (1992) The effect of six weeks of squat, plyometric and squat-plyometric training on power production. *Journal of Applied Sport Science Research* **6**, 36–41.

Alexander R. (1987) The spring in your step. *New Scientist* **114**, 42–44.

American College of Sports Medicine (1984) Position stand on the use of anabolic-androgenic steroids in sport. *Sports Medicine Bulletin* **19**, 13–19.

American College of Sports Medicine (1987) Position stand on the use of anabolic-androgenic steroids in sport. *Medicine and Science in Sport and Exercise* **19**, 534–539.

Anderson T. & Kearney J. (1982) Effects of three resistance training programmes on muscular strength and absolute and relative endurance. *Research Quarterly for Exercise and Sport* **53**, 1–7.

Arvidsson I., Eriksson E., Haggmark T. & Johnsson R. (1981) Isokinetic thigh muscle strength after ligament reconstruction in the knee joint. *International Journal of Sports Medicine* **2**, 7–11.

Asmussen E. & Bonde-Petersen F. (1974) Storage of elastic energy in skeletal muscles in man. *Acta Physiologica Scandinavica* **91**, 385–392.

Atha J. (1981) Strengthening muscle. In Miller D. (ed.) *Exercise and Sport Science Reviews*, Vol. 9, pp. 1–73. Franklin Institute Press, Philadelphia.

Baker D., Wilson G. & Carlyon B. (1994) Periodisation: The effect of manipulating volume and intensity upon strength. *Journal of Strength and Conditioning Research* **8** (in press).

Behm D. & Sale D. (1993) Intended rather than actual movement velocity determines velocity-specific training response. *Journal of Applied Physiology* **74**, 359–369.

Bender J., Pierson J., Kaplan H. & Johnson A. (1964) Factors affecting the occurrence of knee injuries. *Journal of the Association for Physical and Mental Rehabilitation* **18**, 130–134.

Berger R. (1962) Optimum repetitions for the development of strength. *Research Quarterly* **33**, 334–339.

Berger R. (1963) Effect of dynamic and static training on vertical jumping. *Research Quarterly* **34**, 419–424.

Bloomfield J., Blanksby B., Ackland T., & Allison G. (1990) The influence of strength training on overhead throwing velocity of elite water polo players. *Australian Journal of Science and Medicine in Sport* **22**, 63–67.

Bloomfield J., Fricker P. & Fitch K. (eds) *Textbook of Science and Medicine in Sport*, pp. 13, 15, 21, 41, 42, 529. Blackwell Scientific Publications, Melbourne.

Bosco C., Komi P., Pulli M., Pittera C. & Montonev H. (1982) Considerations of the training of the elastic potential of the human skeletal muscle. *Volleyball Technical Journal* **6**, 75–80.

Brylinsky J., Moore J. & Frosch M. (1992) The effect of using a weighted softball on pitching velocity, wrist strength and handgrip. *Journal of Applied Sport Science Research* **6**, 170–173.

Capen E. (1950) The effect of systematic weight training on power, strength and endurance. *Research Quarterly* **21**, 83–93.

Cavagna G., Saibene F. & Margaria R. (1964) Mechanical work in running. *Journal of Applied Physiology* **19**, 249–256.

Chandler J., Kilber B., Stracener E., Ziegler A. & Pace B. (1992) Shoulder strength, power and endurance in college tennis players. *The American Journal of Sports Medicine* **20**, 455–459.

Chinery S. (1984) *In Quest of Size—Anabolics and Other Ergogenic Aids*, p. 7. L and S Research Publishing, Toms River, NJ, USA.

Chromiak J. & Mulvaney D. (1990) A review: The effects of combined strength and endurance training on strength development. *Journal of Applied Sport Science Research* **4**, 55–60.

Chu D. (1992) *Jumping into Plyometrics*, pp. 13–24. Leisure Press, Champaign, IL, USA.

Clarke D., Hunt M. & Dotson C. (1992) Muscular strength and endurance as a function of age and activity level. *Research Quarterly for Exercise and Sport* **63**, 302–310.

Coleman A. (1977) Nautilus vs. universal gym strength training in adult males. *American Corrective Therapy Journal* **31**, 103–107.

Cook E., Gray V. & Savinar-Nogue E. (1987) Shoulder antagonistic strength ratios: A comparison between college-level baseball pitchers and non pitchers. *Journal of Orthopedic Sports Physical Therapy* **8**, 51–61.

Counsilman J. (1986) Sports training programmes: Swimming. In Pearl, B. (ed.) *Getting Stronger*, pp. 149–152. Pearl and Shelter, Bolinas, CA, USA.

Davies B., Elford J. & Jamieson K. (1991) Variation in performance in simple muscle tests at different phases of the menstrual cycle. *The Journal of Sports Medicine and Physical Fitness* **31**, 532–537.

Di Pasquale M. (1987) *Drug Use and Detection in Amateur Sports — Update Four*, pp. 2–18. M.G.D. Press, Warkworth, ON, Canada.

Duda M. (1988) Plyometrics: A legitimate form of power training? *The Physician and Sportsmedicine* **16**, 213–219.

Dudley G. & Djamil R. (1985) Incompatibility of endurance- and strength-training modes of exercise. *Journal of Applied Physiology* **59**, 1446–1451.

Edman K. A. P. (1979) The velocity of unloaded shortening and its relation to sarcomere length and isometric force in vertebrate muscle fibres. *Journal of Physiology* **291**, 143–159.

Ekstrand J. & Gillquist J. (1983) The avoidability of soccer injuries. *International Journal of Sports Medicine* **4**, 124–129.

Ekstrand J., Gillquist J. & Liljedahl S. (1983) Prevention of soccer injuries. *The American Journal of Sports Medicine* **11**, 116–120.

Elko K. & Ostrow A. (1992) The effects of three mental preparation strategies on strength performance of young and older adults. *Journal of Sport Behaviour* **15**, 34–41.

Elliott B., Wilson G. & Kerr, G. (1989) A biomechanical analysis of the sticking region in the bench press. *Medicine and Science in Sports and Exercise* **21**, 450–462.

Fahey T. & Brown C. (1973) The effects of an anabolic steroid on the strength, body composition, and endurance of college males when accompanied by a weight training programme. *Medicine and Science in Sports* **5**, 272–276.

Faulkner J., Claflin D. & McCully K. (1986) Power output of fast and slow fibres from human skeletal muscles. In Jones N., McCartney N. & McComas A. (eds) *Human Muscle Power*, pp. 81–94. Human Kinetics Publishers, Champaign, IL, USA.

Francis C. (1990) *Speed Trap*, pp. 1–4, 58–64, 127–142. Collins Publishers, Sydney.

Fry A. & Kraemer W. (1991) Physical performance characteristics of American football players. *The Journal of Applied Sport Science Research* **5**, 126–139.

Fry A., Kraemer W., Weseman C., *et al.* (1991) Effects of an off-season strength and conditioning programme on starters and non-starters in women's collegiate volleyball. *The Journal of Applied Sport Science Research* **5**, 174–181.

Fry R. & Morton A. (1991) Physiological and kinanthropometric attributes of elite flat-water kayakists. *Medicine and Science in Sports and Exercise* **23**, 1297–1301.

Funato K., Ohmichi H. & Miyashita M. (1985) Electromyographic analysis on utilization of elastic energy in human leg muscles. In Winter D., Norman R., Wells R., Hayes K. & Patla A. (eds) *Biomechanics IX–A*, pp. 60–64. Human Kinetics Publishers, Champaign, IL, USA.

Griffin J. (1987) Differences in elbow flexion torque measured concentrically, eccentrically and isometrically. *Physical Therapy* **67**, 1205–1209.

Grimby G., Gustafsson E., Peterson L. & Renstrom P. (1980) Quadriceps function and training after knee ligament surgery. *Medicine and Science in Sports* **12**, 70–75.

Hakkinen K., Alen M. & Komi P. (1984) Neuromuscular, anaerobic and aerobic performance characteristics of elite power athletes. *European Journal of Applied Physiology* **53**, 97–105.

Hakkinen K., Alen M. & Komi P. (1985a) Electromyographic and muscle fibre characteristics of human skeletal muscle during strength training and detraining. *Acta Physiologica Scandinavica* **125**, 573–585.

Hakkinen K., Komi P. & Alen M. (1985b) Effect of explosive type strength training on isometric force- and relaxation-time, electromyographic and muscle fibre characteristics of leg extensor muscles. *Acta Physiologica Scandinavica* **125**, 587–600.

Hakkinen K., Komi P. & Kauhanen, H. (1986) Electromyographic and force production characteristics of leg extensor muscles of elite weight lifters during isometric, concentric, and various stretch-shortening cycle exercises. *International Journal of Sports Medicine* **3**, 144–151.

Hakkinen K., Komi P., Alen M. & Kauhanen H. (1987) EMG, muscle fibre and force production characteristics during a one year training period in elite weight-lifters. *European Journal of Applied Physiology* **56**, 419–427.

Hakkinen K., Pakarinen H., Alen M., Kauhanen H. & Komi P. (1988) Neuromuscular and hormonal adaptations in athletes to strength training in two years. *Journal of Applied Physiology* **65**, 2406–2412.

Hart C., Ward T. & Mayhew J. (1991) Anthropometric correlates of bench press performance following resistance training. *Sports Training, Medicine and Rehabilitation* **2**, 89–95.

Henneman E., Clamann H., Gillies J. & Skinner R. (1974) Rank order of motorneurons within a pool: Law of combination. *Journal of Neurophysiology* **37**, 1338–1349.

Hickson R. (1980) Interference of strength development by simultaneous training for strength and endurance. *European Journal of Applied Physiology* **45**, 255–263.

Hickson R., Dvorak B., Gorostiaga E., Kurowski T. & Foster C. (1988) Potential for strength and endurance training to amplify endurance performance. *Journal of Applied Physiology* **65**, 2285–2290.

Ikai M. & Steinhaus A. (1961) Some factors modifying the expression of human strength. *Journal of Applied Physiology* **16**, 157–163.

Jones A. (1974) Progressive exercise. *Athletic Journal* **55**, 76–79, 99–100.

Kammerer R. (1993) Drug testing and anabolic steroids. In Yesalis C. *Anabolic Steroids in Sport and Exercise*, p. 305. Human Kinetics Publishers, Champaign, IL, USA.

Kaneko M., Fuchimoto T., Toji H. & Suei K. (1983) Training effect of differing loads on the force-velocity relationship and mechanical power output in human muscle. *Scandinavia Journal of Sport Science* **5**, 50–55.

Komi P. & Bosco C. (1978) Utilization of stored elastic energy in leg extensor muscles by men and women. *Medicine and Science in Sports* **10**, 261–265.

Kretzler H. & Richardson A. (1989) Rupture of the pectoralis major muscle. *The American Journal of Sports Medicine* **17**, 453–459.

Lindh M. (1979) Increase of muscle strength from isometric quadriceps exercises at different knee angles.

Scandinavian Journal of Rehabilitation Medicine **11**, 33–36.

Marey M. & Demeny M. (1885) Locomotion humaine, mécanisme du saut. *Comptes Rendus Hebdomadaires des Séances de l'Académie des Sciences (Paris)* **101**, 489–494.

MacDougall J. D., Sale D. G., Moroz J. R., Elder C. B. & Sutton J. R. (1979) Mitochondrial volume density in human skeletal muscle following heavy resistance training. *Medicine and Science in Sports* **11**, 164–166.

McDonagh M. & Davies C. (1984) Adaptive response of mammalian skeletal muscle to exercise with high loads. *European Journal of Applied Physiology* **52**, 139–155.

McLaughlin T. (1985) Control in lowering the bar. *Powerlifting USA* **8**, 19.

McLaughlin T., Gillman C. & Lardner T. (1977) A kinetic model of performance in the parallel squat by champion powerlifters. *Medicine and Science in Sports* **9**, 128–133.

Mero A., Luhtanen P., Viitasalo J. & Komi, P. (1981) Relationship between the maximal running velocity, muscle fiber characteristics, force production and force relaxation of sprinters. *Scandinavian Journal of Sports Science* **3**, 16–22.

Milner-Brown H., Stein R. & Lee G. (1975) Synchronisation of human motor units: Possible role of exercise and supraspinal reflexes. *Electroencephalography and Clinical Neurophysiology* **38**, 245–254.

Miyashita M. & Kanshisa H. (1979) Dynamic peak torque related to age, sex and performance. *Research Quarterly* **50**, 249–255.

Moritani T. & DeVries H. A. (1979) Neural factors versus hypertrophy in the time course of muscle strength gain. *American Journal of Physical Medicine* **58**, 115–129.

Moritani T., Muro M., Ishida K. & Taguchi S. (1987) Electrophysiological analyses of the effects of muscle power training. *Research Journal of Physical Education in Japan* **1**, 23–32.

Newton R. & Wilson G. (1993) Reducing the risk of injury during plyometric training: The effect of dampeners. *Sports Medicine, Training and Rehabilitation* **4**, 1–7.

O'Shea K. & O'Shea J. (1989) Functional isometric weight training: Its effect on dynamic and static strength. *Journal of Applied Sport Science Research* **3**, 30–33.

O'Shea J., O'Shea K. & Wynn B. (1988) Functional isometric lifting — Part 2: Application. *National Strength and Conditioning Association Journal* **1**, 60–62.

Peterson J. (1982) Strength training: Health insurance for the athlete. In Riley D. (ed.) *Strength Training by the Experts,* 2nd edn, pp. 7–9. Leisure Press, New York.

Pipes T. (1978) Variable resistance versus constant resistance strength training in adult males. *European Journal of Applied Physiology* **39**, 27–35.

Poliquin C. (1988a) Variety in strength training. *Sports* **8**, 8.

Poliquin C. (1988b) Five ways to increase the effectiveness of your strength training programme. *National Strength and Conditioning Association Journal* **10**, 34–39.

Pousson M., van Hoecke J. & Goubel F. (1990) Changes in elastic characteristics of human muscle induced by eccentric exercise. *Journal of Biomechanics* **23**, 343–349.

Rasch P. J. & Morehouse L. E. (1957) Effect of static and dynamic exercises on muscular strength and hypertrophy. *Journal of Applied Physiology* **11**, 29–34.

Rogozkin V. (1976) The effect of the number of daily training sessions on skeletal muscle protein synthesis. *Medicine and Science in Sports* **8**, 223–225.

Rohrs D., Mayhew J., Arabas C. & Shelton M. (1990) The relationship between seven anaerobic tests and swim performance. *Journal of Swimming Research* **6**, 15–19.

Roman W. J., Fleckenstein J., Stray-Gundersen J., Alway S. E., Peshock R. & Gonyea W. J. (1993) Adaptations in the elbow flexors of elderly males after heavy-resistance training. *Journal of Applied Physiology* **74**, 750–754.

Roundtable NSCA (1986) Practical considerations for utilising plyometrics. *National Strength and Conditioning Association Journal* **8**, 14–22.

Rutherford O., Greig C., Sargent A. & Jones D. (1986) Strength training and power output: Transference effects in the human quadriceps muscle. *Journal of Sports Sciences* **4**, 101–107.

Sale D. (1991) Testing strength and power. In MacDougall J., Wenger H. & Green H. (eds) *Physiological Testing of the High Performance Athlete,* 2nd edn, pp. 21–106. Human Kinetics Publishers, Champaign, IL, USA.

Sale D. (1992) Neural adaptation to strength training. In Komi P. (ed.) *Strength and Power in Sport,* pp. 249–265. Blackwell Scientific Publications, Oxford.

Schmidtbleicher D. (1988) Muscular mechanics and neuromuscular control. *Swimming Science V International Series Sport Science*, pp. 131–148. Human Kinetics Publishers, Champaign, IL, USA.

Schmidtbleicher D. & Buehrle M. (1987) Neuronal adaptations and increase of cross-sectional area studying different strength training methods. In Johnson G. (ed.) *Biomechanics X-B*, Vol. 6–B, pp. 615–620. Human Kinetics Publishers, Champaign, IL, USA.

Schmidtbleicher D., Gollhofer A. & Frick U. (1988) Effects of a stretch-shortening typed training on the performance capability and innervation characteristics of leg extensor muscles. In de Groot G., Hollander A., Huijing P. & van Ingen Schenau G. (eds) *Biomechanics XI–A*, Vol 7–A, pp. 185–189. Free University Press, Amsterdam.

Schmidtbleicher D. & Haralambie G. (1981) Changes in contractile properties of muscle after strength training in man. *European Journal of Applied Physiology* **46**, 221–229.

Secher N. (1975) Isometric rowing strength of experienced and inexperienced oarsmen. *Medicine and Science in Sports* **7**, 280–283.

Sharp R., Troup J. & Costill D. (1982): Relationship between power and sprint freestyle swimming. *Medicine and Science in Sports and Exercise* **14**, 53–56.

Stone M., O'Bryant H. & Garhammer J. (1981) A theoretical model for strength training. *Journal of Sports Medicine* **21**, 342–351.

Stromme S., Meen H. & Aakvaag A. (1974) Effects of an androgenic-anabolic steroid on strength development and plasma testosterone levels in normal males. *Medicine and Science in Sports* **6**, 203–209.

Sweet W. (1987) *Sport and Recreation in Ancient Greece.* Oxford University Press, Oxford.

Talag T. (1973) Residual muscular soreness as influenced by concentric, eccentric and static contractions. *Research Quarterly* **44**, 458–469.

Tidow G. (1990) Aspects of strength training in athletics. *New Studies in Athletics* **1**, 93–110.

Todd T. (1987) Anabolic steroids: The gremlins of sport. *Journal of Sport History* **14**, 87–107.

Tuttle W., Janney C. & Thompson C. (1950) Relation of maximum grip strength to grip strength endurance. *Journal of Applied Physiology* **2**, 663–670.

Ward P. (1973) The effect of an anabolic steroid on strength and lean body mass. *Medicine and Science in Sports* **5**, 277–282.

Wilmore J. (1974) Alterations in strength, body composition and anthropometric measurements consequent to a 10-week weight training programme. *Medicine and Science in Sport* **6**, 133–139.

Wilmore J. & Costill D. (1988) *Training for Sport and Activity: The Physiological Basis of the Conditioning Process*, 3rd edn, pp. 3–17, 113–139, 293–312. Wm C. Brown Publishers, Dubuque, IL, USA.

Wilson G. (1991) Stretch–shorten cycle: Nature and implications for human muscle performance. *Journal of Human Muscle Performance* **1**, 11–31.

Wilson G., Elliott B. & Kerr G. (1989) Bar path and force profile characteristics for maximal and submaximal loads in the bench press. *International Journal of Sports Biomechanics* **5**, 390–402.

Wilson G., Elliott B. & Wood, G. (1991a) The effect on performance of imposing a delay during a stretch–shorten cycle movement. *Medicine and Science in Sports and Exercise* **23**, 364–370.

Wilson G., Elliott B. & Wood G. (1992) Stretch–shorten cycle performance enhancement through flexibility training. *Medicine and Science in Sports and Exercise* **24**, 116–123.

Wilson G., Newton R., Murphy A. & Humphries B. (1993) The optimal training load for the development of dynamic athletic performance. *Medicine and Science in Sports and Exercise* **25**, 1279–1286.

Wilson G., Wood G. & Elliott B. (1991b) Optimal stiffness of the series elastic component in a stretch shorten cycle activity. *Journal of Applied Physiology* **70**, 825–833.

Wilson G., Wood G. & Elliott B. (1991c) The performance augmentation achieved from use of the stretch–shorten cycle: The neuromuscular contribution. *Australian Journal of Science and Medicine in Sport* **23**, 97–100.

Wright J. (1980) Anabolic steroids and athletics. *Exercise and Sport Science Reviews* **8**, 149–202.

Wright J. (1982) *Anabolic Steroids and Sports*, Vol. II, pp. 48–54. Sport Science Consultants, Natick, MA, USA.

Young W. (1989) Weight training — the going through the motion syndrome. *Sports Coach* **13**, 35–37.

CHAPTER 10

FLEXIBILITY IN SPORT

Flexibility can be defined as the range of movement in a joint or in several joints. It is developed by stretching the soft tissue, primarily around a joint, and is of great value to the athlete in many sports, because it can improve the overall performance significantly. The purpose of this chapter is to demonstrate the advantages or disadvantages of flexibility in sport and to present, with caution, the methods that will improve an athlete's potential to perform in various sports and events.

VALUE OF STRETCHING

During the past two decades coaches have increasingly realized the value of stretching for their athletes. In some sports, such as swimming and track and field, stretching has been used for over 50 years, but coaches in the majority of sports have not been aware of the specific benefits until recently.

General Benefits

Many coaches and sport scientists now believe that flexibility exercises are of more value than was previously thought. In the past they have been used as part of the warm-up programme for various sports, but their value in technique and increasing the explosive power in a movement has only recently been realized. It is for these reasons that stretching has become an integral part of the modern training programme in a similar way to that of strength and power, speed and mental skills training.

Specific Benefits

IMPROVEMENT IN PERFORMANCE

All well-informed coaches today are aware of the role played by stretching, if high levels of performance are to be reached. Sigerseth (1971) stated that certain skilled performances may be enhanced by increasing or decreasing the range of motion around various joints. Since that time coaches have realized that there are three main areas where improvements can be made and these are as follows:

- Being able to *increase the range of various movements throughout the body has enabled athletes to place themselves into more aesthetic positions* in almost all sports. In many cases these positions are accompanied by a more technically sound performance and as well they are very pleasing to watch, as for example in a high hurdles race, where the competitors stride smoothly over the hurdles rather than partially jumping them; or in a butterfly race, where instead of swimmers 'climbing' out of the water and then sinking back into it, they appear to glide over it. Further, in sport disciplines that are judged, such as gymnastics, diving or ice skating, the participant is expected to reach certain set positions in order to score high artistic marks. Without a high level of flexibility athletes are not able to match their very supple opponents

- It has been hypothesized for some time by observant coaches that a *stretched muscle can produce a greater contractile force than a non-stretched one*. This is because the pre-stretched muscle stores elastic energy and then releases it as it is shortened. Wilson *et al.* (1992) demonstrated that flexibility training significantly increased the elasticity of the musculotendinous unit and in so doing enhanced the utilization of elastic energy. This finding has corroborated the subjective opinions of coaches referred to above and will have a significant effect on the use of the explosive power concept in the future. There is no doubt that in the sports where explosive power is used, athletes can benefit greatly from its development through flexibility training
- When an athlete is able to *increase the range of motion in any skill in a ballistic sport, the potential to produce more force or velocity* becomes possible, because a greater range of movement increases the distance and the time over which a force can be developed (Ciullo & Zarins 1983). This in turn increases the velocity of the racquet, club, bat or projectile, and a more powerful hit, throw or kick can be made. Sports such as tennis, golf, cricket, baseball, football and some field sports are good examples of this

PREVENTION OF INJURY

Flexibility is a component of fitness that is frequently associated with muscular injury. Alter (1988) suggested that stretching exercises may decrease the incidence, intensity and duration of musculotendinous and joint injury and further stated that flexibility is currently seen as one of the best ways of avoiding musculotendinous injuries. There are two mechanisms that account for the strong relationship between the flexibility of the musculature and its predisposition to injury. The first of these (Shellock & Prentice 1985) is based on the effect of flexibility on the range of motion about a joint, while the second is based on the relationship between flexibility and the elasticity of the musculotendinous units (Wilson *et al.* 1991).

RELIEF OF MUSCULAR SORENESS

Muscular soreness can occur immediately after exercise and last for several hours, or be delayed for up to 24 hours or even longer. DeVries (1986) recommended static stretching for both types of soreness. He suggested that a brief period of static stretching (10 min) can be done after a workout, so as to alleviate immediate soreness. If a muscle or group of muscles become sore at a later time, the athlete should again use static stretching with stretch times up to 2 min. This can be repeated two or three times a day.

MUSCULAR RELAXATION

Alter (1988) stated that one of the important benefits of a stretching programme is the promotion of relaxation. When a muscle stays partially contracted for a period of time 'contracture' develops. This syndrome, plus chronic muscle tension, can shorten the muscle and make it less supple. As a result, undue muscular tension can produce excessive muscle tightness. Static stretching combined with a relaxation programme is of great value to alleviate this condition.

RANGE OF FLEXIBILITY

It is important for coaches to understand that, as in the normal population, the range of flexibility within the competitive sporting population is also extensive. Surburg (1983) suggested that flexibility was a continuum and that at one end there was almost no movement, while at the other, there was an excessive amount. The former creates a very restricted range of movement, while the latter causes excessive instability, leading to partial (subluxation) or in some cases, complete dislocation. It is necessary therefore, for the coach to decide the athlete's optimal level of mobility and to make sure that this is attained and then maintained.

Hypermobility

Hypermobile individuals with loose joint capsules, loose ligaments and in some cases abnormally small bony articulating prominences, have commonly been labelled as 'double-jointed' and contortionists who performed in circuses or vaudeville in the past were basically hypermobile. In some sports such as gymnastics, swimming and diving, this can be an advantage, providing it is not extreme. However in contact sports, where the game is played at a high speed and collisions with other players often occur, it can be very dangerous, particularly in contact games such as the football codes.

Hypermobility is not only a problem in sport as it relates to injury, but it can also be very detrimental to technique. Athletes who are partially hypermobile often have too wide a range of movement with back-swings and follow-throughs. This can place them in an awkward position to perform the next shot, or it may take them out of the play in some agility sports for a split second while they are recovering. In highly technique-oriented sports such as swimming, for example, a degree of hypermobility is of value in freestyle or butterfly, but quite detrimental in backstroke, because if the swimmer has a hypermobile shoulder joint, the arm may enter the water directly behind the head, instead of level with the shoulder. The first part of the pulling stroke is then lateral; this in turn creates an equal and opposite movement of the hips, causing a high degree of lateral frontal resistance. The type of action therefore reduces the efficiency of the stroke.

There are various tests for hypermobility. Figure 14.35 demonstrates several of these with the fourth position in each test showing hypermobility. If an athlete needs to decrease the range of movement in one or several joints, an *intensive* strength training programme needs to be undertaken in order to tighten the musculotendinous units, thereby giving more support to the joint itself. If possible this should be done during the adolescent growth spurt, as the athlete will not build up muscle and connective tissue in pre- or post-adolescence as quickly as during adolescence.

Hypomobility

Joint stiffness or unusual soft tissue tightness often occurs in primary mesomorphs. It can be due to abnormally large bony prominences in the joint, very 'tight' joint capsules, or a large and 'bulky' musculature.

With hypomobile or inflexible athletes, stretching exercises must be commenced conservatively and carried out with caution. If this occurs over an extended period of time, their mobility will significantly improve. Each individual should be carefully evaluated and decisions made on which joints should be stretched and to what degree. In contact games such as the tackle football codes, the coach should be aware that shoulder joints need to be 'tight', as do the hip and knee joints. Flexibility exercises to lengthen the musculotendinous units, especially in the areas of the hamstrings, quadriceps and calves, must be carried out carefully, with no exercises being performed which might loosen the ligaments and joint capsules of the athlete.

SPECIFICITY IN FLEXIBILITY

There is a common belief that if athletes are flexible in one joint, then they will have a similar range of movement in others. However, DeVries (1986) stated that 'an individual is a composite of many joints, some of which may be unusually flexible, some inflexible and some average'. Flexibility therefore is specific and depends not only on the 'tightness' of the ligaments, muscles, tendons and joint capsules, but also on the size and shape of the bones and how they are articulated. This is demonstrated in people who have dysplasia, where one or several parts of the body are disproportionately larger or smaller than the others. Examples of this would be a square-shouldered male with a large and protruding acromion process which makes the shoulder joint reasonably inflexible; or a female with a flat back and buttocks. In the first case this individual would make a reasonably poor butterfly swimmer, unless the technique is modified to accommodate this partial handicap, possibly by using side breathing. In the second example, a flat back and buttocks would not assist this person to easily perform a trunk hyperextension manoeuvre in gymnastics, even though levels of flexibility were above average in the other joints.

FACTORS AFFECTING FLEXIBILITY

Age

Corbin and Noble (1980) suggested that flexibility increased in a child until adolescence, when there appeared to be a plateau effect, followed by a steady decrease in mobility as the individual aged. Research by Phillips (1955) and Kirchner and Glines (1957) did not support this finding and both stated that elementary school aged children became less flexible as they grew, reaching a low point between 10 and 12 years of age. From this time on, flexibility appeared to improve slightly until late adolescence. There seems to be no dispute in the literature about the fact that from young adulthood there is a steady decline in flexibility until death, unless an intervention programme aimed at increasing flexibility is carried out.

CRITICAL TRAINING PERIODS

The literature is confusing on this subject, with some researchers maintaining that it is during childhood and early adolescence that the best flexibility training results are obtained, while others disagree with this. Regardless of the exact time for optimal benefit, flexibility exercises can be done at any period in an athlete's life and are not dangerous, provided certain safeguards are adhered to. These will be discussed in detail later in this chapter.

CHILDHOOD AND ADOLESCENCE

Individuals are undergoing rapid growth during childhood and adolescence, and therefore the coach must be careful not to overstress the musculoskeletal system of a young athlete. Early in a child's life, the bones have not as yet fully formed and the bone modelling process is rapidly occurring. This means that cartilage, which is steadily being replaced by bone, is very vulnerable to overuse syndromes and trauma. Well-planned strength and flexibility training will not cause injuries, but overtraining will. Further information on the types of injury which can occur with overtraining will be discussed in the section on the effect of growth on flexibility. It should also be noted that during periods of rapid growth a loss of flexibility can occur, as the bones may grow at a faster rate than the muscles around them. Consequently it is often necessary for children to perform flexibility exercises during the adolescent growth spurt in order for them to maintain reasonable levels of flexibility at this time.

POST-ADOLESCENCE

As the individual ages, muscles, tendons and connective tissue shorten and calcification of some cartilage occurs, with a resultant loss in the range of movement. This usually appears first in the lumbar region, followed by the knees, then in other joints. It can be minimized with a well-planned stretching and strength training programme, provided the individual does not overstress the musculoskeletal system.

Gender

Research by Phillips (1955) and Kirchner and Glines (1957) found that elementary school aged girls were more flexible than boys of a similar age. From adolescence onward, females appear to be more flexible with smaller bones and less musculature than males; however, these observations made by a large number of health professionals, teachers and coaches, have not been conclusively supported by research at this time.

Environmental Conditions

There is general agreement that a warm-up must precede a stretching session. When soft tissue, particularly the musculotendinous unit, is heated, it can promote relaxation which allows safe stretching to be performed. DeVries (1986) stated that flexibility was improved by 20%, by the local warming of a joint to 45°C (113°F) and was decreased by between 10 and 20% by cooling it to 18°C

(65°F). Furthermore, by warming up the body in general and specific joints in particular, there is also less risk of muscular injury.

Psychological Effect

Alter (1988) stated that when team members warm up and stretch together they can serve as models and guides for one another. In a social situation, it is possible for a cohesive and co-operative group to achieve better results than if they had worked individually. Alter (1988) further pointed out, however, that co-action can be detrimental if the element of competition is introduced and that it is important for team members not to compete with one another, as this can be dangerous, and over-stretching will only injure the muscles and joints. Flexibility is a highly individual capacity and must be treated as such by all athletes.

LIMITATIONS TO THE RANGE OF MOVEMENT

When examining the range of movement in any athlete, it is important for the coach to understand the anatomical and physiological limitations that are placed on the individual. The following sections illustrate this point.

Anatomical Limitations

CONNECTIVE TISSUE (SOFT TISSUE)

Connective tissue is widespread in the body and plays an important role in determining an athlete's range of motion, as it covers the end of the bone at each joint like a sleeve. It is also basically responsible for binding together various structures and consists of both fibrous connective tissue (collagen) and elastic connective tissue. Some joints in the body have slightly more of the elastic tissue and this is one of the factors that determines their range of motion.

FASCIA

This is a band of fibrous like tissue which binds many structures in the body. The deep fascia which envelops the muscle is known as the *epimysium* (Fig. 9.4) and within the muscle can be found the *perimysium*, *endomysium* and the *sarcolemma*, all of which bind various components of the muscle. This tissue has limited stretch and soon resists movement.

MUSCLE

The component parts and the contractile nature of skeletal muscle have already been described in Chapter 9 and are only of academic interest in a section on stretching. What is of importance with relation to muscle tissue, is that although it is not able to lengthen of its own accord, it can be stretched externally. By doing this the myofilaments can slide further apart and an elongation of the muscle can occur. When a muscle is stretched under tension, for example, during an eccentric contraction, the myofilaments slide apart and elastic energy is stored in the cross-bridge linkages between the actin and myosin filaments. The greater the muscular tension the more actin and myosin filaments are linked. As a result of this, more elastic energy will be stored.

TENDONS

Generally tendons join muscle to bone and are normally cord-like, but they can also be flat; when flat or ribbon shaped they are known as aponeuroses. Tendons consist of closely packed collagenous bundles which have a longitudinal striation. Their structure ensures that they have little stretch and this quality enables them to transfer a muscular contraction directly to the bone to which they are attached. Nevertheless tendons do possess some elasticity, particularly the longer ones such as the Achilles tendon and are major storage sites for elastic energy (Alexander 1987).

LIGAMENTS

These are strong bands of connective tissue joining bone and their main function is to support a joint. They consist of bundles of collagenous fibres which run parallel to one another and have a structure that is similar to tendons, but they are usually flatter in shape. Their level of stretchability is also similar to that of tendons, in order to allow some limited movement at the joint, but they are strong enough to bind bone to bone, resisting moderate trauma or overstretching.

SOFT TISSUE STIFFNESS

It should be remembered by individuals who conduct stretching programmes that caution must be used at all times. The abovementioned tissues are to a point elastic by nature and are designed to return to their normal length after being stretched. If the force applied is too great, however, and the stretch is overdone, these tissues may rupture and the joint or joints being stretched may become unstable.

BONE TISSUE

It is obvious that the bone structure at the joints plays a restrictive role in flexibility. It is well known that individuals with large bony prominences at the ends of their bones have a finite limit on their joint mobility and any amount of stretching of the connective tissues around the joint will not alter this.

Physiological Limitations

Sense organs or proprioceptors are involved in all movements where precision is required and are found in the muscles, tendons and joints. When stretching, two types of sense organs come into play, namely the *muscle spindles* and the *Golgi tendon organs* (GTOs). These organs pick up changes in the muscle length, or its velocity or force and transmit them by electrical signals to the central nervous system (CNS), where they are processed and the appropriate response is made.

MUSCLE SPINDLES

These are the primary stretch receptors in the muscle which respond to changes in length and rate of stretch. They run parallel to the muscle fibre and are enclosed in a fusiform-shaped spindle, and are known as *intrafusal* fibres. They should not be confused with *extrafusal* fibres which are the contractile units of the muscle itself.

GOLGI TENDON ORGANS

These sensory receptors are located in the tendon close to the musculotendinous junction and respond to force or tension in the muscle. Their function is basically inhibitory and because they have a higher threshold than the muscle spindle, they only come into play after the muscle is vigorously stretched.

STRETCH REFLEX (MYOTATIC REFLEX)

If an individual stretches a muscle or group of muscles with a *ballistic* motion, the muscle spindles come into play and the *stretch reflex* is initiated. The magnitude of this reflex is dependent upon the amount and rate of stretching of the muscle, so that dynamic ballistic stretches invoke the maximal stretch reflex response. When this reflex fires, the muscle which is close to being overstretched suddenly contracts, reducing the extension of the limb. In this way the stretch reflex serves as a mechanism to protect the limb from being overstretched. Individuals should not take part in exercises that are strongly ballistic or bouncy, because this type of action will activate the stretch reflex when the muscle is at full stretch, increasing tension, which should be avoided because a better result will ensue if the muscle is stretched in a relaxed state.

INVERSE STRETCH REFLEX (INVERSE MYOTATIC REFLEX)

This is also known as *autogenic inhibition* and occurs when a *slow* contraction or stretch on a tendon exceeds a critical level. This causes an immediate reflex action which inhibits any further muscular contraction or stretching and the tension is quickly reduced. This reduction of tension acts as a protective mechanism which prevents injury to the muscles and tendons, and is only made possible by the inhibitory impulses of the GTOs, which override the excitatory impulses from the muscle spindles.

The *inverse stretch reflex* can be used, however, if it is carefully controlled, to assist individuals to reach high levels of flexibility. This is done by slowly stretching a muscle group to a point where the tension suddenly dissipates and the muscle relaxes. When this occurs the stretch can be slowly recommenced until the tension reaches another critical point and a further relaxation phase occurs.

Finally, it should be remembered that there is a risk associated with this technique if it is being carried out intensively, because it develops tension in the muscle which may result in soreness and/or injury. Consequently care must be exercised when using the inverse myotatic reflex to achieve extreme ranges of motion.

FLEXIBILITY AND INJURY

There are many causes of sports injuries, but coaches have known for a long time that either a lack of flexibility, or in some cases hypermobility, can cause injury.

Prevention

Moynes (1983) suggested that stretching exercises were of value in the prevention of injury if they were carried out in conjunction with a suitable warm-up and strength training programme. Alter (1988) further stated that more than minimal joint extensibility appeared to be advantageous in some sports, to prevent severe muscle strain and/or joint sprain. In other words there seemed to be an 'ideal or optimal' range of flexibility that will help to prevent muscular injury, particularly in ballistic or collision sports. Hubley-Kozey and Stanish (1984) partially supported this view by suggesting that some athletes, such as gymnasts, must be capable of reaching an extreme range of motion (ROM) without damaging the surrounding tissues.

Many sports, however, do not demand extremely high levels of flexibility, so the coach must 'tailor' the stretching programme to suit each individual. Almost all athletes need a reasonable level of flexibility, which can be of great value to them when they are trying to relax, even though they may not directly need it for their sport. Athletes involved in contact sports, however, must be very careful not to overstretch joints, as they may become unstable and, as a result, easily injured.

DeVries (1986), discussed the phenomenon of muscle soreness which occurred after training, and suggested that certain types of activity were more likely to cause soreness than others. They are as follows:

- Eccentric contractions which will occur in plyometric jumping or downhill running
- Vigorous contractions, carried out while the muscle is in a shortened condition
- Muscle contractions which involve jerky movements or repetitions of the same movements over a long period of time
- Bouncing movements which involve stretching

He further suggested that on many occasions it was not possible to avoid muscle soreness, but recommended that a 10 min period of static stretching can bring about a significant degree of pain prevention.

Rehabilitation

Stretching is frequently used in the rehabilitation of muscle tissue. The muscle must be very slowly returned to its original length with gentle stretching exercises, which will encourage it to re-form in its long state, thus reducing cross-adhesions. At the same time as the above process is occurring, proprioception and tension will be returning.

Where muscle soreness becomes a problem 24–48 h after exercise, gentle *static stretching* should also be used. The athlete should hold each stretch for approximately 2 min and the exercises can be repeated two or three times a day until the soreness subsides.

EFFECT OF GROWTH ON FLEXIBILITY

Childhood and Adolescence

In humans, various systems of the body grow at differing rates and this is the case with the skeletal and the muscular systems, as the former can lead the latter by as much as 6 months (Tanner 1963), thus causing imbalances between the systems. Added to this phenomenon, and mentioned earlier in this chapter, is the bone modelling process which further complicates the individual's training programme. This is because there is still a small amount of cartilage in various parts of the skeleton, especially around the growth plates, which in some cases do not close until late in adolescence.

Problems occur during the many minor growth spurts in a child's life when the long bones grow rapidly and increase the tension of the musculotendinous unit (Leard 1984). This causes tightness around the joints and often places a considerable amount of stress at the epiphyseal attachments. In some cases this causes an avulsion fracture to occur (i.e. the tearing away of a bony landmark to which a muscle is attached) when too much stress is placed on the apophysis (a projection of a bone to which a muscle is attached) by a forceful contraction of a muscle or group of muscles (Watson 1992). Watson (1992) further stated that the most common avulsion fractures in children involve the following muscles and their attachments:

- The forearm flexors attached to the medial epicondyle of the humerus
- The sartorius muscle attached to the anterior superior iliac spine
- The rectus femoris muscle attached to the anterior inferior iliac spine
- The iliopsoas muscle attached to the lesser trochanter of the femur
- The abdominal muscles attached to the iliac crest
- The hamstring muscles attached to the ischial tuberosity
- The patellar tendon attached to the tibial tuberosity
- The Achilles tendon attached to the calcaneus

These injuries are most commonly seen in throwers, sprinters, jumpers, footballers and other agility athletes and occur when a sudden violent contraction is made. With relation to the above problem, and other less specific injuries, Leard (1984) suggested that if stretching exercises were started early in an athlete's career, flexibility should be maintained and many injuries would be prevented.

The reader should also be aware that various musculotendinous syndromes occur from lack of flexibility during childhood and adolescence. Alter (1988) reported that in certain stages of development, the skeleton and the ligamentous and capsular tissues within the joint may not all grow at the same time. This may cause a degree of either hypermobility or hypomobility if there is too little or too much ligamentous tissue at various stages of the child's development. Leard (1984) further pointed out that low levels of flexibility were now thought to be the primary cause of several overuse injuries. These were as follows:

- Tightness of the structures in the popliteal region which prevents full leg extension, was often a characteristic of young athletes with chondromalacia
- Decreased mobility and weakness in the cervical region and the shoulder girdle will sometimes be the predisposing factor which causes medial epicondylitis (little league elbow) and lateral epicondylitis (tennis elbow). Pain in these regions can sometimes be the result of nerve impingement from the neck and can be alleviated if this area becomes more mobile
- Lack of mobility in the thigh flexors and extensors and the lumbosacral region can result in chronic low back pain caused by poor posture

Finally, it is important to understand that with children and adolescent athletes, all muscle groups must be in balance (i.e. antagonists and agonists), both from a flexibility and strength perspective. It must be emphasized again, however, that it is very dangerous to overstretch the immature skeleton, which still has much cartilaginous material in each joint. As the body is very pliable at this time, it may appear that flexibility levels are rapidly improving but there can be long-term deleterious effects on the joints if this is overdone. Coaches should carefully supervise their athletes in order to ensure that no static stretching is done to the point of pain, especially during puberty, when changes are occurring in the musculoskeletal system at a very rapid rate.

Middle and Old Age

Veteran or senior athletes must understand that as they age, their muscles shorten and connective tissue becomes stiffer and tighter. Cartilage steadily calcifies, becomes thinner because of wear and tear and as a result cannot absorb the pressure it could tolerate when the individual was considerably younger. All this leads to a steady reduction of mobility, but if regular stretching is continued, which is not overly stressful, then reasonable levels of flexibility can be maintained. Alter (1990) made an additional interesting point when he stated that 'stretching stimulates the production or retention of lubricants between the connective tissue fibres, thus preventing the formation of adhesions'.

Older athletes should be careful of the knee joints and the lumbar region of the spine when they stretch, especially the L5–S1 joint and the facet joints, which are very susceptible to stress and strain. Osteoarthritis can affect these and other joints and this problem can be exacerbated by ballistic ('bouncy') stretching. Caution must therefore be shown with the type of stretching performed by senior athletes, but if they adhere to a static stretching routine which is not to the point of pain, they should avoid many of the problems which occur in less prudent individuals.

FLEXIBILITY MEASUREMENT

Cureton (1951) was one of the first sport scientists to systematically measure the flexibility of champion athletes and several of the field tests he formulated are still used today. Flexibility testing was at first crude, but has become more sophisticated during the past two decades and because of its importance in sport, will become more so in the future.

Static Testing

Static testing is a method of measurement carried out with the subjects in a non-dynamic situation, meaning that they are not performing a sport skill at the time, but rather having their range of movement assessed in a laboratory environment.

FIELD TESTS

These are tests where there is a small degree of subjectivity in the rating procedure; however, they are useful for coaches in the field. The assessment can be carried out quickly and a rating scale is used in order to give the subject a specific numerical rating for each joint (Fig. 14.35).

Other tests, which sometimes include several joints, have been used for some time and are general indicators of regional flexibility. The most popular, despite its lack of validity (see Chapter 14), is the *sit-and-reach test*, where the subject sits on the floor with the legs extended in front and with the feet pressed against a box which supports a measuring stick. With the legs flat on the floor, the trunk is flexed at the hip joints and the arms are fully extended along the measuring stick. Three other tests which are sometimes used to gauge general flexibility are the *trunk-and-neck extension test, the shoulder rotation test* and the *ankle flexion–extension test*. These tests are fully described in Johnson and Nelson (1979).

LABORATORY TESTS

There are various levels of sophistication in these tests, ranging from the use of a simple goniometer to sophisticated instrumentation. The simplest device for measuring static flexibility is the *goniometer*, which is a protractor with two moveable arms attached to it. It measures the angle between two body segments at the extreme ends of the ROM. The tester must be very careful to locate the axis of the bones that form the joint and be aware that the soft tissue around the joint can influence the accuracy of the measurement.

A more sophisticated goniometer known as the *electrogoniometer or 'elgon'* (Fig. 14.47) incorporates a potentiometer at the axis of the two measurement arms. Changes in the joint angle are recorded as voltage fluctuations, thus providing a real time, analogue display of joint motion. This device may therefore be used to provide measurements of static as well as functional flexibility. Recent advances in elgon technology have permitted the recording of three-dimensional movements without the previous encumbrance to normal athletic performance.

Rather than measure the angle between two body segments, the *Leighton flexometer* (Fig. 14.36), a device containing two rotating and weighted dials, may be used to record the motion of the single, isolated segment with respect to the perpendicular plane. The body segment is moved through its full range of motion and the flexometer records the angular displacement in degrees. With this instrument, it is of paramount importance that other body regions be held rigid, so that only movements of the isolated segment are recorded. Care should also be taken to ensure that the dynamic posture is accurately simulated and that the correct plane of movement is followed. This technique usually requires some passive guidance by the tester.

Functional Testing

The athlete's flexibility during the execution of a closed skill has been generally neglected by coaches and sport scientists. The use of high-speed cinematography or videography to provide a two-dimensional or three-dimensional reconstruction of athletic performance is used extensively in the field of biomechanics in technique analysis. These tools may also be used to measure functional flexibility during activity. It is important to have the subject perform with a minimum of clothing, so that the bony landmarks can be marked, then clearly seen, when each individual film or video is analysed. Such a system is advantageous in that the ROM in various movements which involve a combination of joints may be measured during actual athletic performance, but as yet it has not been fully developed and utilized to its full potential, mainly because of the time and cost involved.

METHODS USED TO INCREASE FLEXIBILITY

Traditional stretching exercises which have been used in sport have been ballistic in nature. Kiputh's (1942) text on swimming was one of the first to present a specialized series of flexibility exercises and this was soon followed by others, especially for track and field athletes. When discussing methods to improve the ROM, DeVries (1986) stated:

> Conventional callisthenic exercises used for this purpose have usually involved hopping, bouncing, or jerky movements in which one body segment is put in movement by active contraction of a muscle group and the momentum then arrested by the antagonists at the end of the range of motion. Thus the antagonists are stretched by the dynamic movements of the agonists. Because momentum is involved, this system has been called the *ballistic method*.

Ballistic Stretching

Ballistic stretching was used for approximately 50 years and was never questioned, until sport scientists and sports medicine specialists began to report that it could lead to injury and muscle soreness.

DISADVANTAGES OF BALLISTIC STRETCHING

Alter (1988) suggested that there were several reasons why ballistic stretching was not the best system to use and these are as follows:

- When connective tissue is rapidly stretched it does not have time to adequately adjust and this can result in soreness or injury
- If a sudden stretch is applied to a muscle, a reflex action occurs which causes the muscle to contract. This then causes muscle tension to increase, making it more difficult to stretch the connective tissue. Further, with the muscle being stretched and contracted at the same time, the likelihood of injury is reasonably high
- It has also been found that a quick stretch does not allow time for neurological adaptation to take place when one compares it to a slow stretch. This in itself will be a limiting factor in the improvement of flexibility

ADVANTAGES OF BALLISTIC STRETCHING

Some coaches still support ballistic stretching because they maintain that many movements in sport are ballistic in nature. Its supporters suggest that it is specific to sport and provided it is done with caution and the athlete does not overstretch, it can be an effective way to increase flexibility. When the sport has a strong agility component and the development of elastic energy is necessary, there is no reason why a certain number of exercises cannot be ballistic in nature, especially if they are very specific to the sport. However, it is of great importance that the musculature is thoroughly warmed up prior to performing ballistic stretching.

Static Stretching

Static stretching involves holding a static position for a period of time after the limb has already been stretched and it has become very popular during the past decade, because it is both effective and relatively safe. Simply put, it involves a slow stretch (to inhibit the firing of the stretch reflex) almost to the point of resistance, where it is then held for 20–30 s or even up to 60 s if necessary. During this time the tension partially diminishes (due to the inverse stretch reflex) and the athlete slowly moves into a deeper stretch and repeats the above.

ADVANTAGES AND DISADVANTAGES OF STATIC STRETCHING

It is difficult to find any good reason why static stretching should not make up the majority of any worthwhile flexibility programme, despite the fact that some coaches feel that sport specific ballistic exercises are better for some sports. Currently there is strong support for static stretching among sport scientists and coaches, first because it gives very good results and second because it results in less muscle soreness and injury. Furthermore, slow stretching allows muscle relaxation to occur as a result of the firing of the GTOs if the stretch is performed over a reasonable time.

COMPARISON OF BALLISTIC AND STATIC STRETCHING

DeVries (1962) compared ballistic and static stretching methods and found that each type resulted in significant improvements in flexibility. He also found that neither system was better than the other in terms of the amount of mobility achieved, but stated that static stretching offers three advantages over the ballistic method. These were as follows:

- 'There is less danger of exceeding the extensibility limits of the tissues involved
- Energy requirements are lower
- Although ballistic stretching is apt to cause muscular soreness, static stretching will not; in fact the latter relieves soreness'

Proprioceptive Neuromuscular Facilitation

Proprioceptive neuromuscular facilitation (PNF) is primarily based on Kabat's (1958) PNF theory which was first adapted for use in physiotherapy, then later in sport. It was hypothesized that an increased ROM was promoted through the principles of successive induction, autogenic inhibition and active mobilization of connective tissues (Holt 1974). Specifically it was suggested that greater muscle relaxation occurs after a significant contraction of the muscle. This may occur as a result of a reduced discharge of the muscle due to increased GTO activity.

There are many different combinations of PNF stretching and these can be found in Holt (1974), Alter (1988) and McAtee (1993). The most common technique which is currently used in sport is as follows.

CONTRACT–RELAX–CONTRACT TECHNIQUE

Sometimes known as Scientific Stretching for Sport (3S), this is the most utilized method of the PNF techniques within the sport community. It was popularized by Holt (1974) and used with good results. For each exercise the muscle is initially placed in a lengthened position, then isometrically contracted against the immovable resistance of a partner for 6 s. This is followed by a *very brief* period of relaxation, after which the athlete contracts the appropriate muscle group, placing the body part into a new position. This movement is aided by the partner with *light pressure,* which allows for a greater ROM to be achieved than in a static stretch (Fig. 10.32). The exercise is then repeated three or four times. It should be noted that a special computer-controlled flexibility system known as FLEX.SYS has been recently developed in order to carry out the exercises without a partner assisting (Fig. 10.1).

ADVANTAGES AND DISADVANTAGES OF PNF

The supporters of PNF stretching claim that this technique increases the range of motion in a shorter time than several of the other techniques. This claim has been strongly supported by research performed by Wallin *et al.* (1985) who reported that PNF stretching techniques increased flexibility to a greater extent than ballistic stretching methods. The second advantage appears to be that there is a *slight* gain in strength at the same time that the ROM is being increased.

However, there are critics of the method who suggest that there is an increased chance of injury if the partner is incompetent and applies too much pressure. If care is taken, however, and the individual assisting the athlete is given verbal instructions, this should not occur.

Other Techniques

ACTIVE STRETCHING

The athlete alone is responsible for the stretching without the assistance of any external force, whether from a partner or from equipment. The individual should carry out this method slowly in order that the stretch reflex is not initiated. There is no need under this method for the athlete to stay at the full range of the stretch for more than 2 or 3 s.

PASSIVE STRETCHING

Where athletes in such sports as gymnastics, diving, skating, track and field and swimming need an extreme range of flexibility in certain joints, the passive stretching system is of great value. When using this technique the athlete stays relaxed and makes no active contribution to the stretch, which should be done slowly and with care, because if it is carried out jerkily or outside the athlete's normal ROM an injury to a muscle

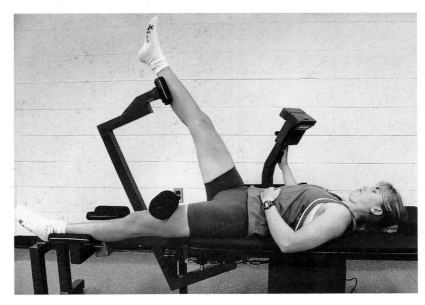

Fig. 10.1 The FLEX.SYS computer-controlled flexibility system (courtesy of FLEX.SYS).

and/or joint could occur. An external force is usually created by a partner (Fig. 10.2); however, it can also be with a piece of equipment. The partner method is well known, but the use of equipment has only developed with the variable resistance strength training machines, which can place the muscle on passive stretch, with a slight change in posture near the end of each repetition (Fig. 10.3). The advantages of this method are as follows:

- It allows the individual to stretch *well beyond* the active limit
- It is effective when the agonist (the muscle group responsible for the movement) is too weak to initiate a movement which will move the limb through the full ROM
- Because this technique is usually carried out in pairs it creates an enjoyable social atmosphere for the participants

In some situations where athletes are attempting to recover the normal range of movement after a soft tissue injury, or wish to increase their flexibility, *performance massage* (King 1993) and light mobilization should be used before passive stretching is carried out. Those athletes who have experienced it, attest to its definite value. As well, performance massage, in combination with light passive stretching, is also being used after strenuous competition or even heavy workouts, in order to relax the athlete as well as contributing to his or her flexibility.

STRETCHING GUIDELINES

During the past decade, informed coaches' attitudes have changed, first with relation to the value of flexibility and second with regard to the way it should be done. The old-fashioned approach was to stretch, often ballistically, to the point of pain and with an inadequate build-up. It is important for coaches to understand that stretching cannot be rushed and that it takes several years of flexibility training for an athlete to become proficient in carrying out these exercises.

As was previously mentioned, flexibility training is now an important part of many sport train-

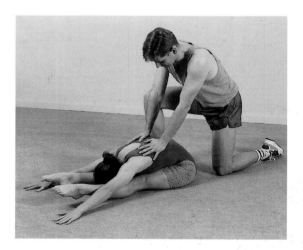

Fig. 10.2 An elite gymnast undergoing passive stretching.

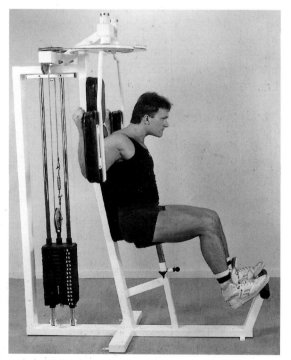

Fig. 10.3 Passive stretching using a variable resistance machine.

ing regimens. It is also used extensively for the purposes of warming up and warming down. The following sections consist of guidelines that should be adhered to if the full benefits from flexibility training are to be obtained.

Preparation for Stretching

The area where the exercises are performed should be reasonably comfortable and warm and non-restrictive clothing which allows the athlete to stretch with ease should be worn. The individual should be in a relaxed state and warmed up before the exercises commence. At least a mild sweat must be reached before the stretching routine is started, otherwise an injury could occur.

Concentration during the Exercises

During a stretching session the athlete must carefully monitor the amount of tension that is developed in the muscles. Each exercise must be commenced in a very relaxed state. Some coaches suggest that athletes develop a mental image of themselves in a particular situation which will help them to relax before each exercise. For example, they may be able to visualize themselves lying in a warm saline bath in which they can float easily in a relaxed situation.

Athletes should also become aware of their breathing pattern and a useful technique is to slow down the breathing rate and increase the depth of each breath for the first five or six breaths in each exercise. A steady light pattern should follow the slightly deeper and longer breathing technique for the remainder of each exercise.

Specificity of the Exercises

When stretching to improve the range of motion for any skill, the individual should carry out the stretch in the same postural position, the same plane of motion and through the same range of movement as the skill, if each or all of these are possible. If *ballistic stretching* is performed, then the stretch should be done in a similar way and at 75–80% of the speed of the skill, but *only after the muscle groups involved have first been warmed up and then stretched by the static method.*

Applying Stretching Principles

In order for the ROM to be improved in any part of the body, various stretching principles must be applied. The actual stretching of the muscle group can be done from *20 to 30 s*; however, this can last for up to *60 s* if several 'small relaxations' are felt during the stretch. Each time one of these occurs the athlete is then able to stretch a little further. Between *four and eight* repetitions can be carried out for each exercise; however, this will depend on the amount of mobility training the athletes have already done during their competitive career.

Furthermore, the number of training sessions per day will be determined by the amount of improvement the athletes wish to make. One session a day, depending on its length, will result in an improvement in flexibility; however, two sessions are needed if any significant improvement is to be made in the short term. One of these is usually done in the morning and the other in the afternoon unless other training arrangements are more suitable. Once the appropriate level of flexibility has been achieved, one training session per week has been shown by Wallin *et al.* (1985) to be adequate to maintain an established level of flexibility. It should also be mentioned that unless warm-up and warm-down stretching sessions are of reasonable duration, they should not be regarded as flexibility training. They are in fact done as a preparation for normal training but in some cases, where a high degree of flexibility is not needed in the sport, they will provide athletes with enough stretchability to enable them to relax when needed. It should be emphasized that some athletes like gymnasts, divers, skaters, some swimmers and those competing in the field events will need specific flexibility training sessions, otherwise they will *never* reach the levels required for their sport.

Intensity of the Stretch

It cannot be stressed too often, that although stretching exercises will produce a degree of discomfort, they should *not cause pain*. If the muscle vibrates or quivers and pain is present, then the athlete should cut down the force applied or limit the ROM. To force a joint past the point of discomfort will *finally result in an injury*.

Dangers Involved in Stretching

The notion that 'some stretching is good, so that more stretching is better' can be quite dangerous to the majority of athletes, especially those involved in collision sports and masters or veteran athletes, because excessive stretching can destabilize their joints, causing ligament or joint capsule injury. Athletes who have had a recent bone fracture, inflammation or infection in or around a joint, or a chronic sprain or strain, should be cautious with their programme.

The athlete should also perform stretching exercises in the correct postural position and not place limbs and the accompanying joints out of alignment. When malalignment occurs and the individual puts considerable pressure on the joint, an injury will almost certainly occur. Moreover, there are certain exercises which middle-aged sports people should not do and several of these have been well illustrated by Alter (1990).

SPECIFIC STRETCHING EXERCISES

In previous parts of this chapter a preference for the *static stretching* technique has been mentioned and much of the following section will be devoted to this; however, the PNF (3S) technique will also be described below.

Specific Guidelines for Static Stretching

In static stretching (SS), the muscle group is held on stretch for a period of *20–30 s*, but can be held

for *60 s* if necessary (Anderson 1980; Beaulieu 1981; Alter 1990). This will basically depend, however, on whether one can utilize the 'small relaxations' that occur during the stretch.

- The *primary* stretch is held for approximately *10 s*, after which a *secondary* stretch is made
- The entire stretch (i.e. both *primary* and *secondary*) will usually take approximately *20–30 s* to execute when the technique has been perfected, but could be slightly less or more depending on whether the desired result has been achieved
- It is very important to hold the *primary* stretch until the inverse stretch reflex occurs and a slight relaxation is felt
- The *primary* and *secondary* stretches must be done very slowly with no pressure or jerkiness. If this occurs there will be a rebound effect from the stretch reflex and some loss of control during the stretch
- At the completion of the stretch the muscle group should be released slowly and under control
- Approximately *four sets* of each exercise should be done during each workout, although this may be too many in the early stages of a flexibility training programme. As was stated earlier in this chapter it can be increased to *eight sets* later in the programme
- It is important to keep agonists and antagonists in balance by stretching each group during a workout. The athlete should also keep each side of the body in balance, unless there is a logical reason not to do so
- There is currently some disagreement as to the order in which the stretching routine should be done. Traditionally exercises have been alternated over the various regions of the body. More recently some sport scientists and coaches have suggested that the athlete should concentrate on one part of the body using several exercises, then move to another, then to another part and so on. There is currently no scientific evidence available which supports one method over the other

- Flexibility training should be carried out each day in either one or two sessions depending on the sport. There should be *at least* 1 day off each week
- It may be of value to use equipment or a partner for support purposes with some exercises. Others can be done quite effectively without them

General Guidelines for PNF Stretching (3S)

In PNF stretching (3S), increased flexibility is gained by using an isometric contraction of the muscles to be stretched for *6 s*, followed by a concentric contraction of the opposite muscle group, with *light pressure* being applied by the partner. The concentric contraction should last approximately *6–10 s* (Fig. 10.32).

Each exercise should be repeated *three* to *four* times during each training session and up to two training sessions per day can be done. At least *1 day* each week should be used for rest and no flexibility training should be carried out.

There is no hard or fast rule with relation to the order of the exercise routine; however most athletes adopt the alternating regional system.

SPECIFIC EXERCISE ROUTINES

Individual Exercises (SS)

No. 1 Neck stretch (Fig. 10.4)

- The athlete sits or stands in a comfortable position
- The head is very *slowly* rolled around through 360°, first in a clockwise direction and then anti-clockwise

No. 2 Tricep stretch (Fig. 10.5)

- The athlete stands upright with one arm flexed behind the head and the hand resting on the upper back. The elbow of the flexed arm should be held with the other hand

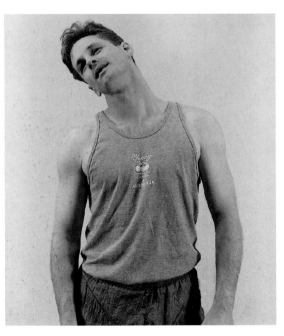

Fig. 10.4 Neck stretch.

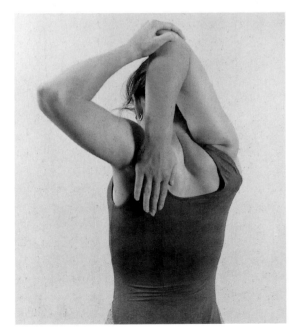

Fig. 10.5 Tricep stretch.

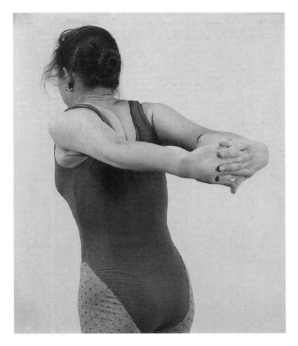

Fig. 10.6 Backward stretch.

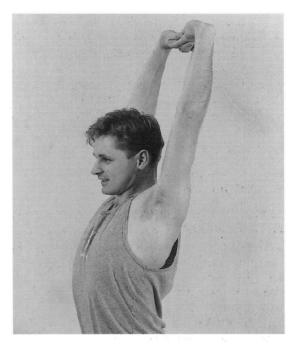

Fig. 10.7 Overhead stretch.

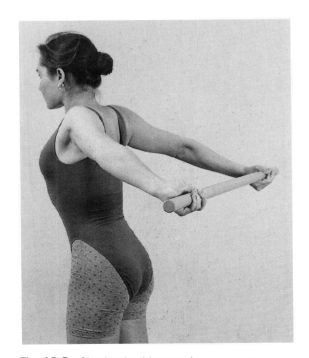

Fig. 10.8 Circular shoulder stretch.

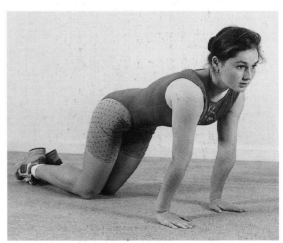

Fig. 10.9 Hand–forearm stretch.

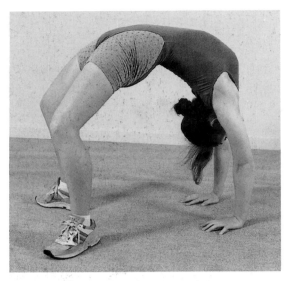

Fig. 10.10 Abdominal and hip stretch.

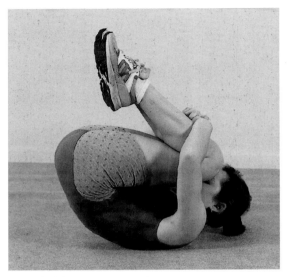

Fig. 10.11 Back roll stretch.

- The athlete then *slowly* pulls the elbow down and behind the head
- After the desired number of repeats has been performed, the other arm should be *slowly* stretched

No. 3 Backward stretch (Fig. 10.6)

- The athlete stands upright and extends the arms behind the trunk and interlocks the fingers
- The arms are then *slowly* raised behind the body

No. 4 Overhead stretch (Fig. 10.7)

- The athlete stands upright and interlocks the fingers above the head with the palms facing upward
- The arms and hands are then slowly pushed up and back

No. 5 Circular shoulder stretch (Fig. 10.8)

- The athlete stands upright and grasps a towel or light pole in front of the hips, using a normal grip
- Keeping the arms straight, the towel or pole

should be *slowly* raised over the head and down to a point where it is just behind the buttocks
- Using the same technique, the towel or pole should then be brought back to the starting position
- When commencing this exercise, the athlete should take a wide grip on the towel or pole, then slowly narrow it as flexibility improves, otherwise an injury could occur

No. 6 Hand–forearm stretch (Fig. 10.9)

- The athlete kneels on the floor with the palms down and the fingers facing away from the body
- The subject then leans *slowly* forward, then back

No. 7 Abdominal and hip stretch (Fig. 10.10)

- The athlete lies on the back with the heels close to the hips and the hands on the floor behind the shoulders
- The subject then *slowly* raises the trunk off the floor, balancing on the feet and hands

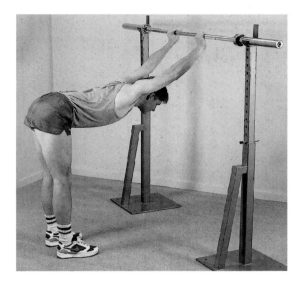

Fig. 10.12 Upper back stretch.

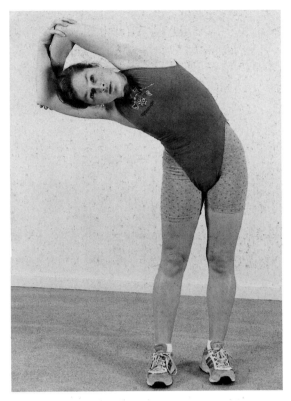

Fig. 10.13 Lateral trunk stretch.

- If the athlete is not flexible enough to raise the forehead from the floor and almost straighten the arms and legs, then a modified version of the exercise can be performed with the forehead resting on the floor

No. 8 Back roll stretch (Fig. 10.11)

- While in a sitting position the athlete holds the knees with the hands and pulls them to the chest
- The subject then *slowly* rolls backwards and forwards several times in a tight tuck
- To develop a tighter tuck, the lower legs can be crossed and pulled towards the chest while rolling back, then placed into the normal position when rolling forward

No. 9 Upper back stretch (Fig. 10.12)

- The athlete grips the bar and moves the feet to a position approximately 1.5 m from it. He/she should then bend at the waist, and extend the arms
- The subject then presses down *slowly* on the bar by pushing the chest towards the floor. It is important to make sure that the head is an extension of the trunk at all times

No. 10 Lateral trunk stretch (Fig. 10.13)

- The athlete stands upright with the legs comfortably apart, and the hands gripping the opposite elbow
- The subject then bends *slowly* sideways from the waist, and gently but firmly pulls the elbow behind the head at the same time
- When the desired number of repeats has been performed, the other side of the body should be stretched

No. 11 Lower back and hip stretch (Fig. 10.14)

- The athlete lies on the back and pulls one leg up, until it is flexed to 90° at the hip and knee joints. The flexed leg should then be gripped above the knee joint with the opposite hand
- The knee is then pulled across the body to the floor and at the same time the head and shoul-

ders are kept flat on the floor. While the leg is being *slowly* pulled across, the head can be turned to the opposite side for more stretch

- When the desired number of repeats has been performed, the other side should be stretched

No. 12 Rotational trunk stretch (Fig. 10.15)

- The athlete stands about 0.5 m from a wall facing away from it, with the feet shoulder width apart
- The subject then turns *slowly* in one direction and places both hands on the wall, then turns in the other direction repeating the same movement

No. 13 Groin stretch - 1 (Fig. 10.16)

- The athlete sits upright, flexes the thighs and legs and brings the soles of the feet together. The legs are then lightly gripped above the ankle and the elbows rest on the inside portion of the thighs above the knee
- The elbows are then used to push the athlete's knees *slowly* to the floor

No. 14 Groin stretch - 2 (Fig. 10.17)

- The athlete sits upright, flexes the thighs and legs and brings the soles of the feet together. The feet are then gripped with the hands and held together

- The subject then leans *slowly* forward as far as possible from the waist without bending the back

No. 15 Groin stretch - 3 (Fig. 10.18)

- The athlete lies on the back, with the thighs and legs flexed, and the soles of the feet together. The feet should also be placed close to the buttocks
- The subject then *slowly* lowers the knees towards the floor while keeping the soles of the feet together

No. 16 Side split stretch (Fig. 10.19)

- The athlete stands with the feet pointed straight ahead
- He/she *slowly* spreads the legs sideways using the hands for balance

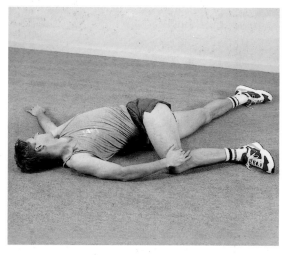

Fig. 10.14 Lower back and hip stretch.

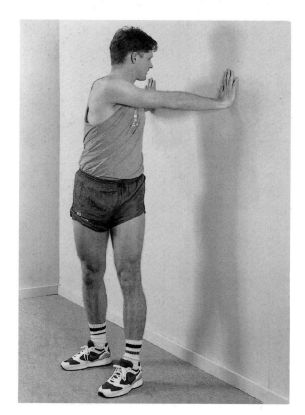

Fig. 10.15 Rotational trunk stretch.

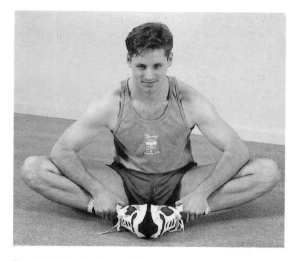

Fig. 10.16 Groin stretch - 1.

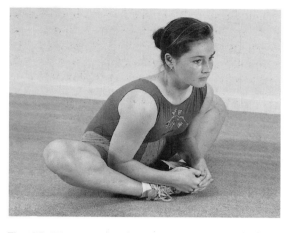

Fig. 10.17 Groin stretch - 2.

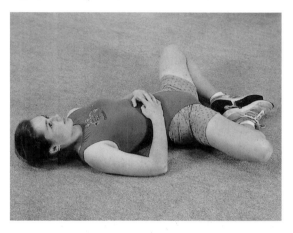

Fig. 10.18 Groin stretch - 3.

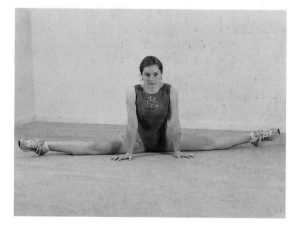

Fig. 10.19 Side split stretch.

- As the athlete becomes more skilled, he/she can keep the toes up and slide sideways on the heels

Note that this exercise should only be performed by a *very* supple athlete.

No. 17 Split stretch (Fig. 10.20)

- The athlete kneels with the legs together and fingers touching the floor close to the knees
- One leg is then slid forward with the body over it, to a position where the knee joint is over the foot. This forward movement partially extends the rear thigh, whose knee joint is resting lightly on the floor
- The front foot is then moved further forward on the heel using the hands for balance
- The athlete continues to move the front foot forward *slowly* while lowering the hips towards the floor. The hands must be used for balance and the trunk should be kept in a vertical position

Note that this exercise should only be performed by a *very* supple athlete.

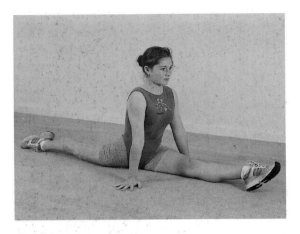

Fig. 10.20 Split stretch.

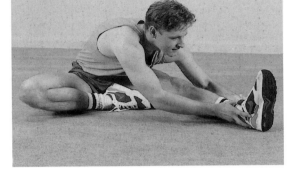

Fig. 10.21 Hamstring stretch - 1.

No. 18 Hamstring stretch - 1 (Fig. 10.21)

- The athlete sits upright with one leg extended and the other leg flexed, with the sole of the foot close to the thigh of the extended limb
- The athlete should then bend at the waist, and slowly lower the upper torso on to the thigh while stretching the extended arms out to grip the ankle. The extended leg must be kept straight at all times
- When the desired number of repeats has been performed, the other limb should be stretched

No. 19 Hamstring stretch - 2 (Fig. 10.22)

- The athlete lies on the back with the legs flexed and the heels reasonably close to the buttocks
- The thigh is then flexed and grasped with one hand above the knee, while the other hand holds the foot. The athlete then *slowly* pulls the limb towards the trunk, which should remain as straight as possible at all times
- When the desired number of repeats has been performed, the other limb should be stretched

No. 20 Hamstring stretch - 3 (Fig. 10.23)

- The athlete stands upright and raises one limb so that it rests on a platform at about hip height
- Keeping both limbs straight, the athlete then

slowly bends forward at the waist and lowers the trunk on to the thigh
- The hands should grip the ankles to assist the trunk flexion
- When the desired number of repeats has been performed, the other limb should be stretched

No. 21 Groin–trunk stretch (Fig. 10.24)

- The athlete stands upright with the feet parallel to a supporting surface
- One limb is then raised sideways onto this surface, with the heel and calf resting on it
- The athlete should then raise the hands above the head and bend *slowly* sideways, lowering the upper trunk towards the raised limb
- When the desired number of repeats has been performed, the other limb should be stretched

No. 22 Quadriceps stretch - 1 (Fig. 10.25)

- The athlete sits upright with one leg flexed and the heel close to the buttock. The other leg is then flexed and the sole of the foot is placed close to the other knee
- The athlete *slowly* leans back using the hands to support the trunk
- When the desired number of repeats has been performed, the other leg should be stretched

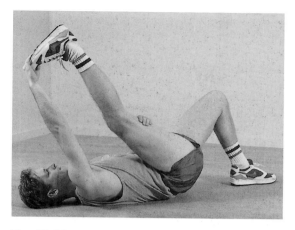

Fig. 10.22 Hamstring stretch - 2.

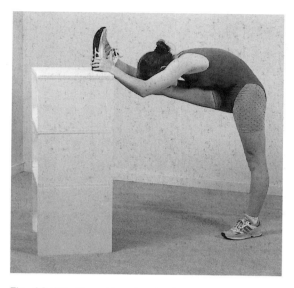

Fig. 10.23 Hamstring stretch - 3.

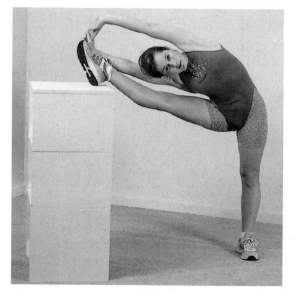

Fig. 10.24 Groin–trunk stretch.

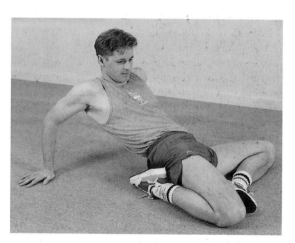

Fig. 10.25 Quadriceps stretch - 1.

No. 23 Quadriceps–ankle stretch (Fig. 10.26)

- The athlete sits on the heels with the toes pointed backwards
- The subject then *slowly* bends backward using the hands to balance the trunk until the shoulders touch the floor

No. 24 Quadriceps–groin stretch (Fig. 10.27)

- The athlete kneels with one foot forward and the other foot back in a similar position to an elementary crouch start. The hands are close to the forward foot
- With the back thigh partly extended behind the body, the hip and thigh are *slowly* lowered towards the floor
- When the desired number of repeats has been performed, the other side of the body should be stretched

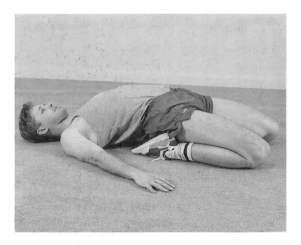

Fig. 10.26 Quadriceps–ankle stretch.

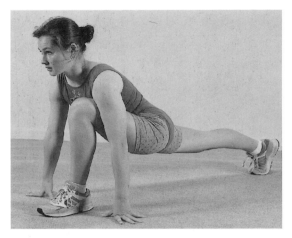

Fig. 10.27 Quadriceps–groin stretch.

No. 25 Quadriceps stretch - 2 (Fig. 10.28)

- The athlete stands partially upright and leans against a vertical surface for support
- The athlete then flexes one leg so that the foot is close to the back of the thigh. The foot is then gripped by the hand on the opposite side of the body
- The foot is then *slowly* pulled upwards
- When the desired number of repeats has been performed, the other limb should be stretched

No. 26 Calf stretch (Fig. 10.29)

- The athlete stands partially upright and leans against a vertical surface for support
- The athlete then places one foot forward and partially flexes the leg at the knee joint, with the other leg being kept extended behind the body
- The hips should then be *slowly* moved forward while keeping the trunk and back limb straight
- When the desired number of repeats has been performed, the other side of the body should be stretched

No. 27 Achilles tendon–ankle stretch (Fig. 10.30)

- The athlete takes up a kneeling position, then moves one foot forward so that the toes are level with the other knee. The arms should then be extended with the hands approximately 0.5 m in front of the shoulders

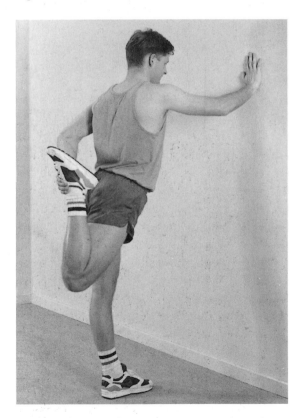

Fig. 10.28 Quadriceps stretch - 2.

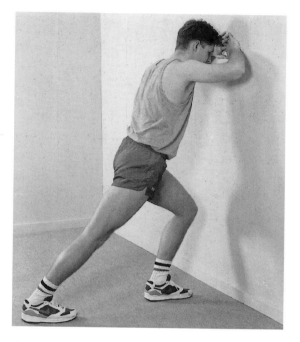

Fig. 10.29 Calf stretch.

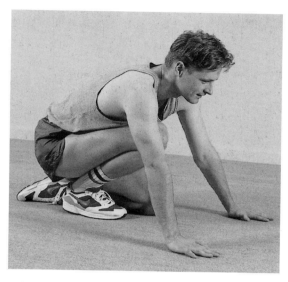

Fig. 10.30 Achilles tendon–ankle stretch.

- The athlete then *slowly* leans forward from the shoulders, keeping the heel of the front foot on the floor
- When the desired number of repeats has been performed, the other leg should be stretched

No. 28 Ankle stretch (Fig. 10.31)

- The athlete sits with one leg extended and the other flexed and just off the floor. One hand should grip the foot and the other should hold the lower leg above the ankle joint
- The athlete then *slowly* rotates the foot, first in a clockwise direction and then anti-clockwise, through the complete ROM. The hand gripping the foot should provide slight resistance
- When the desired number of repeats has been performed, the other ankle is stretched

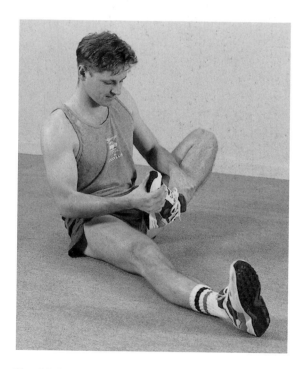

Fig. 10.31 Ankle stretch.

Partner Exercises (PNF)

No. 29 Arm extensor stretch (Fig. 10.32)

- The athlete (a) adopts a long sitting position with the arms extended above the head
- The partner (p) stands behind the athlete with one foot behind the other's buttocks, the knee resting against the athlete's spine and grasps both arms above the wrist joint
- The athlete *slowly* pulls the arms towards the legs and the partner resists, causing an isometric contraction to occur
- After the position has been held for *6 s*, the athlete *slowly* pushes the arms back while the partner assists with light pressure

No. 30 Arm adductor stretch (Fig. 10.33)

- The athlete (a) adopts a long sitting position with the arms abducted to the horizontal plane
- The partner (p) stands behind the athlete with one foot touching the other's buttocks, the knee resting against the athlete's spine and grasps both arms above the wrist joint
- The athlete *slowly* pulls the arms forward and the partner resists, causing an isometric contraction to occur
- After the position has been held for *6 s*, the athlete *slowly* pushes the arms back while the partner assists with light pressure

No. 31 Trunk lateral flexor stretch (Fig. 10.34)

- The athlete (a) adopts a standing position with one forearm flexed at the elbow joint and the trunk slightly bent to one side
- The partner (p) stands on the convex side with one hand on the athlete's waist and the other hand holding the athlete's raised upper arm
- The athlete *slowly* pushes the body towards an upright position while the partner resists, causing an isometric contraction to occur
- After the position has been held for *6 s*, the athlete *slowly* pulls the trunk downwards while the partner assists with light pressure
- When the desired number of repeats has been performed, the other side of the trunk should be stretched

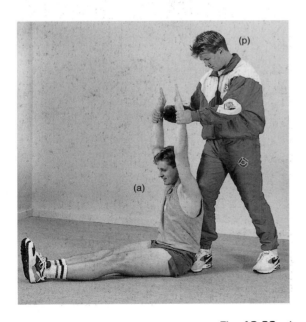
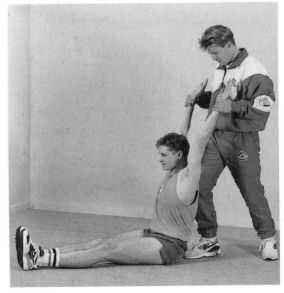

Fig. 10.32 Arm extensor stretch.

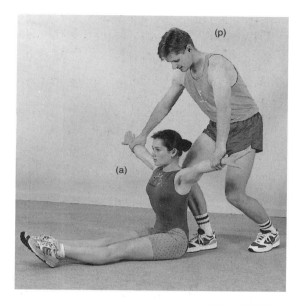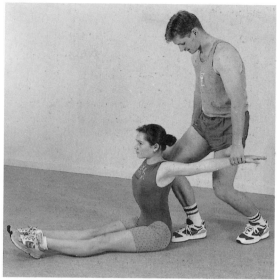

Fig. 10.33 Arm adductor stretch.

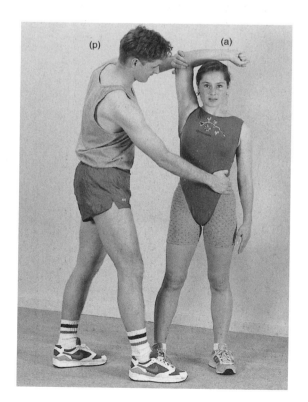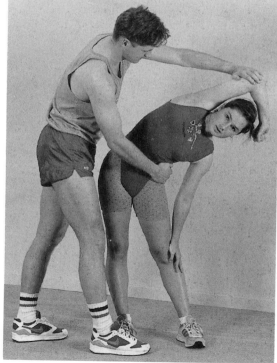

Fig. 10.34 Trunk lateral flexor stretch.

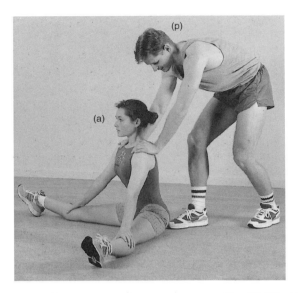
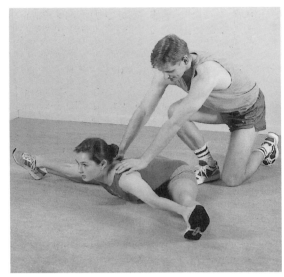

Fig. 10.35 Split pike stretch.

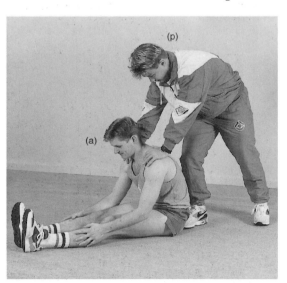
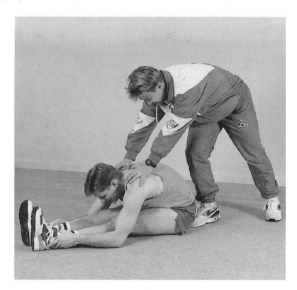

Fig. 10.36 Trunk extensor stretch.

No. 32 Split pike stretch (Fig. 10.35)

- The athlete (a) adopts a sitting position, with a slight forward lean, and the legs extended and spread as far as possible to the side. The hands are placed on top of the legs just above the ankle

- The partner (p) stands behind the athlete with the hands on the other's shoulders
- The athlete *slowly* pushes back while the partner resists, causing an isometric contraction to occur
- After the position has been held for *6 s*, the

athlete *slowly* pulls the trunk forward and downward while the partner assists with light pressure

No. 33 Trunk extensor stretch (Fig. 10.36)

- The athlete (a) adopts a long sitting position, with a forward lean and with the hands grasping the leg above the ankle joint
- The partner (p) stands behind the athlete with one hand on the neck and the other in the middle of the upper back
- The athlete *slowly* pushes back while the partner resists, causing an isometric contraction to occur
- After the position has been held for *6 s* the athlete slowly pulls the trunk forward while the partner assists with light pressure

No. 34 Thigh adductor stretch (Fig. 10.37)

- The athlete (a) lies on the back with the thighs flexed and abducted
- The partner (p) stands in front of the athlete holding the other's legs above the ankle joint
- The athlete *slowly* attempts to adduct the thighs

while the partner resists, causing an isometric contraction to occur
- After the position has been held for *6 s* the athlete *slowly* pulls the legs apart while the partner assists with light pressure

No. 35 Thigh extensor stretch - 1 (Fig. 10.38)

- The athlete (a) lies on the back, with one limb on the floor and the other limb raised in the air. Both limbs must be kept straight throughout the exercise
- The partner (p) kneels on one knee with the opposite foot on the floor and with the shoulder against the back of the athlete's raised leg. The partner grips the leg to be stretched with one hand and the leg which is flat on the floor with the other
- The athlete *slowly* attempts to push the raised limb to the floor while the partner resists, causing an isometric contraction to occur
- After the position has been held for *6 s* the athlete *slowly* flexes the thigh towards the head while the partner assists with light pressure

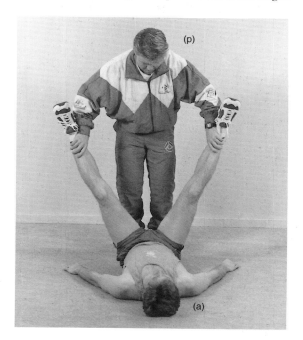 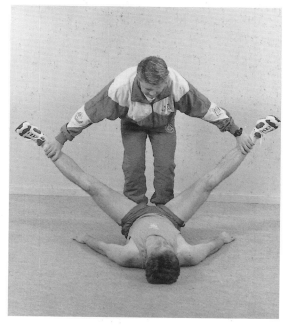

Fig. 10.37 Thigh adductor stretch.

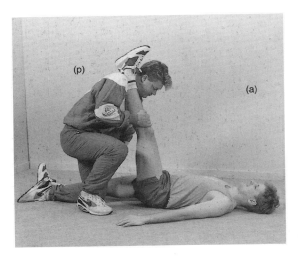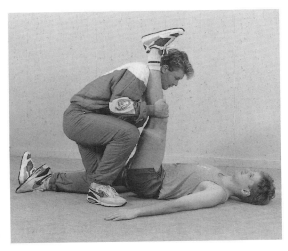

Fig. 10.38 Thigh extensor stretch - 1.

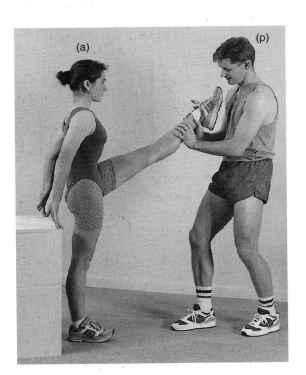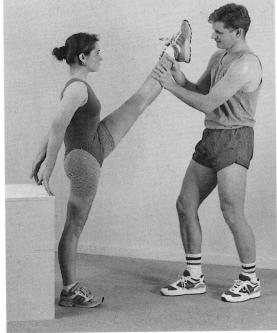

Fig. 10.39 Thigh extensor stretch - 2.

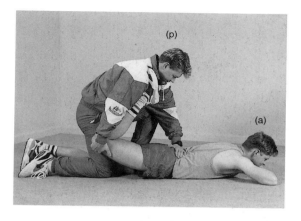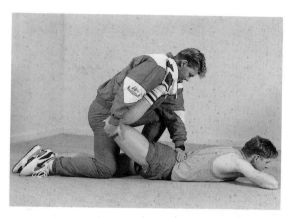

Fig. 10.40 Thigh flexor stretch - 1.

- When the desired number of repeats has been performed, the other limb should be stretched

No. 36 Thigh extensor stretch - 2 (Fig. 10.39)

- The athlete (a) stands on one limb and lifts the other, keeping it straight and to the front. The hands are placed behind the back supporting the body on a table, chair or bench
- The partner (p) stands in front of the athlete, holding the other's leg above the ankle joint with both hands
- The athlete *slowly* attempts to push the raised limb towards the floor, keeping the knee straight while the partner resists, causing an isometric contraction to occur
- After the position has been held for *6 s* the athlete *slowly* flexes the thigh while the partner assists with light pressure
- When the desired number of repeats has been performed, the other limb should be stretched

No. 37 Thigh flexor stretch - 1 (Fig. 10.40)

- The athlete (a) lies prone on the floor with one leg flexed at the knee joint and raised as high as possible
- The partner (p) kneels on one knee, placing it directly beside the athlete's knee, with the other foot level with the athlete's buttocks. The partner grips the athlete's thigh close to the knee

joint, and places the other hand slightly above the buttock
- The athlete *slowly* attempts to push the knee downward while the partner resists, causing an isometric contraction to occur
- After the position has been held for *6 s* the athlete slowly extends the thigh while the partner assists with light pressure
- When the desired number of repeats has been performed, the other limb should be stretched

No. 38 Thigh flexor stretch - 2 (Fig. 10.41)

- The athlete (a) stands on one limb and lifts the other, flexing the leg and placing it up behind the buttocks. The hands are placed on a chair, table or bench in front
- The partner (p) stands behind the athlete and grips the thigh just above the knee of the raised limb and places the other hand slightly above the buttock
- The athlete *slowly* attempts to pull the knee downwards while the partner resists, causing an isometric contraction to occur
- After the position has been held for *6 s* the athlete *slowly* extends the thigh while the partner assists with light pressure
- When the desired number of repeats has been performed, the other limb should be stretched

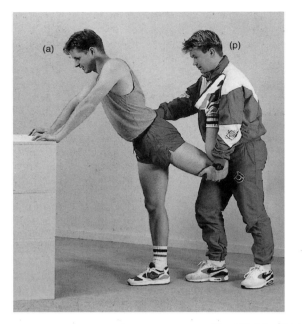 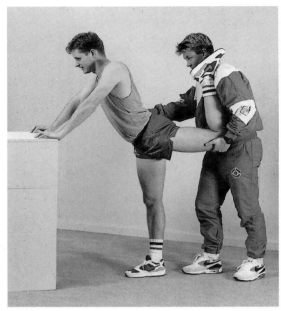

Fig. 10.41   Thigh flexor stretch - 2.

FLEXIBILITY AND SPORT PERFORMANCE

Flexible joints and stretched muscles are of great value in the majority of sports. Stretching exercises will assist an athlete in the following ways:

- By increasing the metabolism in muscles, joints and the surrounding connective tissue
- By increasing both the range and speed of movement around a joint or several joints
- By promoting general muscle relaxation over the entire body
- By increasing the elasticity of the musculotendinous unit and in so doing facilitating the use of elastic energy
- By reducing injury due to the tearing of muscle or its musculotendinous junction

The remainder of this section will discuss the type and amount of mobility which is needed for various sport groups and the specific sports and events within them.

Racquet Sports (Tennis, Badminton, Squash, Racquetball)

From a movement viewpoint, racquet sports are ballistic in nature, and high levels of flexibility are needed in order for athletes to place themselves into positions where they can hit the ball more powerfully, so as to be able to accelerate the racquet through a greater ROM when executing the shot. Furthermore, they will also be able to produce a greater contractile force, because a stretched muscle stores elastic energy and then releases it when it is shortened. High level coaches have begun to realize the value of total body stretching during the past decade, and are now giving more stretching exercises to racquet sports athletes than ever before.

SPECIFIC REGIONS OF THE BODY TO BE STRETCHED

Shoulder girdle

Arm flexion–extension flexibility is an essential capacity of the racquet sports player, as the overhead strokes play an important part in these games. The following exercises should be carried out to achieve this: tricep stretch (exercise no. 2); circular shoulder stretch (5); arm extensor stretch (29); and arm adductor stretch (30).

Trunk

Trunk flexion–extension, lateral flexion and rotation are important movements which are carried out by all racquet sports players. The following exercises should be performed to increase flexibility in the above movements: abdominal and hip stretch (7); upper back stretch (9); lower back and hip stretch (11); rotational trunk stretch (12); trunk lateral flexor stretch (31); and trunk extensor stretch (33).

Pelvic girdle and legs

Any agility athlete must have the thigh, leg and foot flexors and extensors well stretched. The following exercises should be performed to achieve this: groin stretch - 2 (14); hamstring stretch - 1 (18); hamstring stretch - 2 (19); quadriceps stretch - 1 (22); quadriceps–ankle stretch (23); quadriceps stretch - 2 (25); calf stretch (26); Achilles tendon–ankle stretch (27); thigh extensor stretch - 1 (35); and thigh flexor stretch - 1 (37).

Aquatic Sports (Swimming, Waterpolo, Rowing, Canoeing)

The mobility needs of *swimmers* and *waterpolo* players are almost identical, while rowers and canoeists need similar exercises for their shoulder girdles, trunks, pelvis and thighs. Swimmers in particular depend on high levels of flexibility in the shoulder girdle in freestyle and backstroke. This enables them to keep their bodies in a straight line and not 'break' at the hips or roll, which cuts down on lateral frontal resistance and which is the major retarding factor in the great majority of swimmers. Butterfly swimmers should have even more flexibility in the shoulder girdle than freestyle and backstroke swimmers, as they need to be almost hypermobile (Fig. 10.42). This characteristic enables them to stay very 'flat' in the water, thereby avoiding the vertical frontal resistance created by excessive 'rise and fall'. If a butterfly swimmer lacks the amount of flexibility needed to perform at the elite level, then a side breathing technique can be used. A more detailed

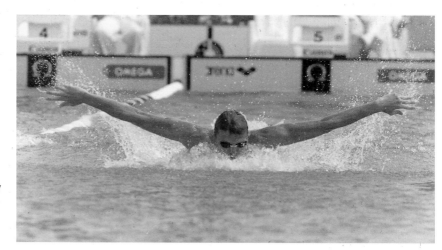

Fig. 10.42 High flexibility levels in butterfly swimmers are essential (courtesy of West Australian Newspapers).

discussion of this point is made in Chapter 4, where the concept of body modification and technique is discussed.

Breast-strokers do not need as high a level of shoulder girdle flexibility as swimmers in the other strokes, but a mobile shoulder girdle will assist them to relax in the recovery phase of the stroke cycle. They do however, need high levels of flexibility in thigh extension and abduction. Finally, all swimmers need above average flexibility in the thigh flexors and extensors, with high levels of plantar- and dorsi-flexion.

It has already been mentioned that backstrokers can be too flexible in the shoulder and elbow joints and that this can cause horizontal frontal resistance. In this situation swimmers must not only modify their technique, but also reduce flexibility levels using strength training exercises. Backstroke swimmers however, do need high levels of trunk hyperextension, which enables them to have their body enter the 'hole' which has already been opened by the hands and head during the start of the race (Fig. 10.43).

Canoeists, particularly those competing in kayaking events, need high levels of flexibility in all the joints, particularly in the shoulder girdle, while *rowers* must have extensive mobility in the thigh, leg and foot flexors and extensors. To have very flexible shoulder girdles is not essential for rowers, but they should be reasonably mobile in the shoulder girdle and trunk in order to relax this portion of the body as much as possible during each stroke.

SPECIFIC REGIONS OF THE BODY TO BE STRETCHED

Shoulder girdle

For freestylers, butterflyers, backstrokers, waterpolo players and kayakists, this region must be well stretched. Rowers can also carry out the same exercises but do not need as many of them. The following exercises should be performed to achieve a high level of mobility in this region of the body: tricep stretch (exercise no. 2); backward stretch (3); circular shoulder stretch (5); arm extensor stretch (29); and arm adductor stretch (30).

Trunk

Swimmers, waterpolo players, canoeists and rowers can profit from flexibility exercises which in-

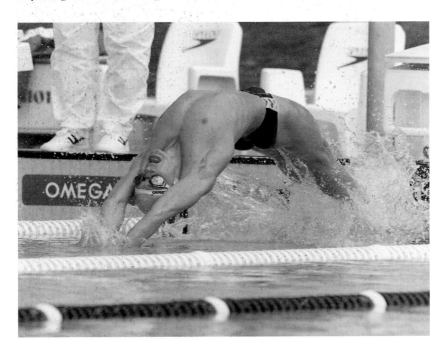

Fig. 10.43 A high level of trunk hyperextension will enable the backstroke swimmer to enter the 'hole' opened by the hands and head (courtesy of West Australian Newspapers).

crease trunk flexion–extension, lateral flexion and rotation. The following exercises should be performed for this purpose: abdominal and hip stretch (7); upper back stretch (9); lateral trunk stretch (10); lower back and hip stretch (11); rotational trunk stretch (12); and trunk extensor stretch (33).

Pelvic girdle and legs

Swimmers, waterpolo players and rowers (and canoeists to a lesser extent), need the thigh, leg and foot flexors and extensors well stretched. The following exercises should be performed to achieve this: groin stretch - 2 (14); hamstring stretch - 1 (18); hamstring stretch - 2 (19); quadriceps–ankle stretch (23); calf stretch (26); ankle stretch (28); thigh extensor stretch - 1 (35); and thigh flexor stretch - 2 (38).

Gymnastic and Power Sports (Gymnastics, Diving, Weightlifting)

Gymnasts and *divers* need the highest level of overall flexibility of any of the sports. It is not possible to attain the aesthetic positions which are needed to gain high marks in the various manoeuvres, unless the body is extremely flexible (Figs 10.44, 10.45). For this reason a wide variety of flexibility exercises need to be carried out and a considerable amount of time spent in mobility training. Furthermore, modern gymnastics and diving have become very ballistic in nature and stretched muscles can produce the contractile force which is needed, because the pre-stretched muscle stores elastic energy which is released as it is shortened. If one asks top level coaches which are the most important physical capacities for gymnasts and

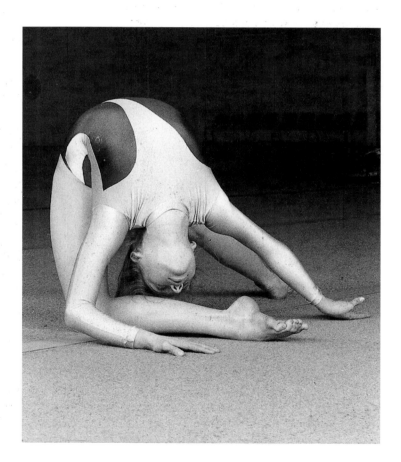

Fig. 10.44 An aesthetic position of a female rhythmic gymnast.

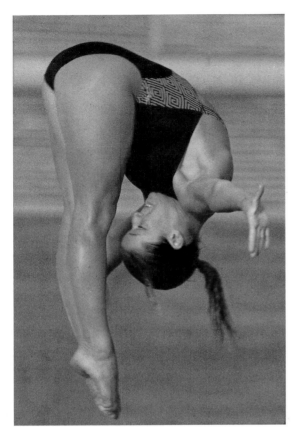

Fig. 10.45 The tuck position can only be attained if the diver has a high level of thigh flexion (courtesy of West Australian Newspapers).

divers to attain, they will state very positively that the development of explosive power and flexibility are essential for elite levels of performance.

When the traditional training routines of weightlifters were examined, high levels of flexibility were not seen to be important. However, Wilson *et al.* (1992) have recently demonstrated the value of flexibility with experienced power-lifters who improved their bench press performance by 5.4% after an 8 week flexibility training period. The above investigators concluded that the improvement was brought about by the additional elastic energy which had been stored in the musculotendinous units as a result of the training programme. Coaches should heed these important findings and strongly consider commencing flexibility training with their weightlifters. However, because they do not need the flexibility levels necessary for gymnasts and divers, weightlifters should only carry out the routines that have been designed for those competitors who take part in the contact field sports.

SPECIFIC REGIONS OF THE BODY TO BE STRETCHED

Neck, shoulder girdle and forearms

It is important for gymnasts and divers to keep the neck supple and the shoulder girdle, hands and forearms very flexible. The following exercises should be performed to achieve this: neck stretch (exercise no. 1); backward stretch (3); overhead stretch (4); circular shoulder stretch (5); arm extensor stretch (29); and arm adductor stretch (30).

Trunk

In gymnastic sports, high levels of trunk flexion–extension, lateral flexion and rotation are essential. The following exercises should be performed to achieve this: abdominal and hip stretch (7); back roll stretch (8); upper back stretch (9); lower back and hip stretch (11); rotational trunk stretch (12), trunk lateral flexor stretch (31); split pike stretch (32); and trunk extensor stretch (33).

Pelvic girdle and legs

All gymnasts and divers must have *very high* levels of flexibility in the thigh, leg and foot flexors and extensors. Extreme thigh flexion is essential if divers are to reach the classic tuck position which is required of them (Fig. 10.45). The following exercises should be performed to achieve this: groin stretch - 1 (13); groin stretch - 2 (14); side split stretch (16); hamstring stretch - 1 (18); split stretch (17); hamstring stretch - 3 (20); groin–trunk stretch (21); quadriceps stretch - 1 (22); quadriceps–ankle stretch (23); quadriceps–groin stretch (24); Achilles tendon–ankle stretch (27); ankle stretch (28); split pike stretch (32); trunk extensor stretch (33); thigh adductor stretch (34); thigh extensor stretch - 1 (35); thigh extensor stretch - 2 (36); and thigh flexor stretch - 2 (38).

Gymnasts and divers will probably need additional specialized exercises in order to reach the levels they need in these sports. They should also carry out passive stretching exercises with a skilled partner or with their coach.

Track, Field and Cycling

For more than 50 years, it has been traditional for coaches in *track* and *field* to give their athletes intensive stretching exercises. Until 10 years ago most of the exercises were of a ballistic nature, but a gradual change has been made towards the static stretching technique in the majority of countries. Because track and field incorporates a large number of individual events, it is not possible to cover each one of these in detail; however, basic stretching exercises for each sports group will be dealt with.

RUNNING, HURDLING AND CYCLING

Good technique in running, whether in sprints or middle distance events, is very dependent on high levels of flexibility. The same statement can also be made for hurdling, only more so, because the trail leg must be almost hypermobile in order for the hurdler to stride over the hurdle rather than to jump over it. Furthermore, because sprinting and hurdling are very ballistic, many athletes are prone to soft tissue damage, usually in the form of muscle belly or musculotendinous unit tears. It is vitally important for the major muscle groups in the leg to be well stretched and in balance, both from an explosive power and a flexibility viewpoint.

Cycling, on the other hand does not have a history of flexibility training when one compares it with the above sports. However, it has been obvious to sport scientists for some time that the heavy thigh musculature of the average high level cyclist needed stretching and this is now being recommended by some of the more enlightened coaches. Not only will flexibility training improve the muscular efficiency of cyclists, but it will assist them to store elastic energy, which is especially important for track cyclists, who need high levels of explosive power.

SPECIFIC REGIONS OF THE BODY TO BE STRETCHED

Shoulder girdle

In modern sprint running and hurdling the arms contribute greatly to the propulsive power of the movement. In middle distance running there is some assistance from the arms but they are also used for balance. Many elite coaches believe that high levels of mobility in the shoulder girdle and trunk assist the athlete to relax during the event and therefore prescribe stretching exercises for both running and hurdling. This is also true for cycling, and stretching should therefore be carried out by this group. The following exercises should be performed to achieve this: backward stretch (exercise no. 3); overhead stretch (4); arm extensor stretch (29); and arm adductor stretch (30).

Trunk

The trunk of the runner, hurdler and cyclist must also be flexible if high levels of relaxation are to be attained while competing. The following exercises should be performed to achieve this: upper back stretch (9); lower back and hip stretch (11); trunk lateral flexor stretch (31); and trunk extensor stretch (33).

Pelvic girdle and legs

Runners, hurdlers and cyclists must also have very high levels of thigh, leg and foot flexion and extension. The following exercises should be performed to achieve these levels: hamstring stretch - 1 (18); hamstring stretch - 3 (20); quadriceps stretch - 1 (22); quadriceps–groin stretch (24); quadriceps stretch - 2 (25); calf stretch (26); Achilles tendon–ankle stretch (27); trunk extensor stretch (33); thigh extensor stretch - 1 (35). The exercises listed below are for hurdlers only: groin stretch - 1 (13); side split stretch (16); split stretch (17); groin–trunk stretch (21); split pike stretch (32); and thigh adductor stretch (34).

FIELD SPORTS (JUMPS)

In the jumps the athlete needs a very high level of flexibility in all regions of the body in order to perform them well.

SPECIFIC REGIONS OF THE BODY TO BE STRETCHED

Neck and shoulder girdle

The following exercises should be performed to attain a high level of flexibility in this region: neck stretch (exercise no. 1); tricep stretch (2); backward stretch (3); overhead stretch (4); and arm adductor stretch (30).

Trunk

The exercises listed below will assist the jumper to attain high levels of flexibility in trunk flexion–extension, lateral flexion and trunk rotation. The following exercises should be performed to achieve these levels: abdominal and hip stretch (7); upper back stretch (9); lower back and hip stretch (11); rotational trunk stretch (12); trunk lateral flexor stretch (31); and trunk extensor stretch (33).

Pelvic girdle and legs

High levels of flexibility are essential in the thigh, leg and foot flexors and extensors for the jumps. The following exercises should be performed to achieve this: groin stretch - 3 (15); hamstring stretch - 1 (18); hamstring stretch - 3 (20); quadriceps stretch - 1 (22); quadriceps–ankle stretch (23); quadriceps–groin stretch (24); calf stretch (26); ankle stretch (28); thigh extensor stretch - 1 (35); thigh extensor stretch - 2 (36); thigh flexor stretch - 1 (37); and thigh flexor stretch - 2 (38).

FIELD SPORTS (THROWING EVENTS)

As for the jumps, field athletes need high levels of flexibility in all regions of the body.

SPECIFIC REGIONS OF THE BODY TO BE STRETCHED

Neck, shoulder girdle and forearms

An extensive range of movement and elastic energy is needed for any good throw, and therefore the neck, forearms and the shoulder girdle in particular need to be well stretched. The following exercises should be performed to achieve this: neck stretch (exercise no. 1); tricep stretch (2); backward stretch (3); circular shoulder stretch (5); hand–forearm stretch (6); arm extensor stretch (29); and arm adductor stretch (30).

Trunk

Because the trunk is an essential part of any ballistic throwing movement, it must be extremely flexible. The following exercises should be performed to achieve this: abdominal and hip stretch (7); upper back stretch (9); lower back and hip stretch (11); rotational trunk stretch (12); trunk lateral flexor stretch (31); and trunk extensor stretch (33).

Pelvic girdle and legs

High levels of flexibility in this region are important for throwers because they are relying on leg power in the initial part of the throw. In order to achieve this, the thigh, leg and foot flexors and extensors must be well stretched. The following exercises should be performed to increase mobility levels in this region of the body: groin stretch - 1 (13); groin stretch - 3 (15); hamstring stretch - 1 (18); hamstring stretch - 3 (20); quadriceps–groin stretch (24); Achilles tendon–ankle stretch (27); ankle stretch (28); thigh adductor stretch (34); thigh extensor stretch - 1 (35); and thigh flexor stretch - 1 (37).

Mobile Field Sports (Field Hockey, Soccer, Lacrosse)

In mobile field of sports, body contact occurs, but it is not as severe as in the contact field sports where whole body tackling, to impede the opponent's progress, is an important feature of the game. Athletes in the mobile field sports need an above average level of flexibility, but do not need to be excessively flexible in any specific region of the body. Like other agility athletes, all players in this group should understand that high levels of flexibility will enable them to accelerate their stick or leg through a greater range of movement, as well as being able to store elastic energy in their propulsive muscles. These two features will enable them to apply more force to the ball as they hit, throw or kick it.

SPECIFIC REGIONS OF THE BODY TO BE STRETCHED

Neck, shoulder girdle and forearms

Movements of flexion and rotation of the neck, as well as flexion–extension of the arm and flexion of the hand are important. The following exercises will assist the athlete to attain this: neck stretch (exercise no. 1); overhead stretch (4); circular shoulder stretch (5); hand–forearm stretch (6); and arm extensor stretch (29).

Trunk

Because the trunk is constantly moving during a game, flexion–extension, lateral flexion and rotation are important movements carried out by all players. The following exercises should be performed to reach the level of flexibility needed by this group: abdominal and hip stretch (7); back roll stretch (8); upper back stretch (9); lateral trunk stretch (10); lower back and hip stretch (11); and trunk extensor stretch (33).

Pelvic girdle and legs

All agility athletes must have thigh, leg and foot flexion–extension in the field sports. To achieve this the following exercises should be carried out: groin stretch - 1 (13); groin stretch - 3 (15); hamstring stretch - 1 (18); hamstring stretch - 2 (19); quadriceps stretch - 1 (22); quadriceps stretch - 2 (25); calf stretch (26); ankle stretch (28); thigh extensor stretch - 1 (35); and thigh flexor stretch - 1 (37).

Contact Field Sports (Rugby, Australian and American Football)

Players in contact field sports need strong joint capsules and musculature around the shoulder, knee and ankle joints so that these joints are not dislocated or easily injured. In the above regions they should have normal levels of flexibility; however, the adductors of the thigh, hamstrings, quadriceps and calf groups should be well stretched and in balance in order to avoid soft tissue injuries. The contact athlete must also be careful not to overstretch the knee or ankle joints

with additional activities such as intensive free-style kicking, which can cause cruciate ligament and knee instability in these joints.

SPECIFIC REGIONS OF THE BODY TO BE STRETCHED

Shoulder girdle and trunk

The following exercises should be carried out for these regions but high levels of flexibility should not be striven for: backward stretch (exercise no. 3); overhead stretch (4); abdominal and hip stretch (7); back roll stretch (8); upper back stretch (9); and lower back and hip stretch (11).

Pelvic girdle and legs

The following exercises will enable the adductors of the thigh, hamstrings, quadriceps and the calf groups to be stretched: groin stretch - 2 (14); groin stretch - 3 (15); hamstring stretch - 1 (18); hamstring stretch - 3 (20); quadriceps stretch - 1 (22); quadriceps–groin stretch (24); quadriceps stretch - 2 (25); calf stretch (26); thigh extensor stretch - 1 (35); and thigh flexor stretch - 1 (37).

Set Field Sports (Golf, Baseball, Cricket)

In set field sports, high levels of mobility are of great value, first because the storage of elastic energy which takes place in the well-stretched muscle will enable the player to hit, throw or bowl with a powerful action, but also because the player will be able to deliver the club, bat or ball in a hit, pitch or throw through a greater ROM. The combination of these two phenomena will enable the individual to perform the skills of these games with considerable explosive power.

SPECIFIC REGIONS OF THE BODY TO BE STRETCHED

Shoulder girdle, trunk and forearms

All the games in this group require very high levels of arm flexion–extension, trunk flexion–extension, lateral flexion and trunk rotation as well as extension of the hands. The following exercises should be performed to achieve this: backward stretch (exercise no. 3); overhead stretch (4); circular shoulder stretch (5); hand–forearm stretch (6); upper back stretch (9); lateral trunk stretch (10); lower back and hip stretch (11); rotational trunk stretch (12); arm extensor stretch (29); and trunk extensor stretch (33).

Pelvic girdle and legs

The thighs and legs are used in the performance of almost all of the skills in the sports in this group, high levels of flexibility are also necessary in thigh, leg and foot flexion–extension. The following exercises should be performed to achieve this: groin stretch - 3 (15); hamstring stretch - 1 (18); hamstring stretch - 2 (19); quadriceps stretch - 1 (22); quadriceps–groin stretch (24); quadriceps stretch - 2 (25); calf stretch (26); Achilles tendon–ankle stretch (27); ankle stretch (28); thigh extensor stretch - 1 (35); and thigh flexor stretch - 1 (37).

Court Sports (Basketball, Netball, Volleyball)

Court sports are highly ballistic, and thus ROM and the storage of elastic energy are very important. As well one needs to be concerned with the prevention of injuries to athletes in this group and 'long' stretched muscles will not be injured as readily as those which are 'bunched' and tight.

SPECIFIC REGIONS OF THE BODY TO BE STRETCHED

Shoulder girdle

Arm flexion–extension mobility is an important capacity for athletes in this group. The following exercises should be carried out to achieve this: overhead stretch (exercise no. 4); circular shoulder stretch (5); arm extensor stretch (29); and arm adductor stretch (30).

Trunk

The court sports player when leaping often twists while in the air and as a result needs not only a high degree of trunk flexion–extension, but also lateral flexion and trunk rotation mobility. The

following exercises should be performed to increase flexibility in the above movements: abdominal and hip stretch (7); upper back stretch (9); lower back and hip stretch (11); rotational trunk stretch (12); trunk lateral flexor stretch (31); and trunk extensor stretch (33).

Pelvic girdle and legs

All agility athletes must have the thigh, leg and foot flexors and extensors well stretched. The following exercises should be performed to achieve this: groin stretch - 2 (14); hamstring stretch - 1 (18); hamstring stretch - 2 (19); quadriceps stretch - 1 (22); quadriceps–ankle stretch (23); quadriceps stretch - 2 (25); calf stretch (26); Achilles tendon–ankle stretch (27); thigh extensor stretch - 1 (35); and thigh flexor stretch - 1 (37).

Martial Arts (Wresting, Judo, Punching and Kicking Sports)

Combatants in many of the martial arts in the past have not been very flexible; however, the past decade has seen a very definite change to this training policy. There is now an understanding of the concept of the storage of elastic energy and the realization that serious injuries can be sustained in the grappling sports if the individual does not have a flexibility level well above average, especially in the upper body. Furthermore, a supple wrestler or judoist is sometimes able to escape from a hold by 'slipping' out of it. It must be understood, however, that high levels of strength and explosive power must accompany this mobility.

SPECIFIC REGIONS OF THE BODY TO BE STRETCHED

Neck, shoulder girdle and trunk

All martial arts combatants require high levels of arm flexion–extension, trunk flexion–extension, lateral flexion and rotation. The following exercises should be performed to increase flexibility in the above movements: neck stretch (exercise no. 1); tricep stretch (2); backward stretch (3); overhead stretch (4); abdominal and hip stretch (7); back roll stretch (8); upper back stretch (9);

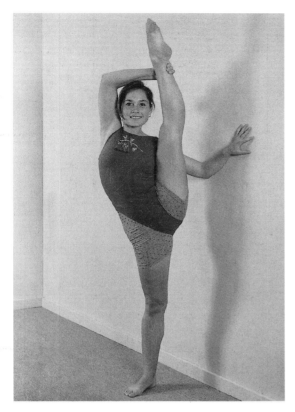

Fig. 10.46 A gymnast performing a highly specialized exercise.

lateral trunk stretch (10); lower back and hip stretch (11); and rotational trunk stretch (12).

Pelvic girdle and legs

Even though the legs only play a supporting role in the majority of the martial arts, participants should have high levels of thigh and leg flexion and extension mobility. The following exercises should be performed to achieve this: groin stretch - 2 (14); hamstring stretch - 1 (18); hamstring stretch - 2 (19); quadriceps stretch - 1 (22); quadriceps–ankle stretch (23); quadriceps stretch - 2 (25); calf stretch (26); thigh extensor stretch - 1 (35); and thigh flexor stretch - 1 (37). The exercises listed below are for participants in the kicking sports only: thigh extensor stretch - 2 (36) and thigh flexor stretch - 2 (38).

ADDITIONAL SPECIALIZED EXERCISES

Where highly specialized exercises are required for elite level performers (Fig. 10.46), such as gymnasts, divers and track and field athletes, the reader should consult texts which contain such exercises. Alter (1990) is a useful reference source in this respect.

CONCLUSION

To conclude this chapter, it should be pointed out that over the past two decades, high levels of flexibility have gradually become *very important* to the majority of athletes, who cannot compete at a high level without them. The three main reasons for increasing the range of flexibility are as follows. First the highly flexible performers are able to place themselves into a more technically correct position in most sports. Where the sport is judged, the competitors are not only expected to be technically correct but are also required to reach certain set positions in order to score high artistic marks. The second reason is that when an athlete wants to increase the ROM in a skill, the potential to produce more force or velocity becomes possible and this is an important factor in many hitting, throwing or kicking sports. Finally, observant coaches have noted for some time that a stretched muscle can produce a greater contractile force than a non-stretched one. This theory has been recently supported by research, which has demonstrated that flexibility training increases the elasticity of the musculotendinous unit and in so doing increases the utilization of elastic energy in the stretch–shorten cycle movement. This finding has very important implications for athletes competing in sports where explosive power is required.

REFERENCES

Alexander, R. (1987) The spring in your step. *New Scientist* **114**, 42–44.

Alter M. (1988) *Science of Stretching*, pp. 7–91. Human Kinetics Books, Champaign, IL, USA.

Alter M. (1990) *Sport Stretch*, pp. 6–18. Leisure Press, Champaign, IL, USA.

Anderson B. (1980) *Stretching*, pp. 12–98. Shelter Publications, Bolinas, CA, USA.

Beaulieu J. (1981) Developing a stretching programme. *The Physician and Sportsmedicine* **9**, 11, 59–69.

Corbin C. & Noble L. (1980) Flexibility: A major component of physical fitness. *The Journal of Physical Education and Recreation* **51**, 23–24, 57–60.

Ciullo J. & Zarins B. (1983) Biomechanics of the musculotendinous unit. In Zarins B. (ed.) *Clinics In Sports Medicine*, Vol. 2, pp. 71–85. W. B. Saunders, Philadelphia.

Cureton T. (1951) *Physical Fitness of Champion Athletes*, pp. 84–93. The University of Illinois Press, Urbana, IL, USA.

DeVries H. (1962) Evaluation of static stretching procedures for improvement of flexibility. *Research Quarterly* **33**, 222–229.

DeVries H. (1986) *Physiology of Exercise — For Physical Education and Athletics*, pp. 462–472, 474–487, 482–488. Wm C. Brown Publishers, Dubuque, IA, USA.

Holt L. (1974) *Scientific Stretching for Sport (3-S)*, pp. 1–8, 12–31. Sport Research, Halifax, Canada.

Hubley-Kozey C. & Stanish W. (1984) Can stretching prevent athletic injuries? *Journal of Musculoskeletal Medicine* **1**, 9, 25–32.

Johnson B. & Nelson J. (1979) *Practical Measurements for Evaluation in Physical Education*, pp. 85–89. Burgess Publishing Co., Minneapolis.

Kabat H. (1958) Proprioceptive facilitation in therapeutic exercise. In Litcht S. (ed.) *Therapeutic Exercise*. E. Licht, New Haven, CT, USA.

King R. (1993) *Performance Massage*, pp. 23–140. Human Kinetics Publications, Champaign, IL, USA.

Kiputh R. (1942) *Swimming*, pp. 38–55. The Ronald Press Co., New York.

Kirchner G. & Glines D. (1957) Comparative analysis of Eugene, Oregon, elementary school children using the Kraus-Weber test of minimum muscular fitness. *Research Quarterly* **28**, 16–25.

Leard J. (1984) Flexibility and conditioning in the young athlete. In Micheli L. *Pediatric and Adolescent Sports Medicine*, p. 198. Little, Brown and Co., Boston.

McAtee R. (1993) *Facilitated Stretching*, pp. 13–92. Human Kinetics Publishers, Champaign, IL, USA.

Moynes D. (1983) Prevention of injury to the shoulder through exercises and therapy. *Clinics in Sports Medicine* **2**, 413–422.

Phillips M. (1955) Analysis of results from the Kraus-Weber test of minimum muscular fitness in children. *Research Quarterly* **26**, 314–323.

Shellock F. & Prentice W. (1985) Warming-up and stretching for improved performance and prevention of sports-related injuries. *Sports Medicine* **2**, 267–278.

Sigerseth P. (1971) Flexibility. In Larson L. (ed.) *Encyclopedia of Sports Sciences & Medicine*, pp. 280–281. Macmillan, New York.

Surburg P. (1983) Flexibility exercise re-examined. *Athletic Training* **18**, 37–40.

Tanner J. (1963) *Growth at Adolescence*, pp. 10–15. Blackwell Scientific Publications, Oxford.

Watson A. (1992) Children in sport. In Bloomfield J., Fricker P. & Fitch K. (eds) *Textbook of Science and Medicine in Sport*, pp. 436–466. Blackwell Scientific Publications, Melbourne.

Wallin D., Ekblom B., Grahn R. & Nordenborg T. (1985) Improvement of muscle flexibility. *The American Journal of Sports Medicine* **13**, 263–268.

Wilson G., Elliott B. & Wood G. (1992) Stretch–shorten cycle performance enhancement through flexibility training. *Medicine and Science in Sports and Exercise* **24**, 116–123.

Wilson G., Wood G. & Elliott B. (1991) An alternative explanation for the occurrence of muscular injury. *International Journal of Sports Medicine* **12**, 403–407.

CHAPTER 11

DEVELOPMENT OF SPEED IN SPORT

Movement speed is an essential physical capacity in the majority of sports, and Dintiman and Ward (1988) stated that 'speed is the most important quality an athlete can possess'. Although this statement is general in nature, and cannot be applied to all sports, it is nevertheless basically correct for most.

Fast movement, or movement speed as it is often called, is a complex phenomenon which is the result of applying force to a mass. In humans it is the movement of a body, or part of it, at a very rapid rate, and requires sufficient driving force to overcome the segmental inertia and the external forces which resist movement. In movement speed then, we have *positive* and *negative* forces, and in order to move faster, we need to increase the positive forces and decrease the negative ones. To achieve this athletes need to develop their explosive power, while at the same time decreasing the resistance to a movement by improving flexibility, as well as increasing their neuromuscular coordination or skill.

TYPES OF SPEED

Speed of Reaction

Speed of reaction is the time it takes from a stimulus to the first movement and this capacity is mainly inherited, but it can be slightly improved by specific training. This chapter will not deal with *reaction speed* or *reaction time*, as this capacity fits more comfortably into the motor control and learning area, but it is important to point out that it is

an essential capacity for many sports, and one that coaches must be capable of improving in their athletes.

Speed of Movement

This is the speed with which muscles can contract to move the limbs quickly. When thinking about speed, the majority of people immediately think of *running speed* or *total body speed*, which is only a part of it. There is no doubt that a high level of running speed is essential for many sports, but *specific limb speed* or very rapid limb movements are also made in many others and must therefore be considered in this chapter.

SPECIFICITY OF SPEED

Contrary to popular belief, speed is quite specific. A fast runner, for example, may have slow upper body movements in other sport skills. Furthermore, specificity relates to the type of task and the direction of the movement (Clarke 1960; Henry 1960). Sinning and Forsyth (1970) also found that speed was reasonably specific to the individual limb as well as to the direction in which it was moved and that there was a low correlation between the speed of movement of the forward and the backward arm swing. It must be understood therefore that it is not possible to generalize that athletes are basically 'fast' simply because they can run quickly or throw a ball at a high velocity. The reason why speed is so specific is that there are many variables which make up any single movement. The specific physical performance determinants of speed are body shape, body composition, proportionality, muscle insertion point, posture, flexibility, explosive power and muscle fibre type, and very few individuals have all of these characteristics in the regions of the body where rapid speed of movement may be needed.

BASIC DETERMINANTS OF SPEED

There are several major factors that, when integrated, go to make up a speedy movement. At this point in the development of sport science, it has not been possible to rate them in order of importance; however, the following information attempts to classify them from the research and anecdotal information that is currently available.

- *Muscle fibre* — there is general agreement that muscle fibres are responsible for rapid and powerful movement. The proportion of fast (FT) to slow (ST) twitch muscle is basic to the generation of high speed, and if FT fibres are fully developed by sprint training then the muscle will reach its full potential to contract with great force and as a result produce a very fast movement (Ackland & Bloomfield 1992). DeVries (1986) also suggested that the differences in the velocity of actin filaments sliding past myosin filaments could account for differences in the speed of muscle contraction
- *Skill* — there is also general agreement that an individual's neuromuscular coordination pattern is a very important factor in executing a skill at a very high speed. The mechanisms by which this can be achieved have not been well investigated, but it is common knowledge among coaches that the development of an efficient and economical technique increases the speed of movement
- *Muscle insertion point* — if the insertion point of a tendon is further away from a joint (axis of rotation), then it will positively affect the muscle function giving the athlete a mechanical advantage, thus making him or her stronger and/or more powerful

- *Lever lengths* — optimal lever lengths need to be developed in order for fast movement to occur. It is necessary for the coach to understand this important physical capacity which has already been discussed in Chapter 7
- *Posture* — the alignment of muscles as they cross the various joints of the body is an important factor in developing power and, in turn, high speeds in many sports. The shape of the bones and the location of the various landmarks to which these muscles are attached, vary greatly between individuals. Some people have almost perfect muscle alignment to gain a mechanical advantage, while others are gravely disadvantaged in comparison
- *Elastic energy* — the storing of elastic energy in the musculotendinous unit is a recent discovery. Stretching routines are partly aimed at increasing the range of movement around a joint, so that the additional range through which the limb will move will create more speed in the movement. Also the stored elastic energy, which is released when a muscle is placed slightly on stretch, gives the performer increased speed (Wilson *et al.* 1992)

EFFECT OF INCREASED STRENGTH AND FLEXIBILITY ON SPEED

Strength and Speed

It is taken for granted by almost all coaches that strength and movement speed are highly related; however, several studies (Clarke 1960; Henry & Whitley 1960; Smith 1961) have claimed that there is little relationship, while others have suggested that there is (Whitley & Smith 1963; Nelson & Fahrney 1965).

The question as to whether speed can be improved by strength training has already been partially answered in the affirmative by Dintiman (1964) and Smith (1964) and there is also strong anecdotal evidence to support this, since strength training has become an important part of athlete preparation wherever power and/or speed are needed. In fact, if one were to suggest to coaches that strength training was not needed for a power and/or speed athlete, the vast majority of them would spurn the advice.

Since plyometric training has developed, and explosive power or ballistic training has become more popular, many coaches feel that these methods are of more assistance in speed development; however, the athlete must have a solid strength base before they can be utilized. Wilson *et al.* (1993) demonstrated the value of both these methods, finding that plyometric and explosive power training gave better results for both speed and agility development than did strength training.

Flexibility and Speed

Many coaches believe that by improving flexibility in athletes, they will cut down negative forces as well as developing elastic energy in the muscles and tendons and that this will improve the athlete's speed. To date there has been no definitive research which *directly* supports high levels of flexibility as being an essential component of speed. However, Dintiman's (1964) study demonstrated that when both strength and flexibility training were used in a sprint training programme, the results were significantly better for the group who used the combination than for the group who used only sprint training. Further, research by Wilson *et al.* (1992) demonstrated that there was an increase in elastic energy as a result of a flexibility training programme. These two studies, although generally supporting a stretching programme have not provided *conclusive* evidence that it is essential for sprinting. There is no doubt that specific research needs to be done; however until this is carried out, athletes who want to increase their movement speed will use flexibility training because of the wealth of anecdotal evidence supporting it.

DEVELOPING SPEED IN CHILDREN

Provided the programme is moderate, pre-adolescent children from 10 years of age onwards, as well as adolescent children, can take part in speed training. Young children should not participate in *heavy* strength training but certainly can be involved if it is moderate. Plyometric or explosive power training is of little value in the younger age group and should be avoided. On the other hand, speed-assisted training is valuable as it conditions the neurological system to very fast movements, so the sooner it is started the better. Young athletes from around 9–10 years of age are often highly motivated and can benefit greatly from an emphasis on skill training. In both speed-assisted and skill training it is also important to constantly emphasize *flow*.

Adolescent athletes can participate in speed training programmes with less caution than those who are pre-adolescent, although this statement should not be interpreted as meaning that speed training for this group can be as vigorous as that undertaken by an adult. During the first half of adolescence it should be a little more intense than during pre-adolescence, but in the second half of adolescence the intensity can be steadily increased. The programme for this group should include strength training, plyometrics, explosive power or ballistic training, speed-resisted training, speed-assisted training and skill training.

SEX DIFFERENCES IN MOVEMENT SPEED

Comparison of sprint times in various sports demonstrates that women are approximately 10% slower than men. DeVries (1986) stated that in controlled arm speed experiments, women were found to be 17% slower than men. However, when the length of the arm was removed as a factor, the difference was only 5%. As speed is very much dependent on strength and power, it is logical that males would have greater movement speed than females, but as more females compete in sport, and training methods for strength and explosive power improve, the gap should be narrowed.

From a training viewpoint there seems to be no reason why females cannot carry out a similar routine to males. They should however be careful to prevent injury by not using too much resistance in strength and/or explosive power training.

PREVENTION OF INJURY IN SPEED TRAINING

The following suggestions will enable the athlete to participate in a speed training programme and avoid injuries which often occur when ballistic activities are carried out:

- No speed training should be commenced unless athletes have a high fitness level, otherwise they will probably sustain an injury early in the programme
- When speed training commences it should be increased gradually and the individual should always 'err on the side of caution'. The programme should commence in the pre-season period and continue for 3–4 months. Before the speed-assisted part is undertaken, the athlete must have a well-developed speed-resisted base on which to build
- The *warm-up session* should be slow and gradual with stretching activities being central to it. When the athlete completes the speed training session there should be a warm-down period, using some stretching exercises which will help to prevent the occurrence of muscle soreness
- It is important to limit the frequency of speed training, which can be dangerous if carried out more than three times in any one week. Power and overspeed activities are the basis of this type of training, and therefore it is easy to sustain an overuse injury from too many training sessions
- The athlete and coach should take as many preventive measures as they can in order to avoid sustaining an injury. These can take the form of orthotics, which may correct any postural deviations the individual has in the feet or legs; scientifically designed shoes, innersoles which will absorb the constant shock of landing; and any other aids that will cut down on the incidence of injury. Furthermore,

the surface on which they train should not be too hard but reasonably resilient. It is also important for athletes to report even the most minor injuries, because these can often be intensively treated without the loss of any training time. However, if they continue to train with a minor injury, it will not be long before it becomes a major one

EVALUATING SPEED IN ORDER TO DESIGN A TRAINING PROGRAMME

Coaches have been evaluating speed using the comparison of sprint times in many sports for most of the 20th century. In sports such as running, swimming, cycling, speed skating, rowing and kayaking, competitive times are available, as well as records of time trials over shorter distances when a 'flying start' is often used. Evaluating a player's speed in games or in some individual contests is much more difficult, but in most cases the movement must be simulated and timed in a laboratory environment. Rather than only using stopwatches to record short sprints, it is best if possible to set up a simple automatic timing device that gives very accurate times. Professional clubs or sports institutes are often able to do this, but it may not be possible for amateur clubs, and in this situation a stopwatch can be used.

Evaluating an athlete's running speed, for example, in order to design a training programme for various sports, is not as simple as just taking a time and making a comparison with other individuals. If the evaluation is done correctly, many factors need to be taken into consideration because a coach needs to have more information than just sprint or movement times in order to increase an athlete's propulsive forces. The following is an example of what should be done to evaluate sprint running:

- Both a *10 m*, from a standing start and a *40 m* or *40 yard (36.6 m) sprint*, either from a standing start, or a run through, should be carried out on a suitable surface
- Stride length and stride rate should then be assessed

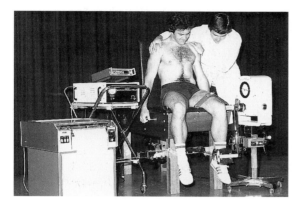

Fig. 11.1 Accommodating resistance testing using the Cybex System.

- Hamstring/quadricep balance should then be evaluated. If a laboratory is available, accurate tests can be administered to the athlete using a Biodex, Cybex, Kincom or other accommodating resistance testing machines (Fig. 11.1). When sophisticated equipment is not available, a variable resistance machine can be used to test both muscle groups by having the subject perform one *maximal contraction* for the leg curl and leg extension exercises (Figs 9.16, 9.17). The ratio of leg curl/leg extension should be 75% or greater
- A high-speed (slow motion) video should also be taken of the athlete's 40 m or 40 yard (36.6 m) sprint. This will isolate technique errors, enabling the coach to assist the athlete to improve his or her technique

When data from the above evaluation have been gathered, the coach will then be in a position to design a programme that will increase the athlete's speed, because information on the individual's stride length, stride rate, muscle power and technique is essential in order to improve performance.

A similar evaluation can also be done for other sports and many coaches in more sophisticated training venues can do this very effectively. It can be carried out with little equipment and careful subjective analysis, because it is better to have some data than none at all.

GENERAL SPEED TRAINING

During the past two decades, speed training programmes have been successfully developed for several sports in which running is a basic skill. More recently however, coaches who have athletes in other sports have been using similar methods to increase the speed of their performers, with very good results. Speed training, like strength, flexibility and mental skills training, has now become an important ingredient in the total programme, particularly where speed of movement is essential in the sport.

The aim of speed training is to condition the athlete to move at high velocity, employing maximal power when needed. In order to do this the neuromuscular system must be conditioned to very fast movements and training needs to be very specific (especially to cadence, posture and skill), with a very high anaerobic component. The basic training programme is as follows.

General Level of Fitness

The athlete must have a reasonably high level of both cardiovascular and musculoskeletal fitness before any programme is commenced. If this is neglected, then there will not be a solid base on which to build a physically demanding programme and there is a strong possibility that an injury will be sustained which will inhibit training.

Strength, Power and Flexibility Training

For any advanced speed training, the athlete *must have* a solid foundation on which to build. This can only be obtained by first taking part in a substantial strength training programme. It is important for both the athlete and the coach to understand that in any sport where power or speed is employed, a general as well as a specific strength base is essential. Several companies now market specialized variable resistance machines, where the athlete is able to strengthen the propulsive

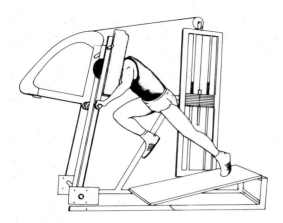

Fig. 11.2 Specific strength training in a sprinting posture using the power driver (adapted from Nautilus, Bloomfield *et al*. 1992).

muscles in specific postural positions (Fig. 11.2). When strength has been gained the individual will be able to take part in the following additional forms of training.

BALLISTIC ACTIVITIES

Many sports require short bursts of speed as well as sudden changes in direction, while athletes are moving at high speed. In other sports, *explosive power* will be needed on impact (Fig. 11.3) or

when propelling an object away from the body. In order for this to occur the athlete must train specifically using explosive kicking, throwing, bowling, punching or tackling movements. Special equipment is now available for these activities in the contact sports in the form of scrummage machines, tackling dummies, contact padding and medicine balls.

PLYOMETRICS

To further develop *explosive power*, plyometrics (see Chapter 9) can be employed by using bounding, jumping, arm swinging, thrusting and throwing actions. It should be emphasized that the number of jumps, thrusts or throws should be carefully monitored and if the athlete feels any overstressing of the propulsive units involved in the various movements, these should be rested.

EXPLOSIVE POWER TRAINING

Chapter 9 has already explained the principles behind the plyometric power system, a very useful method of power training which will be steadily refined over the next few years. Figure 9.32 illustrates the equipment which is used to do this. Athletes should also monitor their training carefully to ensure that overuse syndromes do not develop.

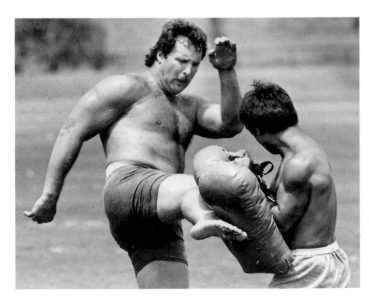

Fig. 11.3 Training for explosive power movements. (Reprinted from Dintiman & Ward 1988 with permission from Human Kinetics Publishers Inc.)

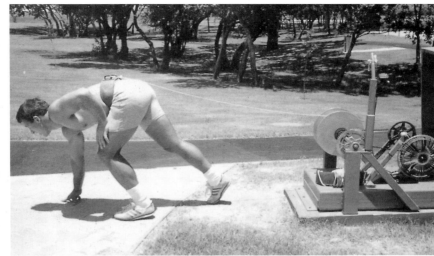

Fig. 11.4 A male athlete using the Diagnostic Power Trainer which creates resistance as he runs. (Reprinted from Dintiman & Ward 1988 with permission from Human Kinetics Publishers Inc.)

FLEXIBILITY TRAINING

Chapter 10 has already dealt with flexibility and its basic value in sport, and its relationship with speed has been further discussed earlier in this chapter. Although no direct research yet supports its use in movement speed training, anecdotal evidence is overwhelmingly in favour of flexibility training.

Speed-resisted Training

Speed-resisted training is a more specific method than that which has been previously discussed in this section. Resistance training, or speed-resisted training as it is known internationally, employs an increased load, or some form of resistance, while the specific skill is being performed. It should only be used in the *pre-season period* and the *early part of the main season* because it will partially interfere with the specificity of a skill or skills which make up the sport or event.

This training method employs the use of a wide variety of equipment and various forms of resistance, which are as follows:

- Running up gradual hills, specially built ramps (4–5° inclines), and stairs; using a power trainer (Fig. 11.4); pulling a specially weighted sled or tyre; running with a small parachute behind; or using weighted shoes

- Cycling in high gear at as fast a cadence as possible, or pulling a sled or tyre behind the cycle
- The use of weight bands or weighted vests, weighted boots or weighted equipment in mobile field games
- Swimming with hand paddles (Fig. 11.5); using pull buoys; towing a sea anchor; or using a speed trainer (e.g. the Sparta Speed Trainer)
- Rowing, canoeing or kayaking using large oars

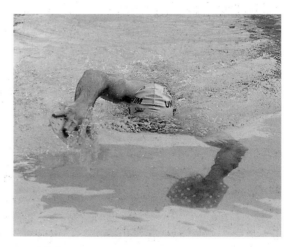

Fig. 11.5 A swimmer performing speed-resisted training using hand paddles.

or paddle blades. Heavy boats, canoes or kayaks are also of assistance in this form of training
- Competing against heavier opponents in the combative sports
- Using very light dumb-bells for boxers (shadow sparring) or for other athletes who use their arms to strike, hit or pump, as in running (Fig. 9.57)

Speed-assisted Training

Speed-assisted training is slightly more specific than speed-resisted training. The aim is to lighten the load or resistance in order to increase the speed of the movement so that the skill is carried out at a faster rate than it would normally be done. The rationale for this type of training is that it conditions the neurological system to *very fast* movements. Speed-assisted, or overspeed training as it is sometimes called, should be done in the *early part of the main season* and *during the mid-season*, steadily replacing speed-resisted training. No training of this type should be carried out during the main competition period.

The speed-assisted training method employs the use of several strategies and types of equipment which are as follows:

- Running on a speeded-up treadmill, down a 2° ramp, or behind a vehicle or motor bike holding onto an extension of it; using surgical tubing to pull the athlete, a method described by Dintiman and Ward (1988, pp. 94–96); towing with the Sprint Master (Fig. 11.6)
- Agility training drills for players in mobile field sports using very rapid sprint and directional changes. To do this sharp commands and shrill whistles should be used
- Cycling in low gear at a fast cadence, on rollers, or riding in the slip stream behind a motor bike while on the cycling track
- Swimming using a sprint towing device or modified flippers
- Rowing, canoeing or kayaking using a *slightly* smaller oar or paddle blade, or with several small holes bored in the blade

Skill Training

Skill training, performed at a very rapid rate, has the greatest effect on the development of move-

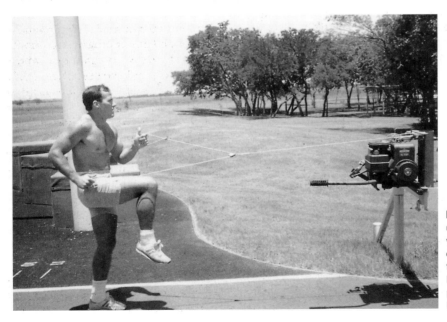

Fig. 11.6 A male athlete using the Sprint Master which enables him to carry out speed-assisted training. (Reprinted from Dintiman & Ward 1988 with permission from Human Kinetics Publishers Inc.)

ment speed and is often neglected by coaches who are more concerned with the building of strength and explosive power. There is no doubt that these physical capacities are essential in developing rapid movement, but the timing or 'flow' which comes from systematic skill training, where a coach is perceptive enough to improve the critical factors that increase speed or velocity, especially in ballistic skills, is important. The question of how one increases the velocity of the bat, racquet or club in the impact area, or generates the greatest velocity just before the release in a throw or bowl, must be dealt with in a holistic way and the components of a speed training programme, discussed above, play an important role in answering the above questions. However, skill is the most important single factor in the attainment of movement speed and this must not be overshadowed by any of the others.

SPORT-SPECIFIC SPEED TRAINING

If an athlete is to reach full potential in a sport and if speed of movement is a necessary component, the speed and velocity demands of the sport must be carefully analysed. This has been done in several sports, and currently there are speed performance norms which have been developed from the data of standard tests for a range of athletes. The more high profile the sport, the more likely it is that it will have these data, whereas minor sports have almost none.

The following material deals with specific training, which will increase the athlete's movement speed.

Racquet Sports

Games such as *tennis, badminton* and *squash* or *racquetball* need training for total body speed as well as specific limb speed.

Total body speed, which includes acceleration and running speed, is essential on a racquet game court. Running speed training that includes strength, power and flexibility activities, combined with speed-resisted and speed-assisted training, should be done.

Specific limb speed can also be improved with strength (Fig. 9.82) and power training as well as speed-assisted and speed-resisted training, but it is skill training which will give the greatest hitting velocities in these games. The coach must constantly look for the technique weaknesses that are hindering the development of power in the various strokes and the combination of a fully co-ordinated high velocity stroke and movement speed training will greatly improve this area of the player's game.

Aquatic Sports

A considerable body of knowledge already exists on the application of movement speed training to *swimming* and this has been partially based on the Dintiman (1979) sprint running programme.

First, specific strength and power exercises, combined with speed-resisted training, are essential. Swimming with hand paddles and pull buoys are almost universally carried out, while a few coaches are now using a speed trainer. Speed-assisted swimming can then be done in the latter part of the early season and during the mid-season. This can take the form of using modified flippers and in some cases, where it is available, a sprint towing device.

In *rowing* and *kayaking* a similar programme is necessary. Strength and power programmes should undergird a speed-resisted programme, where heavy boats or kayaks should be used with slightly larger oar or paddle blades. The speed-assisted programme must be carried out in a light racing boat using slightly smaller oar or paddle blades.

Waterpolo players need total body speed as well as specific limb speed. The first is obtained by methods identical to those used by sprint swimmers, while the second can be developed by specific strength and power, speed-assisted and speed-resisted training and technique coaching.

Gymnastic and Power Sports

Total body speed is not an essential ingredient in *gymnastics* or *weightlifting* except for the run up to the vault in this specialized event. However, some speed training can be done if the coach feels that the gymnast needs it. Training for specific limb speed is of great value to those gymnasts who lack 'snap' in their movements, but the majority of their time should be spent in technique coaching to develop the 'flow' which is essential in their sport.

Track and Field

During the past decade, track *sprinters*, particularly those in the USA, have been using several of the techniques that are common in a strength and power training programme, as well as speed-resisted and speed-assisted training. As this is the case, it is not necessary to outline the running speed training programme in this chapter. However, if track coaches are interested, it can be found in Dintiman and Ward (1988).

Middle and long distance runners may be able to benefit from a total body speed programme, particularly if they have little 'kick' or natural speed for tactical running. In today's highly competitive environment, it is up to the coach to decide if athletes need this capacity in order to improve their performance.

Jumpers and throwers need total body speed as well as specific limb speed. Many track and field coaches are now giving training for both to their athletes as part of their normal programme. Total body speed is now a standard programme but the specific limb speed may need to be formulated by the coach. This is not difficult to do, because there is now a large number of speed-resisted and speed-assisted activities in the literature for jumps and field games athletes. The development of the optimal technique is also up to the coach, who must isolate the critical factors retarding performance and improve on these.

Mobile Field Sports

Sports such as *field hockey, soccer* and *lacrosse* rely on both running speed and specific limb speed. Those coaches who have persevered with a *total body speed* programme have been agreeably surprised with its results. It enables a player to 'burst' with greater speed and power, giving a

dynamic dimension to the performance. For this reason more coaches are concentrating on this particular aspect of training, especially in the early part of the season. As the season progresses, *specific limb speed* is concentrated upon, using simulated techniques from the sport.

Contact Field Sports

Contact field sports, led by *American football*, have seen a heavy concentration on the development of running speed. Dintiman and Ward (1988) have been the major proponents of this move, which has been developed over the past three decades in the USA. As coaches from other contact football codes have visited North America, they have brought back many of the body movement speed techniques that are used there. However, they have not developed the *total body speed* programmes as well as coaches in American football and could benefit from a more systematic application of this regime.

One of the main differences is that coaches in the USA have developed total body speed training techniques for players in different positions. This has probably occurred because they have systematically analysed the game over a long period of time and determined the special skills that are needed in it, such as the need for fast starting, acceleration while already running, increase or decrease in stride length in closed and open running, and speed endurance. The *rugby* codes and *Australian Rules football* would do well to carry out more in-depth studies of the requirements of specific positions in their games and then devise speed training techniques to suit them.

All players in contact football need speed training which should assist them with their acceleration rate, stride length and the rate of their stride for open and closed field running. However they also need *specific limb speed* training using simulated techniques from the sport.

Set Field Sports

Games like *baseball* and *cricket* demand high levels of *total body speed*, but not for long distances. Rapid acceleration from a set position should receive the most emphasis in this pro-gramme. Players must also be aware that specific limb speed is important in hitting, throwing and bowling and this will occur mainly through tech-nique training, although strength, power, flexi-bility, speed-assisted and speed-resisted activities all play a part.

Court Sports

Basketball, netball and *volleyball* have similar demands to the racquet sports, where total body speed and specific limb speed are needed. The section on racquet sports should be referred to for more information.

Martial Arts

Only specific limb speed is needed in *wrestling, judo* and *boxing*. These athletes should mainly use technique training to achieve this; however strength, explosive power and flexibility training, as well as speed-resisted and speed-assisted train-ing, all play an important part. In boxing, slightly heavier gloves and a punching bag can be useful in the early season, then a speed ball and lighter opponents in the speed-assisted phase of training should be used during the mid-season.

CONCLUSION

It must be emphasized again that speed training should be done as a special programme in a simi-lar manner to strength and power, flexibility and mental skills training. The pre-season and early season is the best time for such programmes and a maintenance programme should then be con-ducted to retain them.

This chapter has only dealt with the develop-ment of movement speed and has not covered reaction time training, which is more the domain of the motor control and learning field. Nor has it dealt with endurance speed or the ability to main-tain speed over distances, which are more related to physiology.

In closing, attention should again be focused on the complex nature of speed and the fact that

there are many variables that go to make up a very fast movement. Such factors as posture, pro-portionality, flexibility, fibre type and elastic en-ergy are all interrelated and with skill they must be developed in unison for a very rapid move-ment or movements to occur.

REFERENCES

Ackland T. & Bloomfield J. (1992) Functional anatomy. In Bloomfield J., Fricker P. & Fitch K. (eds) *Textbook of Science and Medicine in Sport*, pp. 13–14. Blackwell Scientific Publications, Melbourne.

Bloomfield J., Fricker P. & Fitch K. (1992) (eds) *Textbook of Science and Medicine in Sport*, p. 18. Blackwell Scientific Publications, Melbourne.

Clarke D. (1960) Correlation between strength/mass ratio and the speed of an arm movement. *Research Quarterly* **31**, 470–474.

DeVries H. (1986) *Physiology of Exercise — For Physical Education and Athletics,* pp. 448–459. Wm. C Brown, Dubuque IA, USA.

Dintiman G. (1964) Effects of various training programs on running speed. *Research Quarterly* **35**, 554–561.

Dintiman G. (1979) *How to Run Faster: A Do-it-yourself Book for Athletes in All Sports*. Champion Athlete, Richmond, VA, USA.

Dintiman G. & Ward R. (1988) *Sport Speed*, pp. 1, 23–101. Leisure Press, Champaign, IL, USA.

Henry F. (1960) Factorial structure of speed and static strength in a lateral arm movement. *Research Quarterly* **31**, 440–447.

Henry F. & Whitley J. (1960) Relationships between indi-vidual differences in strength, speed and mass in an arm movement. *Research Quarterly* **31**, 24–33.

Nelson R. & Fahrney R. (1965) Relationship between strength and speed of elbow flexion. *Research Quarterly* **36**, 455–463.

Sinning W. & Forsyth H. (1970) Lower limb actions while running at different velocities. *Medicine and Science in Sports* **2**, 28–34.

Smith L. (1961) Individual differences in strength, reac-tion latency, mass and length of limbs and their rela-tion to maximal speed of movement. *Research Quarterly* **32**, 208–220.

Smith L. (1964) Influence of strength training on pre-tensed and free arm speed. *Research Quarterly* **35**, 554–561.

Whitley J. & Smith L. (1963) Velocity curves and static strength–action strength correlations in relation to the mass moved by the arm. *Research Quarterly* **34**, 379–395.

Wilson G., Elliott B. & Wood G. (1992). Stretch–shorten cycle performance enhancement through flexibility training. *Medicine and Science in Sports and Exercise* **24**, 116–123.

Wilson G., Newton R., Murphy A. & Humphries B. (1993). The optimal training load for the development of dy-namic athletic performance. *Medicine and Science in Sports and Exercise* **25** 1279–1286.

CHAPTER 12

BALANCE AND AGILITY IN SPORT

Together with capacities such as speed, power, strength and flexibility, the coordination of muscle actions by the central nervous system plays a vital role in successful athletic performance. The ability to accurately coordinate the timing and contraction strength of skeletal muscles is essential in the related capacities of balance and agility. While both are modified by the physical structure of an athlete and may be affected by technique, balance and agility rely primarily on the development of neuromuscular control. According to Tittel (1988) this is particularly important for technical acrobatic sports such as gymnastics, rhythmic gymnastics, diving and figure skating, as well as for such activities as swimming, wrestling, fencing, boxing and ball games.

BALANCE

In all activities, whether stationary or mobile, balance plays an important role. Some activities require *static balance* where a set position has to be maintained for a period of time. In target sports such as archery and shooting, the maintenance of a balanced posture is essential for attaining accuracy, whereas in other sports such as gymnastics and diving, positions which are held without excessive movement demonstrate the athlete's strength and coordination.

Other sports require athletes to remain balanced while in motion. This concept is referred to as *dynamic balance* and the development of this

capacity is essential in highly mobile sports which require the athlete to quickly react to changing circumstances. For this reason, dynamic balance and agility are closely related.

Mechanical Considerations

High levels of balance in a sporting activity are dependent on the following factors:

- The area of the base of support
- The position of the centre of gravity
- The mass (body weight) of the performer

A wide but comfortable positioning of the feet aids the static balance in archery and pistol shooting, while the execution of a stable handstand in diving or gymnastics requires the hands to be placed about shoulder width apart. Thus the area of the base of support is maximized within the ability of the performer to control his or her posture. Obviously, an exaggerated base of support caused by the feet or hands being positioned too far apart can restrict the performance of subsequent movements, and can be aesthetically displeasing.

If the centre of gravity is kept low and within the base of support, it is difficult for an opponent to move the body from a set position. This balanced and stable position is sought in wrestling, for example, when the low centre of gravity and the wide base of support make it difficult for an opponent to shift the line of gravity outside this base. If the opponent achieves this, then balance is lost and the supporting limbs must move to avoid a fall.

These principles are used to good effect in other combative and contact sports. An opponent's balance can be disrupted by pushing or pulling above the centre of gravity, thereby moving it outside the base of support, or below the centre of gravity to take away the base of support, such as in a trip in wrestling, or in a rugby tackle. Using a similar logic, offensive players and ball carriers in contact football should modify their running technique when in close proximity to opponents. By shortening their stride and increasing stride rate, players are able to maintain a more 'compact' and balanced gait which keeps the centre of gravity over the base of support for a greater proportion of time and consequently reduces the effectiveness of a tackle. Training for these players should include drills to reinforce the rapid short steps required in this situation. Furthermore, an opponent's inertia, or resistance to motion is determined by his or her body mass. In contact sports, players of greater mass are more difficult to move and we see evidence for this in the body mass of linemen in American football (see Table 6.4 in Chapter 6).

In certain movements however, the line of gravity will be projected outside the base of support, yet the athlete may still be balanced. This dynamic balance is achieved due to the addition of some external force or load. For example, the ice hockey player shown in Fig. 12.1 would appear to be unbalanced and would fall if this were a static situation. However, the dynamic nature of the movement imposes a centrifugal force on the body. When added to the effect of gravity, the resultant force acts through the base of support to provide a posture in dynamic equilibrium. Slight adjustments to the athlete's posture will be required throughout the execution of this skill as the external force varies in magnitude and direction. The rapid response required to maintain this dynamic balance is reliant upon a well developed and coordinated musculoskeletal system.

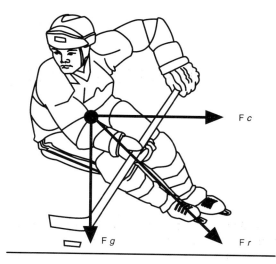

Fig. 12.1 Dynamic balance in ice hockey. The resultant force (F*r*) is the vector sum of the force of gravity (F*g*) and the centrifugal force (F*c*). F*r* passes through the instantaneous base of support provided by the area bounded by the blades of the player's skates.

Neuromuscular Considerations

The control of skeletal muscle activity is reliant upon the supply of information from certain receptors within the body and the correct interpretation of their signals, so that an appropriate movement response is initiated by the brain. With respect to balance or postural control, the structures which provide this information are:

- *Visual receptors* (the eyes) — these provide information on the relative spatial location of objects in the field of view
- *Vestibular apparatus* — this provides the perception of movement of the head through the semicircular canal structures of the inner ear
- *Kinesthetic receptors* — these provide information regarding the relative location of one body part to another, the position of the body in space and an awareness of the body's movements. These receptors include *joint position receptors* (Ruffini endings, Golgi receptors and Paccinian corpuscles) as well as the *muscle*

length and tension receptors (Golgi tendon organs and muscle spindles)

From recent research we know that clear phases exist in the development of static balance among children. Woolacott *et al.* (1989) state that visual dominance in balance control appears to recur at transitional points in human development. During infancy a strong visual dominance is required when learning to sit, crawl, stand and walk.

The ages from 4 to 6 years, however, represent a transitional period when stability often declines temporarily. It is postulated that the child is attempting to integrate the various sensory information from all the above sources, not just the visual cues. In the process of learning to integrate these data, conflict may exist between sensory inputs and balance can suffer. Gradually, however, fine-tuning of the balance control mechanisms leads to adult-like control in which the postural responses occur without a great lag in time.

From 7 to 10 years and beyond, the child becomes more reliant upon kinesthetic and vestibular feedback in balance control. Removal of visual stimuli does not drastically impair balance for these older children and they may practise certain skills with the eyes closed to improve the kinesthetic 'feel' of the performance. Children in these age groups exhibit mature control responses, whereby the amplitude of postural adjustments while maintaining balance diminishes and the levels of muscular activity become less variable.

RAMIFICATIONS FOR MOVEMENT

As the ability to integrate all sensory information improves and the reliance on visual cues for balance control diminishes, the visual system can be freed to concentrate on other tasks such as monitoring opponents and movements of a ball, implement or target. Furthermore, since the kinesthetic information is dealt with at a subconscious level, this frees the brain to process information related to developing strategies and tactics.

In addition to this, reduced reliance on visual information for maintaining balance allows the athlete to perform maximally in poor visual environments, such as under dim or stroboscopic light conditions in artistic pursuits, or during twists, spins and somersaults in gymnastics and diving.

AGILITY

Agility is a difficult capacity to define since it incorporates elements of movement speed, as well as the ability to coordinate changes in direction and modification of the normal locomotion posture. Draper and Lancaster (1985) suggest that there are several types of agility:

- Whole body changes of direction in the horizontal plane, such as in dodging and faking
- Whole body changes of direction in the vertical plane, such as in jumping and leaping
- Rapid movement of body parts, for example, to control implements in sports such as *fencing, tennis, squash* and *field hockey*

Agility is an important capacity for many elite performers to develop. Agile movements of the body can be used to great effect in order to free an offensive player from the opposition. Dintiman and Ward (1988) recognized the importance of agility for *faking and cutting* manoeuvres in *football* and *basketball*. They state that the fake is used to:

- Neutralize the defenders by slowing their movement, breaking concentration and placing doubt in their minds
- Cause the defender to move in a direction away from the player's intended path
- Draw a defender close so that a cut or side step (Fig. 12.2) can be effectively executed

Mastery of all fakes and cuts described by Dintiman and Ward (1988) requires great agility so that the pattern of locomotion can be modified while running at high speed. Good faking skills not only improve the performance of offensive players in contact sports, but also tend to reduce the risk of injury resulting from a hard tackle.

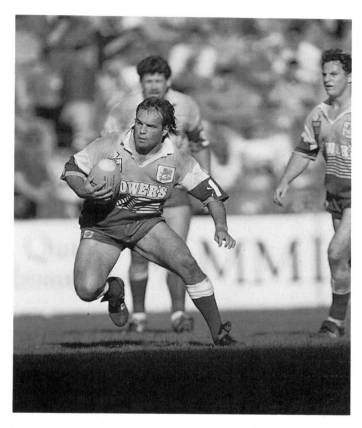

Fig. 12.2 A rugby league player using a side step (from Bloomfield *et al.* 1992).

Agility may also be required in situations where no defensive player is involved. For example, in sports such as *tennis, ice hockey* and *badminton* that involve the striking of a ball, puck or shuttle, the ability to quickly change direction and place oneself into a good position to execute a stroke is of paramount importance to the resulting speed and accuracy of the shot. Furthermore, the execution of a double play in *baseball*, or a catch or run out in *cricket*, often requires great agility to change direction quickly or move the limbs rapidly to intercept a ball.

Improving Agility

Overall, it would appear that agility is a capacity that is highly specific to each particular task. Therefore, the development of strategies to improve agility should be specific to the game or event situation. In the past decade there has been a con-

certed effort to improve agility in the mobile court and field sports, with much more time being spent on set drills in practice. When these have been thoroughly learned they are then integrated into the various moves that are constantly practised in high level sport. The days of the brilliant performer being the only player in the team able to perform cuts, swerves and side steps are long gone, because modern training now incorporates these skills for sports where such moves are needed.

Some tests for evaluating agility (described in Section 3) can also be used to improve this capacity. While many of them have been criticised as being poor tests of agility, their specificity alone makes them appropriate drills for use in the development of this capacity for a particular sport. Because static markers and turning positions are used in these tests, their effectiveness for developing agility among contact sports players is limited. It is often more appropriate to design one-on-one drills so that a player may develop agility and respond to the defensive efforts of a mobile opponent.

Evaluating Agility

Many field tests have been developed in order to evaluate agility. Most are specifically adapted to suit the needs of a particular sport, while others have a more general application. These tests typically involve short sprints and changes in direction, as well as the requirement that the subject accelerates rapidly from point to point on the course. Often equipment that is used in a particular sport will be incorporated into these tests. Several agility tests, both general and specific, are described in Section 3.

CONCLUSION

As with many of the other physical capacities, balance and agility may be modified and they can also be monitored using standardized tests. Intensive practice, however, is needed in sports where players need to change direction fast, or in various games where evasive action is required to avoid contact, so that these manoeuvres can be performed in a flowing and balanced way.

REFERENCES

Dintiman G. & Ward R. (1988) *Sport Speed*, pp. 152–153. Leisure Press, Champaign, IL, USA.

Draper J. & Lancaster M. (1985) The 505: A test for agility in the horizontal plane. *The Australian Journal of Science and Medicine in Sport* **17**, 15–18.

Tittel K. (1988) Coordination and balance. In Dirix H., Knuttgen H. & Tittel K. (eds) *The Olympic Book of Sports Medicine*, pp. 194–211. Blackwell Scientific Publications, Oxford.

Woolacott M., Shumway-Cook A. & Williams H. (1989) The development of posture and balance control in children. In Woollacott H. & Shumway-Cook A. (eds) *Development of Posture and Gait Across the Lifespan*, pp. 77–96. University of South Carolina, Columbia, SC, USA.

CHAPTER 13

TALENT IDENTIFICATION AND PROFILING IN SPORT

The previous chapters in this book have dealt with the various physical capacities of humans in relation to sport performance. This chapter is oriented towards the application of these capacities and how they can be applied when identifying talent and profiling athletes.

During the past 50 years coaches have identified talent and informally profiled athletes, but it was not until the early 1970s that Eastern European countries, especially Russia, East Germany, Hungary, Czechoslovakia and later China, began the systematic programmes that were to help them win a large number of medals internationally in the 1970s and the 1980s. Both Alabin *et al.* (1980) and Hahn (1990) suggest that efficient talent identification procedures play a very important role in modern sport and were a major factor in Eastern Europe's domination of many Olympic sports in the past two decades.

Similar programmes emerged in Western Europe, North America and some Commonwealth countries in the 1980s, but it is extremely difficult for countries that do not have sports institutes or centres of excellence for sport to compete with those that do. Where such sports systems are in operation, sport scientists and sports medicine specialists have been able to form sophisticated testing teams for talent identification and profiling, gathering systematic information from the athletes and integrating it into scientifically based training programmes for the benefit of both individuals and teams.

TALENT IDENTIFICATION

Most talent identification is done at the junior level in sport, although occasionally one hears of individuals who have been advised to change their event or sport when they are already senior athletes. This has occurred because sport science tests have shown that they have certain physical and/or physiological capacities which may enable them to perform at a high level in a particular sport. It is important to point out however, that late identification is occurring less frequently as international competition becomes more intense.

RATIONALE FOR TALENT IDENTIFICATION

As the aggressive sports systems of Eastern Europe have gradually broken down, the stigma of talent identification as being an undesirable practice is fast disappearing. In fact, apart from the use of drugs, which in some of these countries was rampant and cannot be condoned under any circumstances, talent identification was positive in many cases, as young athletes were well catered for both personally and from a sport development viewpoint. Bloomfield (1992) stated that the positive features of such programmes are as follows:

- 'Children are directed towards sports, or particular events, for which they are physically and physiologically best suited. This in turn means that they will probably obtain good results and enjoy their training and participation more
- Because of the nature of the programme, their physical health and general welfare are well looked after
- They are usually the recipients of specialized coaching, which is well supported by the sports medical team and sometimes by a sports psychologist
- The administrators of many of these programmes are now concerned about the vocational opportunities for the athletes after the conclusion of their competitive career and cater for them with high quality secondary or tertiary education or vocational training'

THE TALENT IDENTIFICATION PROCESS

Talent identification can be either very simple or highly sophisticated. One may find, for example, a school basketball coach recruiting players simply because they are tall for their age. Or a school swimming coach, who when walking around the playground, may observe the way children are standing: if they have naturally large pronated feet they may be prospectively good breast-stroke swimmers, as this physical capacity is needed for an efficient kick. Sophisticated programmes on the other hand, are highly oriented towards sport science and medicine, with a comprehensive test battery used to screen the young athletes.

General Talent Identification Screening

Sports systems or institutions within them that have sophisticated screening programmes examine several parameters which relate to junior athletes and construct a general profile of each subject. The following test series illustrates this.

HEALTH STATUS

First a medical examination is usually conducted, during which special attention is paid to the musculoskeletal and cardiovascular systems. Athletes with medical conditions that may at some time in the future limit their training or participation should be very carefully evaluated. Komadel (1988) quoted the diseases that were listed by the Czechoslovak Ministry for Health as contraindications to competition in sport at the highest level. Many Western sports medicine physicians would not totally agree with all of these, citing asthma and diabetes mellitus as diseases that can now be well controlled by high level athletes with the modern drugs which are currently available.

There would be, however, a general endorsement of the abovementioned list by the majority of sports physicians currently working with elite athletes.

HEREDITARY FACTORS

There are important hereditary factors that should be considered in the selection of talented athletes. As yet no systematic research has been carried out in this area, mainly because the parents of current high performance athletes did not have the opportunities to train as intensively, or to be tested as athletes are today and thus there are few comparative data. There is little doubt, however, as Sloane (1985) pointed out, that parents who have a personal interest in their children's activities will strongly support them and this will be of great assistance to them while they develop their basic skills. Even without categorical research, however, subjective observation points to the fact that there is often a strong genetic link between parents and their offspring in various sports.

TIME SPENT IN SPORT

It is important to establish how long each athlete has trained for his or her sport and how much coaching he or she has received. In some instances certain children will have been in a particular sport for a much longer period of time than others and will have already received considerably more specialized coaching. In such cases they may not develop much further with their skills and/or their cardiovascular capacity, if these are important selection criteria.

MATURITY

This important factor must be considered in any talent selection procedure. It is well known that early maturers are often taller, heavier, more powerful and faster than their counterparts during the early to mid teenage years. Many coaches have observed that early maturers have an advantage in junior sport and often neglect their skill development, whereas less physically mature athletes are forced to develop their skills earlier to perform well. The latter group when fully matured may have definite advantages over the early developers, because their physical capacity level is just as high, but their skills are better.

Specific Talent Identification Screening

All talent identification programmes must be concerned with every facet of the particular sport or event. The athletes' functional capacity using various physiological tests must be assessed, as well as their psychological profile. Because this text is oriented towards the physical capacities and technique development of athletes, it is this area which will now be discussed in detail. It is important, however, for the reader to understand that performance in sport is multifaceted and must be approached from many perspectives.

Physical Capacity Screening

SOMATOTYPE (BODY TYPE)

Body type is a general physical capacity which can be a useful indicator of future elite performance.

The *stability during growth* of the somatotype has been discussed by Malina and Bouchard (1991), who suggested that ectomorphy was reasonably stable during growth, but that mesomorphy and endomorphy in adolescent boys were not as predictable. Because boys experience

a marked increase in muscle mass during the adolescent growth spurt as a result of testosterone secretions, it is logical that somatotype variations will occur in this component. However, reasonably accurate forecasts can be made in mesomorphy, from around stage 3.5–4 of pubescent development, when a boy's musculature rapidly develops; that is, at approximately 14–14.5 years of age. The stability of the somatotype components in girls during adolescence is less well understood, but many coaches suggest that adolescent girls from around age 12.5–13 years tend to steadily increase their endomorphy rating as they develop and that this is accompanied by a drop in their power/weight ratio. This decrease can be detrimental for them in weight-bearing ballistic sports such as gymnastics, basketball, netball and volleyball where powerful movements are essential.

The *most suitable body types* for various sports and events have already been discussed in detail in Chapter 5. To be within one component of the mature body type at any time during the adolescent growth period would indicate that the young athlete is generally 'on track' as far as the attainment of an optimal shape is concerned. Well trained coaches are now aware that special intervention programmes using strength and power training and/or nutrition can alter the primary somatotype components over a 1.5–2 year period.

Exceptions to the standard body shape must be carefully considered because coaches and sports scientists report that some high level performers are outside the standard somatotype for a particular sport or event; some examples have been cited in Chapter 5. It must be emphasized again that body type is only a *general* physical capacity and is only useful when combined with several other measures, as it cannot be used as a single criterion in itself.

BODY COMPOSITION

As with somatotype, body composition is only a general indicator of high level performance. The *stability during growth* of an individual's body composition has been reviewed by Malina and Bouchard (1991) who suggested that body fat was not particularly stable from birth to 5 or 6 years, or during adolescence. They also stated, however, that 'the mark of excess fatness (in adults) thus appears to be greater for those who have thicker subcutaneous fat measurements during childhood'.

The *most suitable body composition* for young athletes in various sports has not been systematically documented. However, if they are within 1–2% body fat for a male or 3–4% for a female at around stage 3.5–4 of their pubescent development or when they are close to their peak height velocity (PHV), then they are 'on track' for the optimal body composition that is generally required for that sport or event. It should be noted, however, that the demands of some sports to have low fat levels, for example, in field or court sports, are not as great as in other sports such as gymnastics, where power to weight ratios play a significant role in an athlete's performances. As for body typing, coaches who are trying to predict late adolescent and post-adolescent female body composition, particularly fat mass (FM) for sports such as gymnastics, should 'err on the side of conservatism'. This means that they should select girls who have measures below the accepted optimal FM levels, in order to be as sure as possible that they will not increase their FM to the point where it will greatly affect their power to weight ratio. As a general rule this should be about 2% body fat.

As with body type, intervention programmes that use strength and power training and/or nutrition can be used to assist the individual to reach accepted body composition levels, both for lean body mass and FM for athletes who are reasonably close to the accepted levels.

PROPORTIONALITY

Proportionality can be an important self-selector for various sports and events. Many accurate forecasts with relation to individual and team performances have been made during the past two decades on the measurements of height and body mass alone.

The *stability of height* has not been studied in any detail but reasonable forecasts can be made on existing information and the experience of successful coaches. Malina and Bouchard (1991) and Tanner (1989), when discussing the stability of growth, suggested that until the age of 2 or 3 a child's growth is not particularly constant, but that from 2–3 years to the onset of adolescence, height is reasonably stable and predictable. During adolescence, because of the various spurts and plateaux, it is again unstable, but in the immediate post-adolescent period becomes stable again. At any time during a child's life, height or bone lengths are more constant than body mass.

Predictions of height and body mass (weight) have been made reasonably accurately for some time and Lowery (1978) gave several formulas to estimate height. He also quoted the work of Bayley and Pinneau (Bayer & Bayley 1959) who used skeletal age and tables to forecast growth. Another way to estimate final height and body mass is to determine a subject's skeletal age from an X-ray of the hand and wrist using Greulich and Pyle's atlas (1959), then use growth standards (Tanner 1989) for height and body mass to determine the mature measures. This method has been used by some coaches to forecast final heights and body masses of athletes where these variables are important factors, either when the athlete is too large for the event, such as in gymnastics, or too small, as in the throwing events.

The *proportions of athletes* vary greatly within racial groups and even more so between them, and Chapter 7 has illustrated the fact that certain individuals have very definite leverage advantages over others.

It is important to point out that very little research has been done on the stability of the proportions of the growing child and adolescent. Ackland and Bloomfield (1993) have suggested, however, that various segment widths remain stable throughout adolescence and can therefore be used for predictive purposes. On the other hand they also found that many segment lengths were unstable during adolescence and suggested that these should not be used as prediction criteria in talent identification programmes.

POSTURE

As with proportionality, posture is an important self-selector for various sports and events within them. Chapter 8 has comprehensively discussed the value of certain types of postures which give some competitors very definite advantages over their opponents. However, the *stability of posture* during growth has not been examined in a systematic way and again most of the information has been formulated from anecdotal evidence. The general feeling about posture is that it steadily develops during adolescence and becomes more extreme as the individual ages. Perceptive sport scientists and coaches, however, will be able to identify these developments and forecast with some degree of accuracy what the athlete's ultimate posture will be.

The *posture of athletes*, like that of the normal population, varies greatly. However, there are several postures that give athletes an immense advantage over their competitors. They are as follows:

- Individuals with *inverted feet* or 'pigeon toes' have a speed advantage over short distances when compared to those athletes with conventional foot posture or everted feet (Bloomfield 1979). This characteristic is especially valuable where acceleration is needed over short distances in such games as tennis, squash, badminton and volleyball
- In sprint running events, or in games where very fast running is advantageous, athletes with *partial lordosis accompanied by an anterior pelvic tilt* (APT) are at an advantage. If this characteristic is combined with *protruding* or *'high' buttocks* which are also well muscled, then the athlete is normally a very fast runner, provided that the other physical capacities are present which are important in sprinting (Bloomfield 1979). This posture also appears to assist those individuals who are in jumping-oriented games such as basketball and volleyball, as well as the jumping athletes in the field events (Figs 8.11, 8.13)
- Agility athletes who possess the overhanging knee joint where there is a small degree of flexion at this joint, appear to have an advantage in sprinting and in events where mobility is necessary (Fig. 8.11)

- Distance runners generally have *'flat backs'* with little lordosis, almost no pelvic tilt and flat buttocks. This type of posture assists them to run with a reasonably upright body, which in turn enables them to develop an uncramped stride, thus marginally increasing their stride length (Fig. 8.12)
- Female gymnasts with *lordosis* and an accompanying APT are able to hyperextend their spines more easily than competitors with a flat lower back and buttocks. This postural characteristic also appears to enable them to leap higher than gymnasts who lack this feature
- Various postures assist swimmers in different events. It is well known that *'square-shouldered'* swimmers with long clavicles and large scapulae, particularly the acromion process, have lower levels of flexion–extension movement of the upper limb and shoulder girdle. Foot and leg postures are also important, with *everted feet* or 'duck feet' being very suitable for breast-stroke swimming, while swimmers with *inverted feet* or 'pigeon toes' are able to perform the dolphin, freestyle and backstroke kicks more efficiently

Coaches need to carefully observe the athlete's posture in order to determine whether or not it is advantageous to the performance. Posture can be partially modified using flexibility and strength training, but this must be done at an early stage in the individual's development because changes are difficult to make during late adolescence and early adulthood.

STRENGTH AND POWER

Strength and explosive power in many sports are essential physical capacities and performances in sport have improved at a rapid rate since they became important components of the modern training programme.

The *stability of strength* according to Malina and Bouchard (1991) is reasonably high from year to year, for example, from 11 to 12 years of age, but the correlations decline as the age gap widens. They reported that correlations between 7 and 12 years, and correlations between 12 and 17 years, were low to moderate, with the latter being more highly correlated than the former. One important point which the above authors made, however, was that a composite of strength measures tended to be more stable than specific measures.

Eastern European coaches have suggested for some time that around the PHV period (~14 years of age) in the adolescent male's growth spurt is a reasonably reliable time to make future forecasts on mature strength levels. This has been done particularly well in the sport of weightlifting and can probably apply to other sports.

The *importance of strength and power* in the majority of sports is now well accepted and early identification of high strength and power levels can be very helpful to the coach. Strength and power are closely related to body shape, body composition, proportionality and posture, and therefore the coach can observe the more powerful athletes as they develop during adolescence. Athletes can at an early stage continue to develop this important characteristic as part of the normal training programme if they already demonstrate this capacity, but a special intervention programme may be necessary for the young athlete whose skill levels and other physical attributes are high, but whose levels of strength and power are low. With the modern strength and explosive power training equipment and methods that are now available and which are outlined in Chapter 9, it is possible to develop a strong and powerful athlete, if this training is done during adolescence.

FLEXIBILITY

Flexibility is a very important physical capacity in the majority of modern sports. Very little research has been done with relation to its *stability during growth* and the studies which have been done are mainly of a gross nature with several body segments involved. Malina and Bouchard (1991) reported data from several sources who used the sit and reach test. These showed that in boys the scores were stable from 5 to 8 years, they declined to ages 12–13 years, then increased again to approximately 18 years. The girls' scores were

stable from 5 to 11 years, they increased to 14 years, then gradually flattened out from that time on.

With such variable data currently available, it is difficult to reach any conclusions as to the validity of flexibility as an indicator of future talent. Modern flexibility training methods are so good that reasonably high levels can now be reached by most athletes if their programmes are started either in pre-adolescence or in the early stages of adolescence. Chapter 10 outlines these programmes in detail for a large range of sports.

Finally, if the individual is partially or fully hypermobile (i.e. at levels 3 or 4 in Fig. 14.35), then the coach will be able to determine whether or not this will be detrimental or advantageous for the young athlete when maturity is reached.

SPEED

Speed of movement is an essential physical capacity for high levels of performance in many sports. Again very little research has been done in this area except for running speed, which is only one aspect of speed. However, most coaches are aware at an early stage whether their athlete is fast or slow either in running speed or other movements, because they are continually comparing them with other athletes of similar age.

Finally, speed training techniques are now well developed, and intervention programmes are commonplace in modern training, but young athletes should be at least 10 years of age before they embark on such a programme, if high levels of performance are to be reached by the time they become senior athletes.

RELATIONSHIP OF THE PHYSICAL CAPACITIES OF THE YOUNG ATHLETE TO OTHER CAPACITIES

It is important to again point out that no single physical capacity on its own can be the absolute criterion for success in sport, so the coach should be careful not to place too much emphasis on just one or two variables, but should assess the body as a total unit. It is important for the athlete to have several physical capacities that are basic to a particular sport, but young athletes must also have the other essential physiological, psychological and skill characteristics before they can be regarded as talented.

CONCLUSION

In conclusion, the selection of prospective elite athletes using talent identification is a complex problem. Because there is a dearth of knowledge as to how maturity affects the physical, physiological and psychological make-up of the individual, it is often difficult to ascertain whether the results of tests given early in an athlete's life will be useful predictors for the future. With more longitudinal testing of elite groups, the sport scientist and sport physician will be able to predict future success more accurately, and in so doing make talent identification a more reliable method of choosing future sporting talent. A further important point was raised by Hahn (1990) who stated that: 'Talent identification and talent selection programmes will not of themselves guarantee the emergence of champions. To realize their potential, the people selected must have regular access to top-level coaching, as well as appropriate facilities and equipment. They must (also) have a clear network of support, and, if possible, such additional elements as sport science and sports medicine services.'

PROFILING

Athletic profiling has been carried out by coaches in an informal way for many years. During the past two decades formal profiling has steadily developed, first in Eastern Europe and more recently in Western Europe, North America and some Commonwealth countries. The purpose of this section is to discuss modern sports profiling and how it can aid athletes to produce their best performances.

RATIONALE FOR PROFILING

All high level athletes are unique individuals with many physical, physiological and psychological strengths, otherwise they would not have reached the elite level. Athletes also have weaknesses which need to be known by the coach, who will then be able to take remedial action to strengthen them, because the old adage that 'a chain is only as strong as its weakest link' is true for an athlete as well.

TYPES OF PROFILING

Two types of profiling should be carried out with high level athletes, and these are as follows.

General Profiling

General profiling is done in a de-trained state and administered at the commencement of a season. The results of a series of tests will give the coach a general profile of the athlete.

In order to ascertain the individual's actual status within the group, the above results should be evaluated not only against other high level athletes in the same sport or event, but also against their own team-mates. The most important comparison will be that which is made against other elite athletes in the same sport or event. However, the individual's status within the team or squad is often of interest to the athlete and is certainly of value to the coach.

When the coach has evaluated the test results with the relevant sport scientists and/or the sports physician, the season's training schedule with each individual's strengths and weaknesses in mind can then be planned. Often, this general training plan will also take into consideration skill weakness, so that several team members ranking lower than their team-mates in the various tests will be given an intervention programme in addition to their normal training. It should be kept in mind that general profiling is often more useful for the potential elite athlete in the developmental stages while still at the national junior or youth level, whereas for the senior international level athlete it will not be as valuable.

FREQUENCY OF THE TESTS

Most coaches only profile once each season at this level in order to identify weaknesses. Others have follow-up tests at varying intervals to monitor the general progress of the intervention programmes. Agility athletes in 'closed' sports such as gymnasts and divers are regularly monitored for body composition, because power to weight ratios are crucial factors in their performances.

Specific Profiling

Specific profiling is usually done with elite senior athletes where events are won by very small margins or times, as in aerobic sports such as swimming, rowing, kayaking, running and cycling, where it is important to accurately evaluate the individual's adaptation to the stress of heavy training at regular intervals.

FREQUENCY OF THE TESTS

In some programmes tests are done as regularly as every 2 weeks, but more often a month apart, which fits in well with a 3/1 training cycle. When a major championship is approaching, some coaches request that only the 'key' stress adaptation tests be done at more regular intervals, which could be as often as every week. With athletes who are more skill oriented, specific profiling will only be done approximately every 6 months, because alterations to the athlete's physical capacities take a longer time to occur.

HEALTH STATUS CHECKS

At the commencement of each season a general health evaluation should be conducted by the sports medicine physician. This can also be fol-lowed up in mid-season or at other times which are thought appropriate by the medical and coaching team.

These checks give the sport physician and other specialists such as the nutritionist an opportunity to discuss, both at the team or individual level, various personal health problems which the athletes may have. Young athletes in particular feel that such discussions are very valuable.

SPORT SCIENCE TESTS USED IN PROFILING

Various sports have differing demands, therefore only tests which are highly specific to that sport should be used. It is pointless giving a pistol shooter or archer complex cardiovascular evaluations at regular intervals, because endurance is not an important factor in these events. One should not completely dismiss this point however, because all athletes need a reasonably high physical fitness level to assist them with other more specific skills and mental tasks, even if there is no specific cardiovascular component in their event. However, unless there is a definite need for both endurance and skill in an event, it is often a waste of time and money giving a sophisticated test such as a maximal oxygen uptake ($\dot{V}_{O_2max}$) test to a non-endurance athlete.

Physiological Tests

Physiological tests are selectively used by sport scientists to suit different types of sports or events and fall into the following categories.

CARDIOVASCULAR TESTS

The following tests are normally used in specific profiling:

- Aerobic power tests using specific ergometers to suit the sport or event in which the individual is competing
- Anaerobic power and capacity tests using specific ergometers where mean power output is calculated and total body load measured

BIOCHEMICAL AND HAEMATOLOGICAL TESTS

The following tests are used in order to identify non-adaptation to training:

- Haemoglobin (Hb)
- Blood haematocrit
- Lymphocyte and neutrophil counts
- Ferritin
- Uric acid
- Urea
- Creatine phosphokinase (CPK)
- Testosterone/cortisol levels

Psychological Tests

A large number of psychological variables have recently been isolated which are known to affect sports performance. They are normally used in general profiling and are as follows:

- Aggression
- Anxiety
- Arousal
- Attention
- Cohesion
- Independence
- Personality — extroversion/introversion
- Leadership
- Mood
- Motivation
- Self-concept/self-esteem

Skill Evaluation

During the past decade, coaches and sports biomechanists have been developing skill profiles on both their individual athletes and their games players. With the use of high-speed photography or video, coaches are now able to accurately pinpoint technique weaknesses in their athletes. Some coaches still administer skills tests to their competitors, but much less of this is now being done, mainly because an artificial 'laboratory' environment is created and also because modern technique analysis equipment used in a competitive training situation allows for a more realistic assessment.

When technique errors are located the athlete is placed on a special intervention programme in order to improve one or several skills where the coach feels additional training is needed. This is usually done in separate remedial workouts and not in the scheduled team or squad training sessions.

Physical Capacity Tests

Several physical capacity tests have been mentioned in the talent identification section of this chapter as well as being discussed in detail in the previous chapters of this book.

The following capacities are normally profiled:

- Height and body mass (weight)
- Somatotype and body composition
- Proportionality
- Strength and explosive power
- Speed of movement
- Flexibility
- Posture
- Balance and agility

SETTING UP THE PROFILE

As has been mentioned previously, profiles are normally constructed from data obtained from other elite athletes within the same sport or event. Until recently it has been difficult to obtain international level data for comparative purposes, as there was a dearth of it in published form and because the test protocols sometimes varied from country to country. It is pleasing to note that both these problems are now being overcome and more reliable data are available for comparative purposes.

To develop a profile when one has the data is relatively simple. Norms must first be constructed based on percentile scores, T-scores, Z-scores or deviations from the mean of these data.

Table 13.1 demonstrates flexibility scores of junior swimmers, while Table 13.2 gives physical capacity percentile scores for international women tennis players.

Table 13.1 Shoulder flexion–extension percentiles scores of Australian junior swimmers

Percentile	Males			Females		
	11–12 years (n=15)	13–14 years (n=22)	15–16 years (n=22)	11–12 years (n=20)	13–14 years (n=21)	15–16 years (n=16)
99	271	266	252	268	267	258
95	270	243	242	253	259	257
90	261	240	238	245	248	248
85	260	237	237	244	246	247
80	253	233	236	242	242	246
75	252	230	235	237	240	236
70	250	226	230	236	234	234
65	244	225	234	235	233	233
60	237	224	227	234	232	232
55	236	217	226	233	225	230
50	235	215	226	232	224	229
45	234	214	221	230	216	228
40	233	213	217	225	214	225
35	232	212	215	224	213	207
30	228	211	213	216	212	206
25	225	210	210	213	211	205
20	207	209	206	212	210	191
15	206	208	203	210	206	190
10	205	207	200	209	201	188
5	204	180	190	188	200	161
$\bar{x}$	236	218	216	233	223	220
SD	30	42	16	20	33	35

Scores measured in degrees. (From Bloomfield *et al.* 1983.)

A profile sheet can be used to enter the data then the graph can be constructed from it. Figure 13.1 shows data from an international level male oarsman under *score* and his profile graph under *percentile scores*. Furthermore, the profile should be drawn simply so that athletes can easily understand it, because they should take part in the discussion with the coach and the relevant sport scientist.

EVALUATING THE PROFILE

Physical capacity profiles, whether they be general or specific, are simple to interpret and examples of these profiles are given in Figs 13.2 and 13.3. These are of athletes who were first tested to generally profile them, then at a later time were re-tested to see whether the intervention programme on which they had been placed had improved their physical status. The athlete in Fig. 13.2 is a female gymnast of linear build with low levels of strength and power, but a high level of skill. She had a somatotype which rated **2.5–3.0–3.5** with a percentage fat level of 12.5. She was given a general strength training programme over and above her normal training three times a week for 20 months. During this time her somatotype changed to a **2.0–4.0–3.0** and her percentage body fat was reduced to 9.6. The dotted line on the right-hand side of the original graph shows the other changes which were made during this time.

The subject in Fig. 13.3 had a relatively low cardiovascular fitness level, was slightly overweight and was not particularly strong for his body mass. His somatotype was **3.0–4.5–4.0** and percentage body fat 12.9. After an 18 month training period, which included a moderate diet and three strength training sessions each week in addition to his normal training, his physical status and cardiovascular fitness level had improved significantly. Examples of this can be seen on the

Table 13.2 Percentile scores of international women tennis players

Variable					Percentile					
	10	20	30	40	50	60	70	80	90
Height (cm)	163.0	164.7	165.7	166.5	167.5	168.5	169.5	171.3	173.0
Body mass (kg)	51.6	53.9	56.5	58.7	60.7	62.7	64.8	67.4	70.9
Body composition									
Body density (g/mL)	1.009	1.022	1.031	1.039	1.047	1.055	1.063	1.070	1.075
Body fat (%)	30.3	28.8	26.2	24.1	22.1	20.1	17.9	15.3	11.8
Triceps skinfold (mm)	17.0	16.1	15.5	15.0	14.5	14.0	13.4	12.8	11.9
Subscapular skinfold (mm)	11.0	10.1	9.5	9.0	8.5	8.0	7.4	6.8	5.9
Suprailiac skinfold (mm)	14.4	12.9	11.8	10.8	10.0	9.1	8.1	7.00	5.5
Abdominal skinfold (mm)	14.8	13.2	11.6	10.7	10.1	9.3	7.9	7.2	5.4
Proportionality									
Brachial index	73.2	75.2	76.6	77.8	79.0	80.1	81.8	82.7	84.7
Crural index	98.2	100.2	101.6	102.8	104.0	106.1	108.3	109.7	112.0
Relative sitting height (%)	50.3	51.0	51.6	52.0	52.5	52.9	53.3	53.9	54.6
Flexibility									
Arm flexion–extension (deg)	182.2	189.7	195.1	199.7	204.0	208.2	215.9	224.2	235.7
Forearm flexion–extension (deg)	124.6	129.9	133.7	137.0	140.0	143.0	146.2	150.0	155.3
Foot dorso–plantar flexion (deg)	54.7	58.2	60.8	63.0	65.0	67.0	69.1	71.7	75.2
Leg flexion (deg)	107.0	113.2	117.7	121.5	125.0	128.5	132.2	136.7	142.9
Strength									
Grip strength (kgf)	20.9	23.5	25.4	27.1	28.6	30.1	31.7	33.6	36.2
Arm flexion strength (kgf)	14.2	24.8	32.5	39.0	45.0	51.0	57.4	65.1	75.7
Arm extension strength (kgf)	11.8	21.5	28.5	34.5	40.0	45.5	51.4	58.4	68.1
Leg extension torque SS3 (ft. lbs)	16.4	69.2	107.6	140.0	170.0	200.0	232.4	270.8	323.6
SS7 (ft. lbs)	14.4	54.2	92.6	125.0	155.0	185.0	217.4	255.8	308.6
Power/speed									
Jump and reach (cm)	37.3	39.9	41.8	43.5	45.0	46.5	48.1	50.0	52.6
40 m dash (s)	7.1	6.8	6.6	6.4	6.3	6.1	5.9	5.7	5.4
Agility run (s)	8.7	17.8	17.2	16.7	16.2	5.6	15.1	14.5	13.6

Endomorphy mean = 3.5; mesomorphy mean = 3.5; ectomorphy mean = 3.0.

Male Oarsman

Level: National crew
Age: 22 years

Variable	Score	Percentile scores*
	10 20 30	40 50 60 70 80 90
Height	192 cm	
Body mass	98 kg	
Body composition		
Body density	1.093 g/mL	
Body fat	5%	
Triceps skinfold	7 mm	
Subscapular skinfold	7 mm	
Suprailiac skinfold	4 mm	
Abdominal skinfold	7 mm	
Proportionality		
Brachial index	76	
Crural index	102	
Relative sitting height	53%	
Flexibility		
Arm flexion/extension	216 deg	
Forearm flexion/extension	136 deg	
Foot dorso-plantar flexion	69 deg	
Leg flexion	131 deg	
Strength		
Grip	63 kgf	
Arm flexion	92 kgf	
Arm extension	83 kgf	
Leg extension torque		
Speed setting — 3	382 ft. lbs	
Speed setting — 7	360 ft. lbs	
Power/speed		
Jump and reach	48 cm	
36.6 m dash	5.4 s	
Agility run	17.5 s	

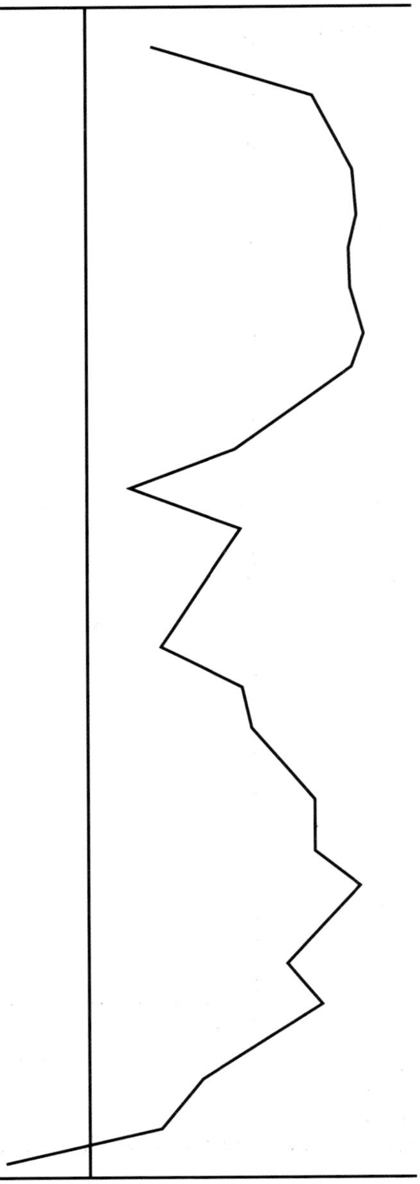

Somatotype:
Endomorphy 1.5; mesomorphy 6.0; ectomorphy 2.5.
* Percentile scores for international level oarsmen.

Fig. 13.1 A profile of an international level oarsman.

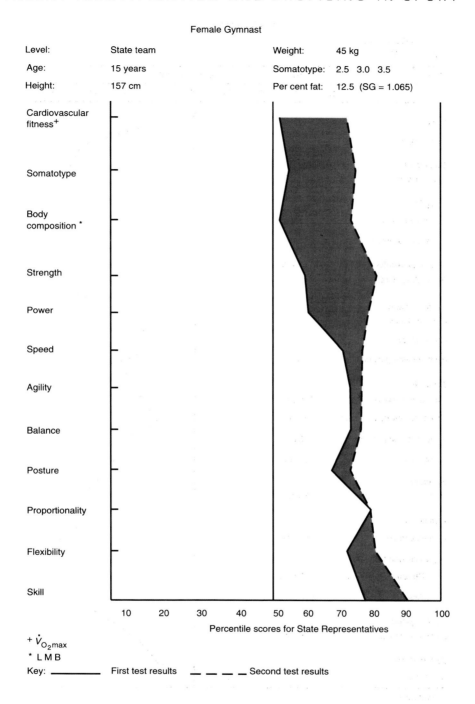

Fig. 13.2 The profiles of a female state level gymnast recorded before and after a 20 month intervention programme (from Bloomfield 1979).

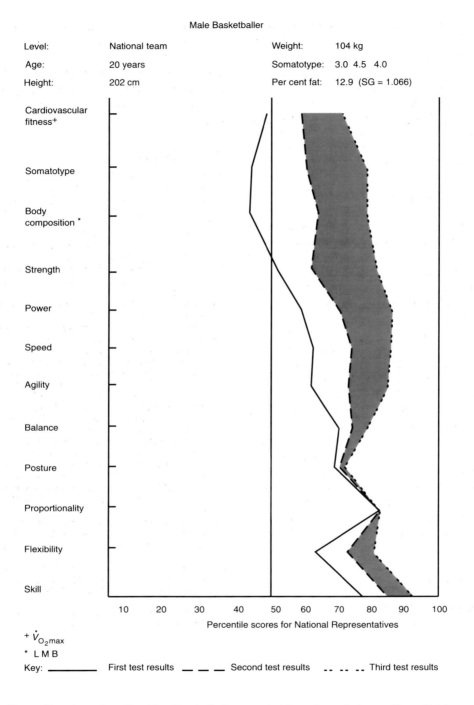

Male Basketballer

Level:	National team	Weight:	104 kg
Age:	20 years	Somatotype:	3.0 4.5 4.0
Height:	202 cm	Per cent fat:	12.9 (SG = 1.066)

Percentile scores for National Representatives

+ $\dot{V}_{O_2 max}$
* L M B

Key: ———— First test results — — — Second test results .. .. .. Third test results

Fig. 13.3 The profiles of a male national level basketballer recorded three times during an 18 month intervention programme.

profile graph which shows his second test, which was done 9 months into his intervention programme, and his third test which was administered 9 months later. Furthermore it is interesting to note that his body type was **2.5–4.5–4.0** at the second test and **2.0–5.0–4.0** at the third, while his percentage body fat measures had changed from 12.9 to 11 then to 9.7% at the third testing session. The other positive changes can be seen on the right-hand side of the graph.

PROGRAMME DEVELOPMENT

After the profile has been evaluated, the decision should be made as to whether the individual needs an intervention programme. Whether one is needed or not, the coach and athlete should confer at this stage, as the status of each team member in comparison with other athletes of a similar level, or the ranking on each variable within the team or squad, should also be known by the individual. In some cases athletes can even take part in the development of their own programme, especially if they are mature individuals.

It is important at this point that a formal intervention programme be devised that is in a printed form. Targets or goals should be realistic and the competitor should be clear as to what these are and how they can be achieved. The coach should also set the time of the next test battery, whether it be 3 or 6 months hence, or at the beginning of the next season. This gives the athlete a target date to be aimed for, rather than a nebulous period over which the programme should be carried out.

CONCLUSION

Until recently, profiling has only been carried out randomly in various institutes and centres of excellence throughout the world. Now that more international sport science literature is available with which to make comparisons between athletes, and more test protocols are becoming internationally standardized, profiling is becoming an important feature of the elite athlete's development.

REFERENCES

Alabin V., Nischt G. & Jefimov W. (1980) Talent selection. *Modern Athlete and Coach* **18**, 36–37.

Ackland T. & Bloomfield J. (1993) Stability of proportions through adolescent growth. *Proceedings of the Annual Meeting of the Australian Sports Medicine Federation*, Melbourne 1993.

Bayer L. & Bayley N. (1959) *Growth Diagnosis.* University of Chicago Press, Chicago.

Bloomfield J. (1979) Modifying human physical capacities and technique to improve performance. *Sports Coach* **3**, 19–25.

Bloomfield J., Blanksby B. & Ackland T. (1983) Anatomical profiles of Australian junior swimmers. *The Australian Journal of Sports Sciences* **3**, 14–20.

Bloomfield J. (1992) Talent identification and profiling. In Bloomfield J., Fricker P. A. & Fitch K. (eds) *Textbook of Science and Medicine in Sport,* pp. 187–198. Blackwell Scientific Publications, Melbourne.

Greulich W. & Pyle S. (1959) *Radiographic Atlas of Skeletal Development of the Hand and Wrist.* Stanford University Press, Palo Alto, CA, USA.

Hahn A. (1990) Identification and selection of talent in Australian rowing. *Excel* **6**, 5–11.

Komadel L. (1988) The identification of performance potential. In Dirix A., Knuttgen H. & Tittel K. (eds) *The Olympic Book of Sports Medicine I,* pp. 275–285. Blackwell Scientific Publications, Oxford.

Lowery G. (1978) *Growth and Development of Children,* 7th edn, pp. 96–97. Year Book Medical Publishers, Chicago.

Malina R. & Bouchard C. (1991) *Growth, Motivation and Physical Activity,* pp. 60–64, 83–84, 96–100, 202–203, 445–458. Human Kinetics Books, Champaign, IL, USA.

Sloane K. (1985) Home influences on talent development. In Bloom B. (ed.) *Developing Talent in Young People,* pp. 440–444. Ballantine Books, New York.

Tanner J. (1989) *Foetus into Man,* pp. 65–70, 178–221. Castlemead Publications, Ware, UK.

SECTION 3

ASSESSMENT OF PHYSICAL CAPACITY

CHAPTER 14

ASSESSMENT OF PHYSICAL CAPACITY

INTRODUCTION

The final section of this book is devoted to a discussion of methods used in the measurement of physical capacities which have been described in Section 2. An overview of many commonly used assessment methodologies is presented here, together with an appraisal of their technical strengths and limitations. This information is vital for students of human movement and physical and health education, as they prepare for a professional career in these fields.

This section of the book may also be used as a reference work for sport and exercise scientists who play a supporting role to coaches in athlete preparation. Full details are given to permit accurate and reliable collection of data for those methodologies which are considered the most appropriate in terms of their validity and reliability. For other methods that are not supported by the authors, appropriate references to source or review publications are given.

While many of the arguments presented for or against the adoption of a particular methodology may be of relevance to the scientist, some coaches with the appropriate background will also benefit from a fuller appreciation of the problems associated with collecting valid and reliable data. Thus it is hoped that by reading this section coaches may gain an increased understanding of the role and requirements of the sport scientist.

KINANTHROPOMETRY

The quantification of human morphology is a fundamental requirement for the assessment and monitoring of high performance athletes and talented juniors alike. Many of the parameters measured under the banner of kinanthropometry are also used in the determination of other physical capacities, such as body composition, body type and proportionality. Furthermore, these fundamental measures may be employed to normalize or equate data for populations of varying size or age, in the assessment of other physical capacities and in the biomechanical analysis of technique.

One serious concern which has plagued scientists in this field for many years has been the lack of a universally adopted protocol for kinanthropometric assessment. Many different measurement procedures and landmarks have evolved in various schools of physical anthropology around the globe and this has added to the problem. The International Society for the Advancement of Kinanthropometry (ISAK) was founded in 1986 with the aim of fostering a united approach to the study of kinanthropometry. The techniques adopted in this chapter are consistent with those prescribed by the ISAK Working Group on Standards and Instrumentation and supported by the Laboratory Standards Assistance Scheme of the Australian Sports Commission (adopted for use in Australia in 1993).

ANATOMICAL CONVENTIONS

A description of body landmarks and other sites for measurement requires a standard reference system. This helps to alleviate confusion, especially when the body is oriented in a posture other than standing. The relative location of parts of the body may be accurately defined using the following terminology for a subject standing in the anatomical position, as shown in Fig. 14.1.

- *Sagittal plane* — a vertical plane which divides the body into left and right portions. The mid-sagittal plane is that which runs centrally through the body to create equal left and right parts. The term *medial* refers to relative locations that are closer to this mid-sagittal plane, as opposed to *lateral* which means away from this plane

- *Coronal plane* — a vertical plane that is perpendicular to the sagittal plane and which divides the body into front and rear portions. The term *anterior* refers to relative locations which are closer to the front of the body, while *posterior* means toward the rear

- *Transverse plane* — a horizontal plane that is perpendicular to both sagittal and coronal planes and which divides the body into upper and lower portions. The term *superior* refers to relative locations which are toward the top of the head, while *inferior* means toward the soles of the feet

- With respect to limbs, which may be oriented in many positions in relation to the trunk, it is often useful to employ the terms *proximal* and *distal*. Proximal refers to relative locations toward the trunk, while distal means toward the extremity

LANDMARKS

A decision must be made initially as to whether both sides of the body are to be measured or whether one side will be sampled. Apart from studies of body asymmetry, it is more common for the latter strategy to be adopted. However, it must also be decided whether to measure on the right side, the left side, the preferred side or the non-preferred side of the body. The logical strategy will depend on the nature of the study or subject population, but for most situations it is usual to measure on the right side. This procedure is supported by the ISAK Working Group on Standards and Instrumentation.

It is very important that sites be rechecked after their initial marking, since movement of the skin over the skeleton may alter the relative position of the mark when pressure is released. Marking should always be performed with a fine to medium point, non-permanent pen or pencil.

The following do not constitute an exhaustive list of landmarks, but are those required for the measurements that are generally used in sport science and medicine. They also form the basis for locating other measurement sites such as those for skinfolds and girths, which will be elaborated

upon in later sections of this chapter. The landmarks and methods for their location are described below and shown in Fig. 14.2, with the assumption that the right side of the body is to be measured. Furthermore, some sites like those for maximum bone breadths do not actually need marking, since they may be easily relocated by palpation of the site.

- *Orbitale* — inferior margin of the orbit (see Fig. 14.2)
- *Tragion* — the notch superior to the tragus of

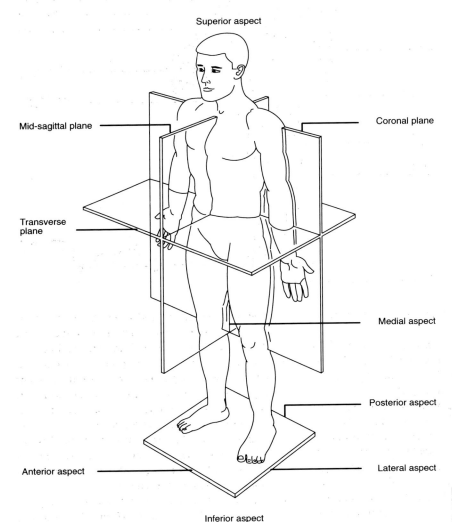

Superior aspect

Mid-sagittal plane

Coronal plane

Transverse plane

Medial aspect

Posterior aspect

Anterior aspect

Lateral aspect

Inferior aspect

Fig. 14.1 A standard reference system for anatomical relationships.

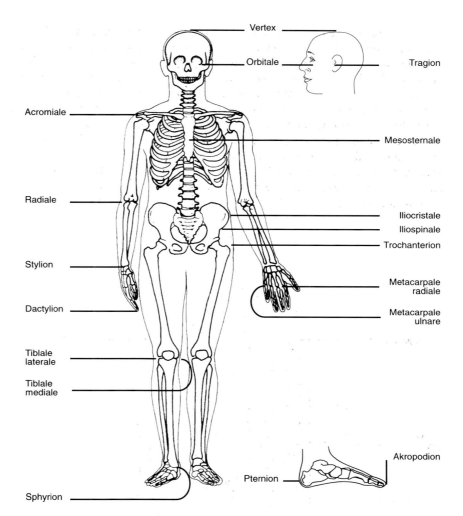

Fig. 14.2 Anatomical landmarks.

the ear at the superior aspect of the zygomatic arch

- *Vertex* — the most superior point on the skull in the mid-sagittal plane, when the head is held in the Frankfort plane. That is, when the orbitale and tragion are horizontally aligned
- *Acromiale* — the point at the most superior and lateral border of the acromion process when the subject stands erect with arms relaxed and hanging vertically. *Marking*: Holding the marking pencil as a straight edge, depress the tissue on the lateral aspect of the acromion process and identify its most superior and lateral border with the left thumb nail.

Remove the pencil and re-establish the location with the nail of your left index finger. Mark the site with a horizontal line and recheck

- *Radiale* — the point at the most proximal and lateral border of the head of the radius. *Marking*: With the subject's arm in a mid-pronated position, palpate the junction between the lateral humeral epicondyle and the head of the radius to establish the most proximal border of the radius. Re-establish the site with the nail of your left index finger. Mark the site with a horizontal line and recheck
- *Stylion* — the most distal point on the styloid process of the radius. *Marking:* The subject's

arm remains in mid-pronation. Palpate the space between the distal radius and the proximal aspect of metacarpal one to find the styloid process. Establish the most distal border of this process with the nail of your left index finger. Mark with a horizontal line and recheck

- *Metacarpale radiale* — the most lateral aspect of the distal head of the second metacarpal
- *Metacarpale ulnare* — the most medial aspect of the distal head of the fifth metacarpal
- *Dactylion* — the most distal point of the third digit of the hand
- *Mesosternale* — a point over the sternum in the mid-sagittal plane at the mid level of the fourth chondrosternal articulation. *Marking*: Using both hands, place the index fingers on top of the subject's clavicles approximately 10 cm apart, and your thumbs in the space below the first rib (the first intercostal space). Move the index fingers in position to replace the thumbs, then reposition the thumbs down to the second intercostal space (thus identifying the second rib). This procedure is repeated twice more until the fourth rib is identified. Keeping the left hand in position, estimate the mid-point and mark over the centre of the sternum. Recheck the location of the site
- *Iliocristale* — the most lateral aspect of the iliac crest
- *Iliospinale* — the inferior surface of the anterior superior iliac spine (ASIS). *Marking*: Palpate the iliac crest anteriorly with your left hand to identify the ASIS, then with the thumb nail, establish the inferior surface. Mark with a horizontal line and recheck
- *Trochanterion* — the most superior aspect of the greater trochanter of the femur. *Marking*: Position the subject so that the feet are together and pointing forward with body weight evenly distributed. Stand behind the subject and place the left hand on the subject's left hip to provide stability. Applying firm pressure, palpate the greater trochanter of the right femur with the palm and thumb of your right hand. Locate the most superior aspect with firm palpation and establish the position of the landmark with the nail of the index finger of your left

hand. Mark with a horizontal line and recheck
- *Tibiale laterale* — the most superior aspect of the lateral tibial condyle. *Marking*: Direct the subject to stand on a box so that you can palpate the junction between the lateral femoral and tibial condyles. Using firm pressure, establish the most superior point on the tibia (which should be approximately one-third of the distance from the anterior aspect moving posteriorly) with the nail of your left index finger. Mark with a horizontal line and recheck
- *Tibiale mediale* — the most superior and medial aspect of the medial tibial condyle. *Marking*: Direct the subject to sit on the box and cross the right leg over the left so that it is horizontal and presents the medial aspect of the leg toward you. Firmly palpate the junction between the medial femoral and tibial condyles and establish the location of this landmark with the nail of your left index finger. Mark and recheck
- *Sphyrion* — the most distal border of the medial malleolus of the tibia. *Marking*: With the subject seated as above, palpate the medial malleolus and locate its distal border with the nail of your left index finger. Mark and recheck
- *Pternion* — the most posterior point of the calcaneus
- *Akropodion* — the most anterior point of the foot, which may be the first or second digit

EQUIPMENT

The following equipment would be regarded as the minimum requirement for a complete anthropometric assessment of athletes (Fig. 14.3). Full descriptions of these instruments and their relative merits may be found in Ross and Marfell-Jones (1991) and Carter and Ackland (1994). This list is by no means exhaustive, but does reflect many of the commonly used instruments which are currently available.

- Length assessment — stadiometer, anthropometer (Siber-Hegner GPM or Harpenden), segmometer
- Body mass assessment — a beam type bal-

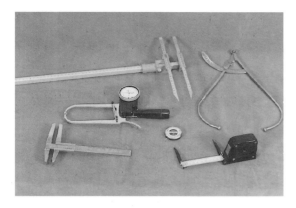

Fig. 14.3 A complete set of standard anthropometric equipment with the exception of a stadiometer and balance or electronic scales.

ance scale with a range of 0–150 kg and calibrated to 0.1 kg

- Breadth assessment — anthropometer (Siber-Hegner GPM or Harpenden), bone caliper (Holtain or Mitutoyo), wide-spreading caliper (Siber-Hegner GPM or Holtain)
- Girth assessment — anthropometric tape (Lufkin Executive diameter tape, Keuffel and Esser Whyteface tape or any other steel tape with clearly marked and calibrated metric units and no wider than 7 mm)
- Skinfolds — skinfold calipers (Harpenden, Slimguide, Skyndex, Lange, TEC or Lafayette)
- Other equipment — anthropometric box (a 50 × 40 × 30 cm box is extremely useful for anthropometric measurement)

MEASUREMENTS

For all of the following measurements, subjects should wear only bathers (preferably two piece for women) or light shorts and no footwear. Unless stated to the contrary, all scores are recorded to the nearest 0.1 cm. Where time permits, measurements should be made in triplicate and the median score selected. That is, each group of measures should be attempted once, then the whole group measured twice more. In this way the measurer is less likely to be influenced by pre-

vious scores. However, if time is a limiting factor the mean of two measures is acceptable. Nevertheless, it is always advisable to attempt triple measurements for girths and skinfolds, since the technical error in these measures is generally greater than that for lengths and breadths.

Body Mass

Check that the scale is at the zero mark, then direct the subject to stand in the centre of the platform. The mass is recorded to the nearest 0.01 kg.

Direct and Projected Lengths

STANDING HEIGHT (STRETCH STATURE)

Direct the subject to stand erect with heels, buttocks and shoulders pressed against the upright portion of the stadiometer. The heels should be touching and the arms should hang by the sides in a natural manner. Lower the headboard so that it touches the vertex of the head. Place your thumbs at the level of the orbitale and index fingers at the level of the tragion and align the subject's head in the Frankfort plane. Place the remaining fingers under the mastoid process of the temporal bone and gently but firmly stretch the vertebral column. Instruct the subject to 'look straight ahead and take a deep breath' then read the score from the stadiometer scale while stretching the subject.

A right-angle set square held by an assistant may be used as a substitute for a stadiometer. A scratch line is made on a paper scale attached to the wall when the subject is being stretched. The distance from the floor to this scratch line can be measured using a segmometer or anthropometer.

SITTING HEIGHT

A small bench is placed at the base of the stadiometer. The subject sits with the thighs projected horizontally (legs may be crossed to achieve this position) with the buttocks and shoulders pressed against the upright portion of the stadiometer. Align the head in the Frankfort plane and follow the instructions for standing height for this measurement. Subtract the height of the box from the resulting score to obtain sitting height.

ACROMIALE–RADIALE LENGTH (ARM LENGTH)

The subject stands erect with the arms extended downward and palms pressed against the side of the thigh. Anchor the end pointer of the segmometer to the acromiale and move the housing pointer to the radiale as shown in Fig. 14.4.

RADIALE–STYLION LENGTH (FOREARM LENGTH)

Subject stands as above. Anchor the end pointer to the radiale and move the housing pointer to the stylion.

MID-STYLION–DACTYLION LENGTH (HAND LENGTH)

First mark the mid-stylion by wrapping an anthropometric tape firmly around the wrist distal to the styloid processes of both radius and ulna. Draw a line on the palmar surface of the wrist at the level of the styloid processes. Then anchor the end pointer at the mid-stylion mark and move the housing pointer to the dactylion.

ACROMIALE–DACTYLION LENGTH (UPPER LIMB LENGTH)

Measure directly from acromiale to dactylion or sum the arm, forearm and hand lengths.

ILIOSPINALE HEIGHT (LOWER LIMB LENGTH - 1)

Direct the subject to stand close to and facing the measurement box so that the feet project beneath its horizontal surface. Place the end pointer of the segmometer on this surface and move the housing pointer up to the iliospinale. Add the height of the box to this score to obtain iliospinale height.

TROCHANTERION HEIGHT (LOWER LIMB LENGTH - 2)

Direct the subject to stand close to the measurement box so that the lateral aspect of the right leg touches the box. Place the end pointer on its horizontal surface and move the housing pointer up to the trochanterion. Add the height of the box to this score to obtain trochanterion height (Fig. 14.5).

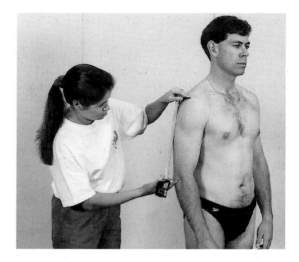

Fig. 14.4 Measurement of acromiale–radiale length (arm length).

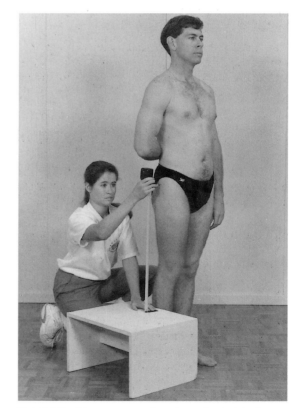

Fig. 14.5 Measurement of trochanterion height (lower limb length - 2).

TROCHANTERION–TIBIALE LATERALE LENGTH (THIGH LENGTH)

Direct the subject to stand on the measurement box. Anchor the end pointer on the trochanterion and move the housing pointer to the tibiale laterale.

TIBIALE LATERALE HEIGHT (LEG LENGTH - 1)

With the subject still standing on the box, place the end pointer on its horizontal surface and move the housing pointer up to the tibiale laterale.

TIBIALE MEDIALE–SPHYRION LENGTH (LEG LENGTH - 2)

Direct the subject to sit on the box and cross the right leg over the left so that the right tibia is horizontal. Anchor the end pointer on the tibiale mediale and move the housing pointer to the sphyrion.

AKROPODION–PTERNION LENGTH (FOOT LENGTH)

Direct the subject to stand on the measurement box. Using an anthropometer, anchor the fixed end to the akropodion and move the sliding end to the pternion.

ARM SPAN

Direct the subject to face the wall with the arms extended horizontally so that the left dactylion touches a corner and the right stretches out maximally. Mark the position of the right dactylion and measure the distance from the corner.

Breadths

BIACROMIAL BREADTH

The subject stands with arms relaxed by the side. From behind the subject and with the pointers of the anthropometer angled upward at 45°, measure the distance between left and right acromion processes. Firm pressure is applied to the acromion process during the measure.

TRANSVERSE CHEST BREADTH

Direct the subject to sit on the measurement box with hands resting on the knees. The anthro-pometer is angled downward at about 30° as the breadth of the chest is measured at the mesosternale level, taking care to avoid the pectoral and latissimus dorsi muscle contours. Moderate pressure is required on the pointers and the measure is taken at the end of a normal expiration (end tidal).

BIILIOCRISTAL BREADTH

The subject stands with arms relaxed by the side. While standing in front of the subject and with the pointers angled upward at 45°, measure the distance between left and right iliocristale. Firm pressure is applied during the measurement.

BIEPICONDYLAR HUMERUS BREADTH

Direct the subject to raise the arm forward to the horizontal position and flex the forearm to 90°. Point the arms of the bone caliper upward at about 45° and measure the greatest distance between lateral and medial epicondyles of the humerus. Firm pressure on the arms of the caliper is required for this measurement (Fig. 14.6).

BISTYLOID WRIST BREADTH

The subject should be seated with the right hand

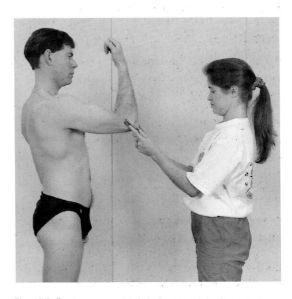

Fig. 14.6 Measurement of biepicondylar humerus breadth.

flexed over the right knee to about 90°. Bisect the angle at the wrist with the arms of the bone caliper and measure across radius and ulna styloid processes. Moderate pressure is required during this measurement.

HAND BREADTH

Direct the subject to place the right hand firmly with palm down on a flat surface with the fingers together. Without excess pressure on the caliper, measure across metacarpale radiale and ulnare using the bone caliper.

BIEPICONDYLAR FEMUR BREADTH

With the subject seated so that the leg is perpendicular to a horizontal thigh, palpate the femoral epicondyles. Angle the bone calipers downward at about 45° and, applying firm pressure, measure across the femoral epicondyles.

ANTERIOR–POSTERIOR CHEST DEPTH

With the subject seated with arms by the side, a wide-spreading caliper is positioned horizontally at the level of the mesosternale. The posterior arm of the caliper is positioned on the nearest verte-

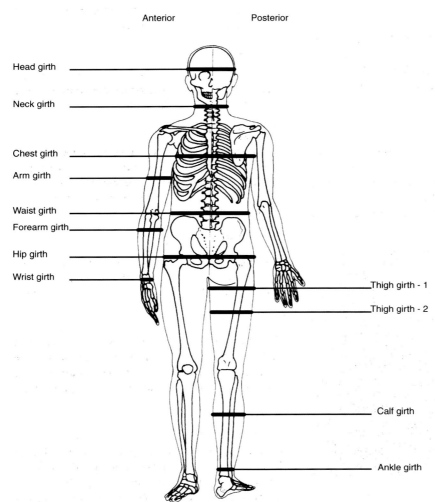

Fig. 14.7 Standard sites for girth measurements.

bral spinous process. Using only light pressure, measure this distance at end tidal.

Girths

The locations of girth measurement sites are shown in Fig. 14.7.

HEAD GIRTH

With the subject seated and the head in the Frankfort plane, place the tape horizontally around the head immediately superior to the glabella (portion of the frontal bone between the supraorbital ridges). Apply firm pressure to flatten the hair.

NECK GIRTH

The subject remains seated with the head in the Frankfort plane while the tape is placed around the neck, perpendicular to the long axis and at a level immediately above the larynx. Measure without constricting the skin.

RELAXED ARM GIRTH

Direct the subject to stand with the right arm hanging naturally by the side. Mark the mid distance between acromiale and radiale landmarks. Place the tape around the arm at this level (perpendicular to the shaft of the humerus) and draw the

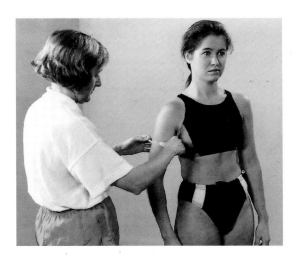

Fig. 14.8 Measurement of relaxed arm girth.

tape together with sufficient tension so that the skin is not constricted (Fig. 14.8).

FLEXED ARM GIRTH

Direct the subject to raise the arm forward to the horizontal, supinate and flex the forearm to 45°. Place the tape around the arm and encourage the subject to isometrically contract the forearm flexors and extensors. Move the tape to the greatest girth and measure without constricting the skin.

FOREARM GIRTH

With the subject's arm supinated and placed by the side, move the tape to the maximum forearm girth and draw together with sufficient tension so that the skin is not constricted.

WRIST GIRTH

Move the tape down to the minimum girth at the wrist (distal to the styloid processes) and measure without constricting the skin.

CHEST GIRTH

Pass the tape horizontally around the subject's chest at the level of the mesosternale. The subject may now lower the arms to a comfortable position by the sides. Measure chest girth at the end of a normal expiration.

WAIST GIRTH

Place the tape horizontally around the waist at the level of the minimum girth. Measure without constricting the skin.

HIP GIRTH (GLUTEAL GIRTH)

The subject should stand erect with feet together. Place the tape horizontally around the hips at the level of the greatest posterior protuberance of the buttocks. Measure without constricting the skin.

THIGH GIRTH - 1

Direct the subject to stand erect with the feet slightly apart and weight equally distributed. Pass the tape around the leg and slide up using a cross-handed technique to a horizontal position 2 cm below the gluteal fold. Draw the tape together with sufficient tension so that the skin is not constricted.

THIGH GIRTH - 2 (MID-THIGH GIRTH)

Measure and mark the mid-position between trochanterion and tibiale laterale landmarks. Place the tape horizontally around the thigh at this level and measure without constricting the skin.

CALF GIRTH

With the subject standing on a measurement box, place the tape horizontally around the leg at the maximum girth. Draw the tape together with sufficient tension so that the skin is not constricted.

ANKLE GIRTH

Move the tape down to the minimum girth which is just superior to the ankle. Measure without constricting the skin.

Skinfolds

For each of the following skinfolds, the caliper is held in the right hand and the fold lifted and held by the thumb and index finger of the left hand. This skinfold, which does not include muscle, includes a double layer of skin as well as the underlying adipose tissue and must be held throughout the measurement. The caliper must be applied at right angles to the fold so that the pressure plate is 1.0 cm from the left thumb and index finger. A reading is taken 2 s after the application of the caliper and the score recorded to the nearest 0.1 mm (Harpenden caliper) or 0.5 mm (Slimline caliper).

Skinfold thicknesses vary considerably if the site is not precisely marked as specified in the following descriptions and shown in Fig. 14.9. Extreme care should therefore be taken in the location of the skinfold sites so as to achieve accurate results.

TRICEPS SKINFOLD

The triceps site is located at the mid-position between the acromiale and radiale landmarks on the most posterior aspect of the arm when the forearm is supinated. A vertical fold is lifted by the left thumb and index finger so that the landmark is midway

between the lower edges of the thumb and index finger. The caliper jaws are applied 1 cm below the marked site, to a similar depth on the fold as the left thumb and index finger (Fig. 14.10).

BICEPS SKINFOLD

This site is also located at the mid-position between the acromiale and radiale landmarks but at the most anterior aspect of the arm when the forearm is supinated. A vertical fold is lifted by the left thumb and index finger so that the landmark is midway between the lower edges of the digits. The caliper jaws are applied 1 cm below the marked site, to a similar depth on the fold as the left thumb and index finger.

SUBSCAPULAR SKINFOLD

This site is marked at the inferior angle of the scapula when the subject is standing erect with the arms by the side. Place the left index finger on the mark and the thumb a sufficient distance inferior to this point so as to lift an appropriate fold. An oblique fold (downwards laterally) is lifted and the caliper applied 1 cm lateral to the left index finger and thumb, perpendicular to the line of the fold.

ILIAC CREST SKINFOLD

Direct the subject to place the right arm across the chest. A mark is then made immediately superior to the iliac crest in the mid-axillary line (the most lateral aspect). Place the left thumb on the mark and the left index finger a sufficient distance superior to this point so as to lift an appropriate fold. Lift an oblique fold (downwards anteriorly) with the left hand and apply the caliper 1 cm anterior to the left index finger and thumb.

SUPRASPINALE SKINFOLD

To locate this site, first project an imaginary line from the iliospinale landmark to the right anterior axillary border (armpit). Mark a point on this imaginary line at a level that is horizontal to the iliac crest (~7 cm above the iliospinale for adults). Lift an oblique fold (downwards medially at about 45°)

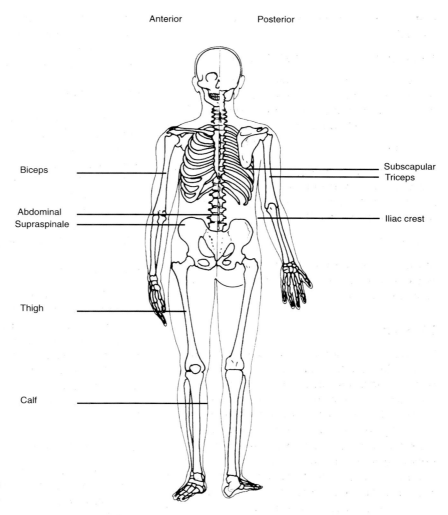

Anterior   Posterior

Biceps

Subscapular
Triceps

Abdominal
Supraspinale

Iliac crest

Thigh

Calf

Fig. 14.9 Standard sites
for skinfold measurements.

at this site and apply the caliper 1 cm medial to
the left index finger and thumb (Fig. 14.11).

ABDOMINAL SKINFOLD

The site for this skinfold is 5 cm to the right side
of the mid-point of the umbilicus. Lift a vertical
fold with the left index finger and thumb at the
site and apply the caliper 1 cm inferiorly.

FRONT THIGH SKINFOLD

With the subject seated, the site for the front thigh
skinfold is located on the anterior thigh, at the

mid-position between the inguinal crease and the
most anterior aspect of the patella. A fold is lifted
parallel to the shaft of the femur at the site and
the caliper applied 1 cm distal to the left index
finger and thumb. Where this fold is difficult to
obtain, have the subject support the hamstring
musculature to relieve tension from the skin. An
assistant may also help to raise the fold with
fingers positioned 1 cm distal to the caliper jaws.

MEDIAL CALF SKINFOLD

This site is located on the medial aspect of the leg
at the level of the greatest girth. The subject may

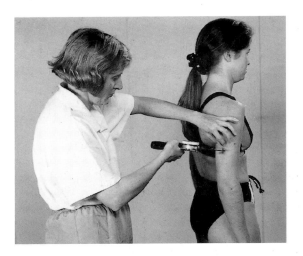

Fig. 14.10 Measurement of triceps skinfold.

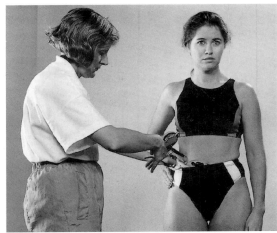

Fig. 14.11 Measurement of supraspinale skinfold.

raise the right leg to rest on a measurement box to assist the measurer. A vertical fold is then lifted at the site and the caliper applied 1 cm distal to the left index finger and thumb.

PRECISION AND ACCURACY

Several features related to the preparation for, and execution of, data collection combine to help ensure that accurate measurements are recorded. These features include: the training and assessment of testers; provision of a data entry assistant; thoughtful preparation of a data entry sheet or computer spreadsheet; availability of precise and calibrated equipment; efficient design of the work station; and grouping of measurement tasks.

Examples from the Kinanthropometric Aquatic Sports Project (KASP; Carter & Ackland 1994) will be used to illustrate these points. The data collection sheet shown in Fig. 14.12, as well as the identical data entry computer spreadsheet used in KASP, were divided into six sections. Following the space allocated to demographic information, the data sheet reflected the measurements required at five stations: skinfolds, lengths, girths, breadths and other. The apportionment of measures to each station was designed to equate the time taken for measurement at each station and to limit changing of instruments, while the order in which the variables were to be measured reflects the desire to maximize work efficiency.

Space is available at each group of variables for triple measurements to be recorded and boxes with decimal points are provided for the scores. This removes any ambiguity related to the precision of the measure and helps to avoid transcription errors. It should be noted that for KASP the computer spreadsheet program automatically determined the mean of two measurements or the median of three and as a result no final or summary score facility was needed on the data sheet in Fig. 14.12.

Prior to testing at the 1991 World Swimming Championships, all personnel were thoroughly trained and assessed. A test–re-test protocol was used to determine the reliability of each measurer, while their precision was determined from the technical error of measurement (TEM). An experienced criterion anthropometrist was chosen to set the standard for measurement and the scores obtained by each measurer on a group of subjects were compared to those from the criterion anthropometrist, using the following formula:

$$\text{TEM} = (\ (x_2 - x_1)^2/2n)^{0.5}$$

where   TEM = the absolute technical error of measurement for a particular

KINANTHROPOMETRIC AQUATIC SPORTS PROJECT

Subject Name (last, first) ______________ , __________ Subject ID#

Sport ID# Events (1°, 2°, 3°) 1° 2° 3°

Country Ethnicity Sex (2=F, 1=M) Projection box + const

Date of birth Year Month Day

Year Month Day Checker ID#

Triceps sf
Subscapular sf
Biceps sf
Iliac crest sf
Supraspinale sf
Abdominal sf
Front thigh sf
Medial calf sf

Acromiale-radiale
Radial-stylion
Midstylion-dactylion
Iliospinale b.ht
Trochanterion b.ht
Trochanterion-tibiale laterale
Tibiale laterale ht
Tibiale mediale-sphyrion tibiale

Arm girth relaxed
Arm girth fully flexed and tensed
Forearm girth maximum
Wrist girth distal styloids
Chest girth mesosternale
Waist girth minimum
Hip (gluteal) girth
Thigh girth (1) 1cm gluteal line
Thigh girth (2) mid tro-tib lat
Calf girth maximum
Ankle girth minimum

Biacromial breadth
Biiliocristal breadth
Transverse chest breadth
Foot length (ac-pt)
Humerus breadth cm
Wrist breadth (bistyloid) cm
Hand breadth cm
Femur breadth cm

Body mass
Stature (stretch)
Sitting height
A-P chest depth
Head girth
Neck girth
Span

Fig. 14.12 Data collection proforma used in the Kinanthropometric Aquatic Sports Project (courtesy of Carter & Ackland 1994).

variable

x_2 = the score obtained by the measurer

x_1 = the score obtained by the criterion anthropometrist

n = the number of replicated pairs.

The percentage TEM may then be calculated as follows:

$$\%TEM = 100 \, (TEM/M_1)$$

where M_1 = the mean of the criterion anthropometrist's measurements for that variable.

In general, one expects skinfold measurements to have a %TEM of about 5%, breadths and the larger girths slightly higher than 1%, with other variables slightly less than 1%. The KASP personnel were required to meet these standards prior to joining the measurement team.

BODY TYPING

The Heath–Carter somatotype method (Carter & Heath 1990) is described in Chapter 5 and may be calculated using either a graphical solution (Fig. 14.13) or a computer-generated solution (Drinkwater *et al*. 1994). In this section the graphical method will be illustrated, since it provides a 'first principles' view of the assessment process. Similarly, the location of a particular somatotype rating on the somatochart (Fig. 14.14) may be made graphically, or X–Y coordinates may be generated via a computer program for subsequent plotting (Carter & Marfell-Jones 1994).

ANTHROPOMETRIC MEASUREMENTS

Record the following information on the data sheet in Fig. 14.13:

- Skinfolds — triceps, subscapular, supraspinale and calf skinfolds
- Bone breadths — biepicondylar humerus and femur breadths
- Girths — flexed arm and calf girths
- Stretch stature
- Body mass

RATING PROCEDURE

Endomorphy

- Sum the three skinfolds (triceps, subscapular and supraspinale)
- Apply the dimensional scaling factor to calculate a value for the proportional sum of three skinfolds
- Circle the closest value in the table and then circle the rating value for that column

Mesomorphy

- Mark the subject's height on the height scale with an arrow and then, in the row below,

circle the numeral closest to the measurement obtained
- For each bone breadth, circle the figure in the appropriate row that is nearest to the measurement value
- Subtract triceps skinfold (T) from biceps girth and calf skinfold (C) from calf girth *before* circling the figure in the appropriate row which is nearest to the calculated value. (Note: change skinfold measures from millimetres to centimetres before subtracting)
- Considering the breadth and girth rows only, calculate the algebraic sum of column deviations (D) from the circled height column; positive deviations to the right, negative deviations to the left of the height column. (See for example, the calculations in Fig. 14.15, where $D = +9 + (-2) = +7$)
- Considering the height measurement, a correction (K) is necessary when the subject's height is not identical to the circled height numeral. Referring to Table 14.1, the correction factor is negative if the subject's height is greater than the circled value, or positive if less than the circled value
- Calculate mesomorphy rating using the following formula:

$$\text{Mesomorphy} = D/8 + K + 4.0$$

- Circle the closest rating value, being conservative if the calculation falls midway between values

Ectomorphy

- Use the nomogram in Fig. 14.16 to determine the ratio of height to the cubed root of body mass and then record this value
- Circle the closest numeral on the scale, then circle the rating value corresponding to that column

HEATH-CARTER SOMATOTYPE RATING FORM

Name: _____ Sex: _____ Date: _____

Age: _____

Skinfolds (mm)

triceps	=
subscapular	=
supraspinale	=
Sum 3 skinfolds	=
x ($\frac{170.18}{Ht}$)	=
calf	=

HEIGHT CORRECTED SUM OF 3 SKINFOLDS (mm)

Upper limit	10.9	14.9	18.9	22.9	26.9	31.2	35.8	40.7	46.2	52.2	58.7	65.7	73.2	81.2	89.7	98.9	108.9	119.7	131.2	143.7	157.2	171.9	187.9	204.0
Mid-point	9.0	13.0	17.0	21.0	25.0	29.0	33.5	38.0	43.5	49.0	55.5	62.0	69.5	77.0	85.5	94.0	104.0	114.0	125.5	137.0	150.5	164.0	180.0	196.0
Lower limit	7.0	11.0	15.0	19.0	23.0	27.0	31.3	35.9	40.8	46.3	52.3	58.8	65.8	73.3	81.3	89.8	99.0	109.0	119.8	131.3	143.8	157.3	172.0	188.0
Endomorphy	½	1	1½	2	2½	3	3½	4	4½	5	5½	6	6½	7	7½	8	8½	9	9½	10	10½	11	11½	12

Height (cm)	139.7	143.5	147.3	151.1	154.9	158.8	162.6	166.4	170.2	174.0	177.8	181.6	185.4	189.2	193.0	196.9	200.7	204.5	208.3	212.1	215.9	219.7	223.5	227.3
Humerus breadth (cm)	5.19	5.34	5.49	5.64	5.78	5.93	6.07	6.22	6.37	6.51	6.65	6.80	6.95	7.09	7.24	7.38	7.53	7.67	7.82	7.97	8.11	8.25	8.40	8.55
Femur breadth (cm)	7.41	7.62	7.83	8.04	8.24	8.45	8.66	8.87	9.08	9.28	9.49	9.70	9.91	10.12	10.33	10.53	10.74	10.95	11.16	11.36	11.57	11.78	11.99	12.21
Biceps girth - T^1 (cm)	23.7	24.4	25.0	25.7	26.3	27.0	27.7	28.3	29.0	29.7	30.3	31.0	31.6	32.2	33.0	33.6	34.3	35.0	35.6	36.3	37.0	37.6	38.3	39.0
Calf girth - C^2 (cm)	27.7	28.5	29.3	30.1	30.8	31.6	32.4	33.2	33.9	34.7	35.5	36.3	37.1	37.8	38.6	39.4	40.2	41.0	41.7	42.5	43.3	44.1	44.9	45.6
Mesomorphy	½	1	1½	2	2½	3	3½	4	4½	5	5½	6	6½	7	7½	8	8½	9						

Body mass (kg) Upper Limit	39.65	40.74	41.43	42.13	42.82	43.48	44.18	44.84	45.53	46.23	46.92	47.58	48.25	48.94	49.63	50.33	50.99	51.68
Mid-point	and	40.20	41.09	41.79	42.48	43.14	43.84	44.50	45.19	45.89	46.32	47.24	47.94	48.60	49.29	49.99	50.68	51.34
Lower limit	below	39.66	40.75	41.44	42.14	42.83	43.49	44.19	44.85	45.54	46.24	46.93	47.59	48.26	48.95	49.64	50.34	51.00
Ectomorphy	½	1	1½	2	2½	3	3½	4	4½	5	5½	6	6½	7	7½	8	8½	9

HT/³√body mass =

Anthropometric Somatotype

Endomorphy	Mesomorphy	Ectomorphy

Rater: _____

1 Biceps girth corrected for fat by subtracting triceps skinfold

2 Calf girth corrected for fat by subtracting calf skinfold

Fig. 14.13 Heath–Carter somatotype rating form (courtesy of Carter & Heath 1990).

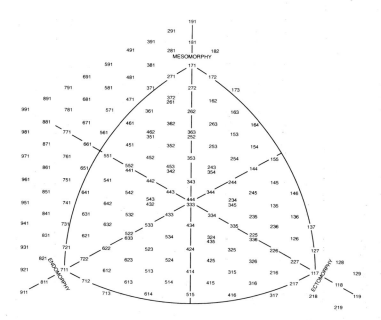

Fig. 14.14 Somatochart (courtesy of Carter & Heath 1990).

Table 14.1 Height correction values (*K*) for mesomorphy assessment

Difference in height (mm)	K	Difference in height (mm)	K
1	0.01	11	0.14
2	0.03	12	0.16
3	0.04	13	0.17
4	0.05	14	0.18
5	0.07	15	0.20
6	0.08	16	0.21
7	0.09	17	0.22
8	0.11	18	0.24
9	0.12	19	0.25
10	0.13		

HEATH-CARTER SOMATOTYPE RATING FORM

Name: **B.A.** Age: **20** Sex: **M** Date: **25-10-93**

$$D = \frac{+7}{8} = .875$$
$$-.07$$
$$.805$$
$$+4.000$$
$$4.805$$

HEIGHT CORRECTED SUM OF 3 SKINFOLDS (mm)

Skinfolds (mm)
- triceps = 6.4
- subscapular = 7.1
- supraspinale = 4.6
- Sum 3 skinfolds = 18.1
- $\times \left(\dfrac{170.18}{Ht = 178.3}\right)$ = **17.3**
- calf = 5.2

Endomorphy

	½	1	1½	2	2½	3	3½	4	4½	5	5½	6	6½	7	7½	8	8½	9	9½	10	10½	11	11½	12
Upper limit	10.9	14.9	18.9	22.9	26.9	31.2	35.8	40.7	46.2	52.2	58.7	65.7	73.2	81.2	89.7	98.9	108.9	119.7	131.2	143.7	157.2	171.9	187.9	204.0
Mid-point	9.0	13.0	(17.0)	21.0	25.0	29.0	33.5	38.0	43.5	49.0	55.5	62.0	69.5	77.0	85.5	94.0	104.0	114.0	125.5	137.0	150.5	164.0	180.0	196.0
Lower limit	7.0	11.0	15.0	19.0	23.0	27.0	31.3	35.9	40.8	46.3	52.3	58.8	65.8	73.3	81.3	89.8	99.0	109.0	119.8	131.3	143.8	157.3	172.0	188.0
Endomorphy	½	1	(1½)	2	2½	3	3½	4	4½	5	5½	6	6½	7	7½	8	8½	9	9½	10	10½	11	11½	12

Mesomorphy

- Height (cm) = 178.3
- Humerus breadth (cm) = 7.2
- Femur breadth (cm) = 9.75
- Biceps girth - T¹ (cm) = 33.1
- Calf girth - C² (cm) = 33.8

	½	1	1½	2	2½	3	3½	4	4½	5	5½	6	6½	7	7½	8	8½	9
Height (cm)	139.7	143.5	147.3	151.1	154.9	158.8	162.6	166.4	170.2	174.0	(177.8)	181.6	185.4	189.2	193.0	196.9	200.7	204.5
Humerus breadth (cm)	5.19	5.34	5.49	5.64	5.78	5.93	6.07	6.22	6.37	6.51	.65	6.80	6.95	7.09	(7.24)	7.38	7.53	7.67
Femur breadth (cm)	7.41	7.62	7.83	8.04	8.24	8.45	8.66	8.87	9.08	9.28	.49	(9.70)	9.91	10.12	10.33	10.53	10.74	10.95
Biceps girth - T¹ (cm)	23.7	24.4	25.0	25.7	26.3	27.0	27.7	28.3	29.0	29.7	30.3	31.0	31.6	32.2	(33.0)	33.6	34.3	35.0
Calf girth - C² (cm)	27.7	28.5	29.3	30.1	30.8	31.6	32.4	33.2	(33.9)	34.7	35.5	36.3	37.1	37.8	38.6	39.4	40.2	41.0
Mesomorphy	½	1	1½	2	2½	3	3½	4	4½	(5)	5½	6	6½	7	7½	8	8½	9

Ectomorphy

- Body mass (kg) = 69.2
- HT/³√body mass = **43.4**

	½	1	1½	2	2½	3	3½	4	4½	5	5½	6	6½	7	7½	8	8½	9
Upper Limit	39.65	40.74	41.43	42.13	42.82	(43.48)	44.18	44.84	45.53	46.23	46.92	47.58	48.25	48.94	49.63	50.33	50.99	51.68
Mid-point	mid	40.20	41.09	41.79	42.48	43.14	43.84	44.50	45.19	45.89	46.32	47.24	47.94	48.60	49.29	49.99	50.68	51.34
Lower limit	below	39.66	40.75	41.44	42.14	42.83	43.49	44.19	44.85	45.54	46.24	46.93	47.59	48.26	48.95	49.64	50.34	51.00
Ectomorphy	½	1	1½	2	2½	(3)	3½	4	4½	5	5½	6	6½	7	7½	8	8½	9

Anthropometric Somatotype

Endomorphy	Mesomorphy	Ectomorphy
1½	5	3

Rater: **T.A.**

1 Biceps girth corrected for fat by subtracting triceps skinfold
2 Calf girth corrected for fat by subtracting calf skinfold

Fig. 14.15 A somatotype assessment using the graphical method.

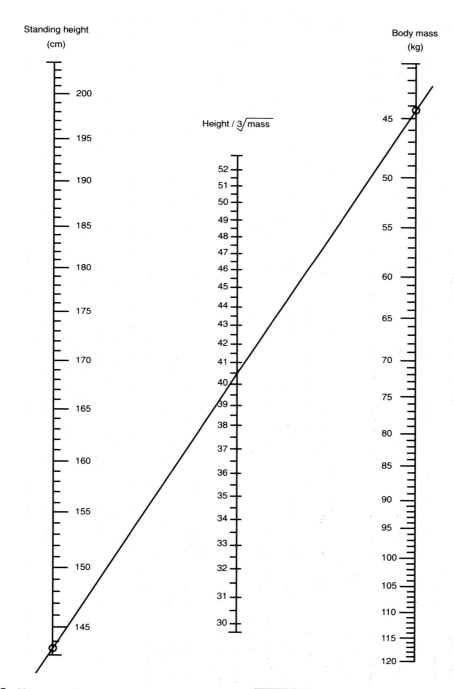

Fig. 14.16 Nomogram for determining the ratio of height to $\sqrt[3]{\text{body mass}}$.

BODY COMPOSITION

Indirect techniques for the assessment of body composition are classified into five groups for discussion:

- Weight-for-height indices
- Densitometry
- Skinfolds
- Tissue fractionation
- Other techniques

This section deals with the advantages and limitations of each methodology in order to support the value judgement made in Chapter 6, with regard to the 'best' technique for use in the discipline of sport science. Some of the methods lack validity and standardization, while others are prohibitive in terms of the cost of instrumentation. The most practical, valid and reliable methods are described in full, while other methods are discussed to reveal their inherent flaws.

WEIGHT-FOR-HEIGHT INDICES

Weight–height indices have been used for many years in an attempt to determine the 'ideal weight' for an individual. The best known of these indices are the weight–height index (W/H), and Quetelet's index and more recently, the body mass index (BMI; W/H^2), the Khosla-Lowe index (W/H^3), the Benn index (W/H^b, where b is an allometric exponent) and the inverse ponderal index ($H/W^{1/3}$). They all provide a measure of ponderosity which should *not* be construed as meaning *adiposity*. Further discussions related to these indices may be found in Ross *et al*. (1986).

For an individual of any given stature, body mass may vary according to the amount and density of lean body tissue as well as fat. This fact was clearly demonstrated by Behnke *et al*. (1942) who reported that 70% of a sample of American college football players were classified as 'overweight' using weight-for-height indices. These players were rated as unsuitable for military service and classified as 'bad risks' by standard life insurance tables.

Indices of weight and height have been universally employed by scientists and clinicians for the following reasons:

- *Epidemiological validity* — significant correlations between weight-for-height indices and other measures of adiposity, morbidity or mortality have been reported in the literature and supplied as evidence of epidemiological validity. Such information was generally gathered on large cross-sectional samples
- *Precision and reliability* — the measurements of height and body mass are among the most accurate and reliable of all anthropometric dimensions. Mean inter-measurer differences for height in the Fels Longitudinal Study, reported by Gordon *et al*. (1988), ranged from 1.4 mm for the 20–55 year age group, to 2.4 mm for the 5–10 year age group
- *Ease of measurement* — the recording of height and weight requires minimal operator training and is not reliant upon very costly or technical instrumentation
- *Patient comfort* — minimal discomfort to, or co-operation from, the patient is associated with these measurements

While the above reasons are legitimate in a practical sense, they do not qualify as a scientific rationale for the use of weight–height indices as measures of body composition. Much emphasis is placed on the results of epidemiological studies but, with only an elementary knowledge of statistics, it is clear that a highly significant relationship may be achieved with a relatively low correlation coefficient. Thus the ability to predict adiposity from these indices for an individual is correspondingly low. These relationships in epidemiological studies have typically been low but significant.

In a sample of 94 obese and non-obese boys and girls, Houtkooper (1986) used the BMI to predict adiposity with respect to a criterion measure based on densitometry. Only 53% of the variance in adiposity was predicted by the BMI for this population, compared to 85% by anthropometry. Furthermore, Dietz (1987) reinforced the fact that weight-for-height indices reflected lean body tissue development as much as fatness, by reporting similar correlations for frame size and skinfolds with the BMI. Therefore, the use of such indices in epidemiological studies may be justified to predict mean values for a population, but not to predict individual adiposity.

DENSITOMETRY

The ability of humans to float in water without the aid of propulsive movements of the limbs is related to the density of constituent tissues as well as to the buoyancy attributed to entrapped air. It is commonly observed that obese people float more easily than those with linear or muscular builds. These principles of buoyancy were first observed by Archimedes (287–212 BC) and form the basis for this widely used method of monitoring change in human body density.

It is important to understand that body weight itself provides no valid indication of body composition, as is illustrated in the following example. In anatomical terms the body can be divided into a simple two-compartment model: the first compartment is the lean body mass (LBM) while the second compartment is fat mass (FM).

Subject A in Fig. 14.17 is composed of a high proportion of LBM with a total body mass of 90 kg and a density of 1.082 g/mL. The LBM comprises bone, muscle, connective tissue and organs. A certain proportion of fat is necessary to support normal function and is included as a separate compartment. For subject B, the inner and intermediate circles encompass tissue similar to A in density and composition but differ in mass by 23 kg. The outer circle circumscribes an accumulation of 25 kg of excess fat and so the density of this 90 kg individual is 1.035 g/mL.

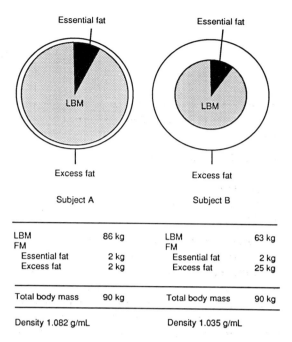

LBM	86 kg	LBM	63 kg
FM		FM	
Essential fat	2 kg	Essential fat	2 kg
Excess fat	2 kg	Excess fat	25 kg
Total body mass	90 kg	Total body mass	90 kg
Density 1.082 g/mL		Density 1.035 g/mL	

Fig. 14.17 Tissue composition for two individuals of similar body mass (from Bloomfield *et al.* 1992).

Determining Net Hydrostatic Weight

Two main problems exist with the densitometry measurement: the recording of net body weight in water (hydrostatic weight); and the estimation of entrapped air within the lungs, trachea, bronchioles and gastrointestinal tract. For the measurement of net hydrostatic weight, a tank of water similar to that shown in Fig. 14.18 is required. For patient comfort and hygiene the water should be filtered, chlorinated and heated to approximately 30°C and a submersible seat is suspended from a solid foundation above the tank. This seat should not entrap any air and therefore if tubular materials are used in its construction, holes must be drilled in the material to allow water to fill the cavity to the level of the surrounding tank water.

The submersible seat should also be supported by a pulley arrangement which enables patients of varying size to be positioned correctly in the tank. A force-measuring device (spring scale, load cell or strain gauge) is fitted to the top of the chair

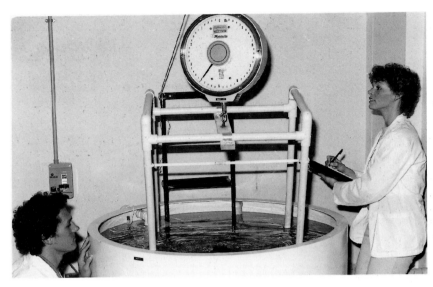

Fig. 14.18 Measurement of gross hydrostatic weight.

in series with the overhead point of attachment, for either instantaneous or continuous recording of weight.

The protocol listed in Table 14.2 together with the water density data in Table 14.3 should be adopted for the measurement of gross hydrostatic weight (W_{gross}). Having determined this value, the following formula may be used to calculate body density (D_b):

$$D_b = \frac{W_a}{W_a - W_{net}/D_w - (RV + C)}$$

where W_a = weight of the body in air
W_{net} = gross weight in water (W_{gross}) – weight of the seat (W_{seat})
D_w = density of water
RV = correction factor for the residual volume
C = a constant volume which represents the entrapped air in the intestinal tract (~100 mL BTPS).

Determining the Volume of Entrapped Air

Residual volume (RV) is defined by Jensen (1976) as the quantity of air remaining in the lungs fol-

lowing a maximal expiration and several methods have been proposed for its estimation. A constant value for RV may be assumed, or alternatively, RV may be estimated as a fixed proportion (30%) of forced vital capacity (FVC). Residual volume is 20–25% of total lung capacity (TLC); however, this proportion increases to approximately 40% in the aged. Further variations in the proportion of RV to TLC may be due to gender, training, body size, altitude, body position and disease (Matthews & Fox 1976).

When observing changes in individuals over time however, the RV should be measured accurately, since it plays a substantial role in the calculation of body density. The accurate measurement of RV may be accomplished using a closed circuit nitrogen/oxygen dilution method (Wilmore 1969). This system requires the patient to breathe pure oxygen within a closed and nitrogen-free spirometry system until nitrogen equilibrium is reached. Having achieved this equilibrium, RV may be calculated by measuring the variation in nitrogen concentration and the volumes of gases involved at the commencement and cessation of the test, using the equation below. It should be noted that the concentration of N_2 at the mouth when exhaling is assumed to accurately reflect the alveolar concentration of N_2.

Table 14.2 Protocol for the measurement of hydrostatic weight

Procedure	Rationale/annotation
Record body weight in air (W_a) to the nearest 0.01 kg.	Subject to wear a light swimsuit only which does not entrap any air.
Turn filtration system off.	To avoid turbulent currents which may affect recordings.
Record water temperature and determine water density (D_w)	Variations in water density influence body weight in water (see Table 14.3).
Direct the subject to enter the tank as gently as possible and stand on the floor of the tank away from the seat. Record the weight of the seat (W_{seat}) to the nearest 0.01 kg.	The added buoyancy given to the seat with the subject in the tank must be taken into account when recording (W_{seat}).
Instruct the subject to sit on the seat, then with lungs full of air, to practise submerging completely and responding to pre-arranged signals to surface.	Three practice trials with air-filled lungs help to instil confidence in the subject.
Instruct the subject to forcefully and fully exhale while submerging, then hold a steady position until the signal to surface is given (~5 s). Record the weight of the subject plus seat, to the nearest 0.01 kg.	Maximal exhalation is the critical factor in this technique.
Repeat the above procedure a further nine times.	Subjects learn to expel more air with each additional trial.
The average of the last three trials is used to provide the submerged weight of the subject plus seat (W_{gross}).	This is done provided all three trials are perceived as valid.

$$RV = \frac{V_{O_2}\,(E_{N_2} - I_{N_2})}{A_i N_2 - A_f N_2} - DS \cdot \text{BTPS factor}$$

where
- RV = residual volume
- V_{O_2} = initial volume of O_2 in the breathing bag
- E_{N_2} = percentage of N_2 at equilibrium
- I_{N_2} = percentage of N_2 initially in the breathing bag
- $A_i N_2$ = percentage of N_2 initially in alveolar air when breathing room air
- $A_f N_2$ = percentage of N_2 in alveolar air at the end of the test
- DS = dead space of mouthpiece, valve and sensing element of the N_2 analyser
- BTPS factor = wedge spirometer conversion factor.

Buskirk (1961) has also proposed the addition of a constant 100 mL to the RV estimation to ap-

Table 14.3 Density of water at various temperatures

Temperature (°C)	Density (g/mL)
18	0.9986
20	0.9982
22	0.9978
24	0.9974
26	0.9968
28	0.9963
30	0.9957
32	0.9950
34	0.9943
36	0.9936

proximate the volume of entrapped gas in the gastrointestinal tract.

Common Methodological Problems

In practice, several components of the densitometry technique present problems with certain subjects. Many are unable to exhale maximally during trials and this constitutes the primary source of error within this methodology. Alternatives have been suggested, including the estimation of body density without fully submerging the head (Donnelly & Sintek 1986) or full immersion with maximum inspiration (Weltman & Katch 1981). However, a more accurate measurement may be possible by the simultaneous recording of W_{gross} and lung volume, with submerged patients breathing continuously through a spirometer. In such a technique the effects of hydrostatic pressure on lung volumes must be accommodated.

Furthermore, many overweight subjects will experience positive buoyancy when fully submerged and this requires some modification of the methodology. A weighted belt may be placed around the abdomen of patients for the recording of W_{gross}, provided the belt is attached to the seat (beneath the water) during the measurement of W_{seat}. This allows the force measurement device to record positive values for W_{gross} and W_{seat}.

Data Treatment

The relative amounts of LBM and FM may be estimated with the adoption of a number of assumptions. The density of FM is assumed to be a constant 0.90 g/mL and LBM a uniform density of 1.10 g/mL in this methodology. For the latter to be true, it is assumed that the constituent tissues of LBM are in constant proportions and that these tissues have constant densities.

Research from the Brussels Cadaver Study (Martin 1984; Martin et al. 1986) does not support these assumptions. Using the data from seven female and six male unembalmed cadavers, the investigators reported a range of muscle mass from 41.9 to 59.4%, bone mass from 16.3 to 25.7% and the mass of other lean tissues from 24.0 to 32.4% of total body mass (Clarys et al. 1984; Martin et al. 1986). Furthermore, Martin (1984) provided evidence of the human variability in bone density. With data from 25 embalmed and unembalmed cadavers, Martin demonstrated variation in density between skeletal elements from 1.164 g/mL for the pelvis to 1.570 g/mL for the mandible.

Standard deviation values varied from 0.037 to 0.100 g/mL.

Investigations spanning the past decade into the effects of osteoporosis also provide evidence to refute the assumption of a constant lean body tissue density. On reviewing the literature in this area, Bailey et al. (1986) reported that bone loss may begin as early as age 20 and generally increases more rapidly from age 40. Bone loss for males after the age of 40 years varied from 0.05 to 0.75% per year, while for women these values were doubled.

In the light of such evidence, it is now generally believed that the accurate measurement of body density should be used for monitoring changes in the composition of an individual, rather than for attempting to predict the proportion of FM. Test–re-test reliability coefficients for this method have been reported above $r = 0.94$ by Katch and Katch (1983).

SKINFOLDS

A caliper may be used to measure the thickness of a compressed double fold of skin together with the entrapped subcutaneous adipose tissue. Skinfold thickness may be measured at a number of sites throughout the body, but this form of body fat assessment assumes the following:

- That the skinfold has a constant compressibility
- That skin thickness is a constant proportion of the fold
- That fat constitutes a constant proportion of adipose tissue
- That the ratio of subcutaneous to internal fat deposits remains fixed
- That inter-individual fat patterning is consistent

The validity of these assumptions has been partially refuted by Martin et al. (1984) using data from the Brussels Cadaver Study. The compressibility of the skinfold, for example, depends upon the age and body size of the subject, as well as the state of hydration of the tissues. Furthermore, measurement errors due to tester inaccuracy and poor site location often lead to spurious skinfold results. Burkinshaw *et al.* (1973), for example, reported errors averaging 2 mm for inexperienced observers when sites were not landmarked, while Bray *et al.* (1978) reported inter-observer differences from 11.0 to 21.6% for skinfold measurements on obese patients.

The use of skinfolds to estimate the quantity of adipose tissue incorporates a low technology method which requires a high degree of operator competence and a full appreciation of the underlying assumptions. To minimize some of the problems identified by Martin *et al.* (1984), it is generally recognized that a minimum of eight sites be sampled: two from the upper limb; four from the trunk; and two from the lower limb. This provides an adequately representative sample of the fat distribution across the range of individual fat patterns.

The ability of observers to select the correct site and the ease with which the skinfold may be lifted and separated from the underlying tissue, varies considerably among subjects with different body builds. These are, however, critical elements of the technique which must be addressed if valid measures are to be recorded.

Data Treatment

Data from skinfold measurements have been used in a variety of ways to estimate body composition. It is common for skinfold values to be included as independent variables in formulae that attempt to predict body mass proportions. These prediction strategies, however, used criterion measures derived from densitometry transformations. Thus, the limitations of both densitometry and skinfold methodologies are incorporated in these regression equations.

Most regression equations for the prediction of the proportion of FM using skinfolds are derived using multiple linear regression analyses and therefore are population-specific. That is, they may be applied, with due caution, to individuals who are similar in age, gender and body type to the criterion population.

These body composition prediction strategies are

therefore of little clinical or scientific value and it is now commonly believed that the skinfold measures should be used directly for comparison without modification, with the exception of some dimensional scaling. The individual skinfold scores may be summed and the result used for comparative purposes over time or between populations.

The O-scale System

The O-scale system (Ward *et al.* 1989) provides a method of comparing individual skinfold results with a normative data base from more than 20 000 observations categorized by age and gender. Individual adiposity ratings are determined from nine standard intervals (stanines) which provide divisions at the percentile equivalents of P4, 11, 23, 40, 60, 77, 89 and 96. Unlike other systems that provide arbitrary labels to define obesity, the O-scale system presents an unbiased description of adiposity and physique in comparison with a healthy standard.

The essential measures to be recorded in this system are age, gender, height, body mass and six skinfolds (triceps, subscapular, supraspinale, abdominal, front thigh and medial calf). From these data the adiposity (A) and proportional weight (W) ratings may be calculated as shown below.

Initially, the arithmetic sum of the six skinfolds (S6SF) is dimensionally scaled to account for individuals of varying size using the equation:

$$pS6SF = S6SF\,(170.8/Ht)$$

where $pS6SF$ = the proportional sum of six skinfolds (mm)
Ht = the subject's height (cm).

The A rating is then determined by reference to the normative data shown in Tables 14.4 and 14.5 (Ward *et al.* 1989).

The W rating is determined by geometrically scaling the subject's weight to a common height in order to produce a proportional weight (pWt) as follows:

$$pWT = Wt\,(170.18/Ht)^3$$

Table 14.4 The O-scale adiposity ratings for male subjects

Age (years)	Stanine threshold values								
	1	2	3	4	5	6	7	8	9
6	43.0*	47.4	57.4	63.0	70.0	80.9	92.7	121.0	
7	40.2	44.6	51.2	59.0	70.9	83.0	99.5	131.0	
8	41.2	45.7	50.7	56.8	65.4	77.6	99.5	137.9	
9	43.6	47.1	50.9	55.9	64.2	77.7	105.2	172.4	
10	45.1	47.1	53.7	59.1	65.4	83.7	129.1	183.2	
11	41.5	45.1	50.8	58.4	68.3	90.9	154.7	193.2	
12	37.6	43.1	47.0	53.4	65.7	89.3	126.6	188.9	
13	34.8	40.2	44.9	51.7	62.7	86.1	116.4	166.5	
14	34.7	37.2	43.4	49.3	57.3	70.9	103.5	146.1	
15	33.5	35.7	42.1	47.0	55.9	69.0	100.8	146.1	
16	32.3	35.4	40.4	44.6	53.3	63.1	79.4	126.7	
17	32.3	35.4	39.5	44.7	53.3	62.4	79.4	107.8	
18–19	31.5	34.3	41.7	47.6	57.0	70.3	87.3	109.3	
20–25	35.0	40.9	48.1	57.8	71.5	89.0	109.0	130.0	
25–30	38.3	45.5	54.5	66.8	81.8	99.5	119.3	144.0	
30–35	41.9	49.8	60.3	72.2	87.3	103.9	121.3	145.5	
35–40	43.9	53.0	62.3	73.9	88.1	102.5	121.9	143.0	
40–45	46.0	53.9	64.2	74.6	87.5	102.5	121.0	142.5	
45–50	44.7	55.2	64.8	76.3	90.5	106.8	123.4	147.0	
50–55	47.2	56.3	66.3	75.7	87.8	105.0	121.0	140.0	
55–60	46.9	56.8	65.8	76.4	87.5	101.1	115.9	136.0	
60–65	47.3	53.9	64.8	74.5	87.2	98.3	116.8	134.3	
65–70	43.0	53.0	60.5	71.6	84.3	92.9	104.8	121.5	

* Proportional sum of six skinfolds (mm).

where Wt = the subject's weight (kg)

Ht = the subject's height (cm).

The W rating is then determined by reference to normative data shown in Tables 14.6 and 14.7 (Ward *et al.* 1989).

When used in combination, the A and W scales provide a significant description of the physique and composition of the individual. The A rating may be regarded as a fatness rating with respect to the population, while the pS6SF score may be used for intra-individual comparisons over time. The W rating is not a fatness rating, but rather one of ponderosity, and together with the A rating, may be used to indicate musculoskeletal development.

TISSUE FRACTIONATION MODELS

In 1921, Matiegka first proposed the idea of estimating four components of body weight from anthropometric measurements. These measurements, which related to the tissue weights being predicted, were used to estimate a skin plus subcutaneous adipose tissue component, skeletal weight, muscle weight and the remaining organs and viscera component. A limited sample of cadavers was used to create the prediction formulae.

Later, Drinkwater and Ross (1980) introduced a departure model for the estimation of four body mass components: adipose tissue, bone, skeletal muscle and a residual consisting of organs and viscera. Using the unisex phantom stratagem (Ross & Wilson 1974), anthropometric variables were geometrically scaled to a reference stature and Z-scores were created with respect to phantom values for each variable. To estimate adipose tissue mass, Drinkwater and Ross (1980) used skinfold values from five sites: the triceps, subscapular, abdominal, front thigh and medial calf

Table 14.5 The O-scale adiposity ratings for female subjects

Age (years)	Stanine threshold values								
	1	2	3	4	5	6	7	8	9
6	46.8*	56.1	61.7	69.5	77.9	96.7	128.6	144.0	
7	44.3	47.4	60.2	68.3	76.1	91.8	113.2	140.0	
8	43.7	49.2	63.9	69.8	81.4	94.5	111.7	143.2	
9	45.4	53.4	66.1	73.2	87.7	98.6	111.7	143.3	
10	49.2	59.6	67.6	78.6	98.3	109.7	143.2	173.5	
11	51.9	56.4	66.5	75.6	96.4	108.8	150.0	173.4	
12	53.0	59.3	66.5	77.8	98.7	111.4	153.0	175.6	
13	46.7	56.9	67.9	77.4	97.7	114.9	153.0	165.5	
14	46.7	60.9	69.0	81.9	99.6	113.4	147.4	164.8	
15	49.4	62.6	72.4	85.4	99.6	113.2	145.3	162.1	
16	53.8	65.0	76.2	90.3	101.1	112.0	142.4	158.1	
17	62.1	69.4	78.3	92.8	106.5	117.6	141.4	156.4	
18–19	63.4	70.5	78.5	90.2	103.4	118.2	135.9	155.7	
20–25	64.0	72.5	81.2	92.0	104.2	118.9	138.0	164.0	
25–30	65.2	74.1	82.2	93.0	107.9	122.9	141.0	169.2	
30–35	64.1	72.0	81.9	94.6	108.0	126.0	144.3	172.2	
35–40	64.5	73.9	85.5	97.9	112.1	131.7	148.0	178.4	
40–45	69.5	80.5	90.3	102.4	120.7	140.9	161.1	187.3	
45–50	72.5	83.2	97.7	110.5	125.7	141.8	165.1	194.0	
50–55	70.0	84.5	96.2	112.5	127.8	144.8	168.3	196.5	
55–60	46.9	90.1	102.6	115.7	130.5	152.8	169.9	198.2	
60–65	78.3	85.3	96.8	114.6	130.6	146.4	166.0	194.0	
65–70	74.3	84.8	97.0	110.4	130.7	140.7	153.4	164.6	

*Proportional sum of six skinfolds (mm).

skinfolds. Z-scores were derived for each component according to the general formula:

$$Z = 1/s \cdot (V \cdot (170.18/b)^d - P)$$

where Z = the phantom proportionality score
s = the phantom standard deviation for variable V
V = the variable score
b = measured stature
d = a dimensional exponent equal to 1 for lengths, 2 for areas and 3 for weights
P = the phantom value for variable V.

Having derived the mean proportionality score (Z-score) for each subgroup of measures, the tissue mass was estimated using the following formula:

$$M = \frac{(Z \cdot s + P)}{(170.18 / b)^3}$$

where M = the mass of the component tissue
Z = the obtained mean proportionality score
s = the phantom standard deviation for that tissue mass
P = the phantom value for that tissue mass
b = the measured stature.

When applied to the data from the Brussels Cadaver Study (Drinkwater 1984), however, the model underestimated body weight by 6.3% and severely underestimated adipose tissue weight by 51.6% for 13 unembalmed cadavers.

Kerr (1988) then proposed an alternative five-way fractionation model in such a way that the component weights of the skin, adipose tissue, muscle, bone and residual tissues could be estimated from anthropometric dimensions. This model also deviated from that of Drinkwater and Ross (1980), whereby the calculation of the pro-

Table 14.6 The O-scale proportional weight ratings for male subjects

Age (years)	Stanine threshold values								
	1	2	3	4	5	6	7	8	9
6	55.2*	56.8	59.9	62.6	64.8	66.7	69.6	73.9	
7	49.5	55.1	56.7	59.8	63.2	35.2	67.5	69.3	
8	49.8	54.2	55.8	57.9	60.5	63.4	66.7	67.8	
9	49.4	53.3	55.1	57.4	59.7	62.5	66.1	69.1	
10	50.1	53.1	54.3	59.5	59.5	66.8	66.0	71.9	
11	48.1	50.4	53.5	55.8	59.6	63.3	70.2	75.7	
12	46.3	50.6	52.8	54.9	58.3	62.2	67.3	74.4	
13	46.2	48.8	51.4	54.2	57.2	61.6	67.0	73.2	
14	46.6	48.8	51.3	54.2	57.3	60.8	64.5	71.3	
15	46.8	49.2	51.4	54.3	57.5	61.2	66.8	71.7	
16	47.1	49.8	52.7	55.3	57.3	61.4	66.8	71.7	
17	47.9	50.8	53.5	56.3	59.3	62.4	67.5	71.8	
18–19	49.5	52.8	56.4	59.0	62.5	64.5	67.8	70.8	
20–25	51.3	54.8	57.8	61.8	65.6	69.4	74.6	80.1	
25–30	53.1	56.2	59.8	63.2	67.5	71.4	76.4	84.3	
30–35	53.8	57.7	61.2	64.6	68.7	73.2	78.3	85.2	
35–40	55.2	58.6	61.8	65.4	69.7	73.8	79.0	86.2	
40–45	55.6	59.1	62.7	66.4	69.7	73.8	78.9	86.0	
45–50	55.6	59.6	63.5	66.8	70.8	75.0	79.7	86.8	
50–55	55.9	59.9	63.4	66.6	70.7	74.8	79.6	86.3	
55–60	56.6	60.4	63.5	66.7	71.3	76.1	80.7	87.8	
60–65	55.9	60.3	63.3	66.3	70.5	74.8	79.8	87.3	
65–70	53.0	57.5	62.1	66.5	69.5	73.9	77.8	81.3	

* Proportional weight (kg).

portionality score for each tissue mass could be scaled according to any required dimension, not just stature. A similar strategy was applied to the prediction formula for tissue mass.

Under this new model, Kerr (1988) used values for six skinfold sites, adding the supraspinale skinfold to the five proposed by Drinkwater and Ross. However, the scaling variable of stature was again chosen for the estimation of adipose tissue mass. This model proved more accurate when validated against the Brussels cadaver data. Adiposity was underestimated by 3.6% for the female cadavers and overestimated by 5.8% in males.

This prediction is no worse than that from regression equations and the solution is not population-specific nor dependent upon the assumption of constant density of the FM and LBM compartments (Kerr 1988). Nevertheless, while the prediction of adiposity using this latest approach provides a closer estimate than previous attempts,

it still does not provide a sufficiently accurate technique for monitoring individual fluctuations in body composition.

OTHER TECHNIQUES

Myriad technologies and methods have been employed to estimate body composition *in vivo*. Methodologies such as Potassium-40 counting, helium dilution and inert isotope dilution (Behnke & Wilmore 1974) require costly and sophisticated equipment. Other electrical and electronic devices have also been employed, giving rise to estimates of body fat from the medical imaging technologies of radiographic analysis, ultrasound, computed tomography and magnetic resonance imaging. In most cases however, these images provide site-specific information which must then be extrapolated to account for whole body tissue compartments.

Table 14.7 The O-scale proportional weight ratings for female subjects

Age (years)	Stanine threshold values								
	1	2	3	4	5	6	7	8	9
6	53.1*	54.4	57.4	60.2	63.8	66.7	71.3	72.9	
7	51.3	53.8	56.2	57.6	60.8	64.1	68.9	72.8	
8	51.7	54.3	55.8	57.3	59.8	62.7	66.6	71.6	
9	49.9	52.0	54.4	56.6	59.7	63.2	67.7	72.2	
10	47.6	51.2	53.2	55.8	60.0	63.7	71.1	75.8	
11	46.6	49.3	52.0	53.8	58.2	65.0	70.7	74.7	
12	46.2	49.2	51.8	54.8	59.6	63.9	72.8	80.2	
13	46.0	49.8	52.2	56.3	59.9	65.3	71.8	77.0	
14	46.3	50.2	53.3	56.7	60.3	64.8	71.8	78.0	
15	47.2	50.3	54.2	57.2	60.5	64.3	71.0	76.3	
16	47.3	52.2	55.3	57.7	60.8	63.8	70.8	75.0	
17	49.0	52.8	55.8	58.4	61.6	64.4	70.0	75.3	
18–19	51.8	54.8	57.5	60.4	63.5	66.8	71.0	77.8	
20–25	52.2	55.2	57.6	60.8	64.2	68.3	72.9	80.0	
25–30	52.5	55.2	57.7	61.0	64.8	68.9	74.8	83.0	
30–35	52.3	55.3	58.5	61.5	64.8	69.1	74.8	84.5	
35–40	53.1	56.2	58.8	62.4	66.3	70.7	76.7	88.0	
40–45	54.4	57.6	60.8	63.8	68.1	73.2	80.2	89.2	
45–50	55.2	58.7	62.0	65.2	69.8	74.6	82.3	91.8	
50–55	54.2	57.8	62.2	65.3	69.6	74.3	82.7	93.0	
55–60	55.5	59.1	62.5	66.8	72.8	78.1	84.4	95.5	
60–65	56.3	59.0	63.8	67.4	71.9	77.5	85.4	93.5	
65–70	53.3	58.7	65.3	69.2	74.8	78.8	84.3	91.7	

* Proportional weight (kg).

Two similar techniques which have received increased attention are based on the differing dielectrical properties of fat and lean tissues of the body (Segal *et al.* 1985) and are known as total body electrical conductivity (TOBEC) and bioelectrical impedance analysis (BIA). The TOBEC method uses uniform current induction to estimate LBM from the magnitude of the body's electrical conductivity. Bioelectrical impedance analysis however, is a localized method that attempts to measure resistance to the flow of electrical current through the body (Harrison 1987). An estimate of fat-free mass (FFM) is then calculated after normalizing for stature (Guo *et al.* 1987) as follows:

$$FFM = C \cdot S^2/R$$

where C = a constant
S = stature
R = electrical resistance.

Fat mass is then derived from total body mass by the subtraction of estimated FFM.

Although the reliability is reportedly high (Houtkooper *et al.* 1989), investigations of the validity of these methods have not involved acceptable criterion values. Lukasaki (1988) and Segal *et al.* (1988), for example, reported a close association between body conductivity methods and estimates of percentage body fat in adults. The close association of an estimate with another estimate cannot be construed as a validation. Furthermore, the regression equations used to predict FM from these methodologies are population-specific and thus cannot be confidently applied to all athletic populations.

Research into the factors that affect the recorded electrical resistance in the BIA technique has been recently reported. Variations in diet, hydration, ethnicity and diseased states affect the body's electrolyte balance, which in turn influences the FM estimate (Malina 1987; Hutcheson *et al.* 1988). To date, there is no compelling evidence that TOBEC or BIA should be used for the accurate monitoring of individual body composition status.

CONCLUSION

After reviewing the available indirect methodologies, a value judgement needs to be made as to the 'best' technique for a particular application. Clearly however, those strategies based on indices of weight and height can be dismissed as unacceptable techniques for the estimation of an individual's body composition, together with many of the techniques in the 'other' subgroup, due to the lack of established validity.

Densitometry provides a possible method of accurately and reliably monitoring body density, pro-

vided the observer is prepared to spend the time during assessment and build the apparatus needed to precisely account for all variables in the density formula. No transformations or modifications of this density score should be made as this only introduces further error, based upon erroneous assumptions.

Finally, for those observers with the required level of skill, the measurement of skinfolds from at least eight sites will provide a useful method of monitoring body fat. These values should *not* be transformed into estimates of percentage body fat via regression equations since they are population-specific and are derived from other indirect methods. Skinfold values should be summed, dimensionally scaled to stature and compared over time, or used in the O-scale strategy when an individual is compared with the general population or average data for a sporting population.

PROPORTIONALITY

In Chapter 7 the problem of comparing the proportions of one individual with those of another, or to a set of normative data, was identified. Using raw scores from anthropometric measures alone does not permit an evaluation of proportionality since these scores are dependent, to some degree, on the size of the individual. Two methods have been proposed to address this problem. The first is the *somatogram*, initially proposed by Behnke *et al.* (1959) and later modified by Behnke to a form described in Behnke and Wilmore (1974). A second method, known as the *unisex phantom stratagem*, was devised by Ross and Wilson (1974) as a metaphorical model for assessing human proportionality.

THE SOMATOGRAM

The somatogram strategy was refined by Behnke to provide a graphical representation of a body's proportions using girth measurements. Typically, data for 11 girths are required (Fig. 14.19) together with k values for each individual measure which are assigned for the *reference man* or *reference woman*. Each measured girth (g) is divided by the appropriate k value (Table 14.8) to obtain the d value ($d = g/k$). Then, the sum of the g values divided by the sum of the k values provides a reference score (D; i.e. $\Sigma g/\Sigma k = D$), which is used to create each positional plot on the somatogram.

For example, a value for the percentage deviation from D for the biceps girth in Fig. 14.19 is calculated as follows:

$$d\,(\text{biceps}) = g\,(\text{biceps})/k\,(\text{biceps})$$
$$= 37.5/5.29$$
$$= 7.09$$

$$D = \Sigma g/\Sigma k$$
$$= 6.51$$

Table 14.8 Girth measurement k values for a reference man and reference woman aged 20–24 years

Girth measure	Reference man k	Reference woman k
Shoulder	18.47	17.51
Chest	15.30	14.85
Abdominal	13.07	12.90
Hips	15.57	16.93
Thigh	9.13	10.05
Biceps	5.29	4.80
Forearm	4.47	4.15
Wrist	2.88	2.73
Knee	6.10	6.27
Calf	5.97	6.13
Ankle	3.75	3.70

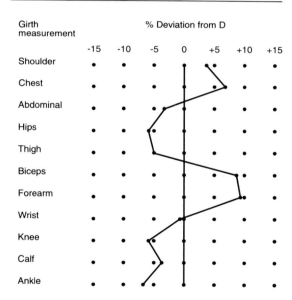

Fig. 14.19 Somatogram of a male weightlifter aged 30 years.

therefore,

$$\% \text{ deviation from } D = (7.09-6.51)/6.51 \cdot 100$$
$$= 8.9\%.$$

Similar values are calculated for the other girths and the somatogram created. In this example, the shape of the subject (a male weightlifter) is clearly abnormal compared with the proportions of the reference man. This young weightlifter has proportionally larger shoulder and chest girths, as well as biceps and forearm girths, than the reference man.

THE UNISEX PHANTOM

Ross and Marfell-Jones (1991) describe the *phantom* as a calculation device, not a normative system, based on a hypothetical unisex reference human with defined mean *(P)* and standard deviation *(S)* values for over 100 lengths, breadths, girths, skinfold thicknesses and fractional masses. The original data were derived primarily from the collation of anthropometric information by Garrett and Kennedy (1971), whereupon reported mean values for males and females were geometrically adjusted to a standard stature. The resulting phantom *P* and *S* values are distributed normally, unimodally and symmetrically. Selected phantom specifications for the anthropometric variables described in this chapter are presented in Tables 14.9 and 14.10.

Phantom Z-scores may be calculated using the formula:

$$Z = \frac{1}{S} \left[V \left(\frac{170.18}{H} \right)^d - P \right]$$

where Z = the phantom Z-score
S = the phantom standard deviation for variable V

Table 14.9 Phantom specifications for selected body mass, length and breadth variables

Variable	P*	S†
Body mass (kg)	64.58	8.60
Standing height (cm)	170.18	6.29
Sitting height (cm)	89.92	4.50
Direct lengths (cm)		
Acromiale–radiale (arm)	32.53	1.77
Radiale–stylion (forearm)	24.57	1.37
Mid-stylion–dactylion (hand)	18.85	0.85
Acromiale–dactylion (upper limb)	75.95	3.64
Iliospinale height (lower limb - 1)	94.11	4.71
Trochanterion height (lower limb - 2)	86.40	4.32
Trochanterion–tibiale laterale (thigh)	41.37	2.48
Tibiale laterale height (leg - 1)	44.82	2.56
Tibiale mediale–sphyrion (leg - 2)	36.81	2.10
Akropodion–pternion (foot)	25.50	1.16
Arm span	172.35	7.41
Breadths (cm)		
Biacromial	38.04	1.92
Transverse chest	27.92	1.74
Biiliocristal	28.84	1.75
Biepicondylar humerus	6.48	0.35
Bistyloid wrist	5.21	0.28
Hand	8.28	0.50
Biepicondylar femur	9.52	0.48
Anterior–posterior chest	17.50	1.38

*P = phantom mean value.
†S = phantom standard deviation value.

Table 14.10 Phantom specifications for selected girth and skinfold variables

Variable	P*	S†
Girth (cm)		
Head	56.00	1.44
Neck	34.91	1.73
Relaxed arm	26.89	2.33
Flexed arm	29.41	2.37
Forearm	25.13	1.41
Wrist	16.35	0.72
Chest	87.86	5.18
Waist	71.91	4.45
Hip	94.67	5.58
Thigh - 1	55.82	4.23
Thigh - 2	—	—
Calf	35.25	2.30
Ankle	21.71	1.33
Skinfolds (mm)		
Triceps	15.4	4.5
Biceps	8.0	2.0
Subscapular	17.2	5.1
Iliac crest	22.4	6.8
Supraspinale	15.4	4.5
Abdominal	25.4	7.8
Front thigh	27.0	8.3
Medial calf	16.0	4.7

*P = phantom mean value.
†S = phantom standard deviation value.

V = the subject's score on variable V

H = the subject's stature

d = a dimensional exponent which is consistent for a geometrical similarity system, $d = 1$ for lengths, breadths, girths and skinfolds; 2 for all areas; 3 for masses and volumes

P = the phantom mean score for variable V.

Using data collected at the World Aquatics Championships in Perth, 1991 (Carter & Ackland 1994), Fig. 14.20 displays proportionality differences between male and female competitors. These differences in proportion are shown for length, breadth, girth and skinfold measures, with Z-score data plotted for each gender group separately. Upon inspection of this figure, clear differences can be identified not only between gender groups, but

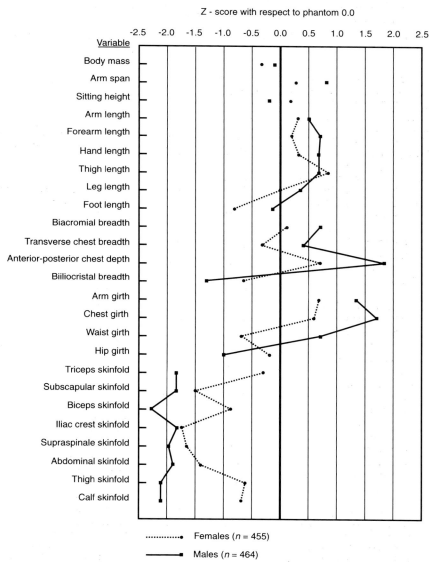

Fig. 14.20 Proportionality differences between aquatic sportsmen and sportswomen.

also between the phantom mean score and aquatic athletes in general (see especially the skinfold scores).

In a second example (Fig. 14.21), male waterpolo players from the KASP study (Carter & Ackland 1994) who play in the specialized positions of centre forward (CF) and goalkeeper (GK) are compared directly with the offensive and defensive wing players (OTH). Rather than using the phantom mean Z-scores as the basis for plotting, as in Fig. 14.20, the data for OTH in Fig. 14.21 are used to create the zero line, and Z-score differences are

then plotted for the specialized positions.

With respect to the data in Fig. 14.21, Ross *et al.* (1994) reported that CF were proportionally heavier than OTH, and had proportionally larger arm spans, leg lengths and waist girths. The GK however, were proportionally lighter and had a shorter sitting height than OTH. Furthermore, although GK were taller than OTH in absolute dimensions, they were proportionally smaller in biacromial and transverse chest breadth and possessed smaller arm, forearm, chest and waist girths.

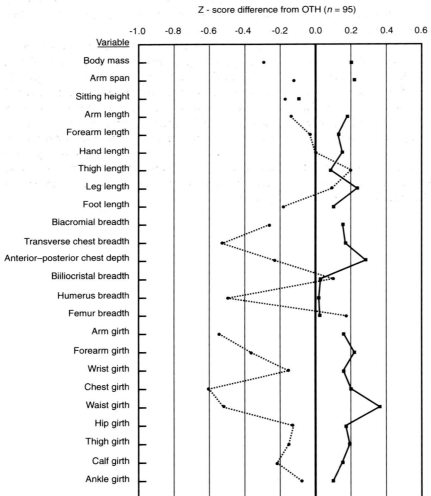

Fig. 14.21 Proportionality differences among male waterpolo players by position.

POSTURE

Static posture is usually assessed subjectively in the standing position using a rating chart as a guide for observers. The form shown in Fig. 14.22 is based on the New York Posture Rating Test (Adams *et al.* 1975) and may be used as an effective screening tool. The alignment of body segments when viewed from the posterior and lateral perspectives is examined by a trained observer. Observers may use a plumb bob, clear grid screen or other devices such as the scan-a-graf to aid in their subjective evaluations.

The subject stands erect in a natural posture (not rigidly in the anatomical position, for example) approximately 3 m in front of the observer. For each of the 13 posture areas shown in Fig. 14.22, the subject is given a score from one to five, based on the sketches on the rating form. Only whole numbers are permitted.

With respect to the condition of the longitudinal arch of the foot, the subject is required to step onto a chalk board after the feet have been moistened. The subsequent imprint of the feet is assessed and scored for this item.

More objective tests which focus on a particular postural deformity rather than mass screening, include medical imaging techniques using radiography and computerized tomography. In addition, special photographic techniques such as Moiré Topology have been developed for the accurate assessment of scoliosis and other spinal postural disorders.

Instrumentation and methodologies for measuring *dynamic posture* are not generally available; however, these may eventually be developed in association with the biomechanical techniques of cinematography and electrogoniometry which are discussed in Chapter 3. In the field of occupational biomechanics, several quasi-static techniques have been used to quantify dynamic postures in the work environment and these have been reviewed by Chaffin and Andersson (1984).

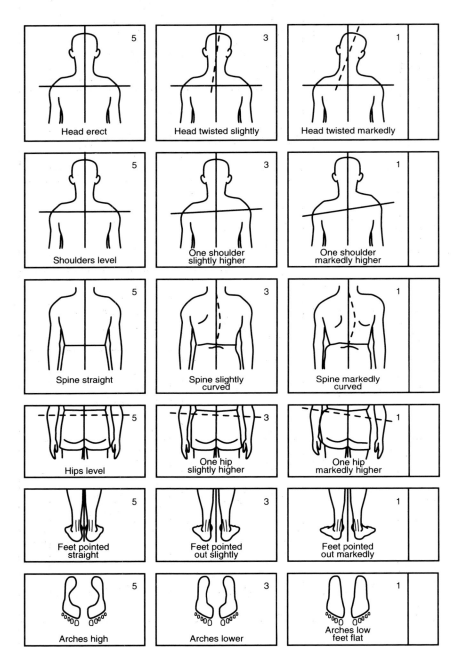

Fig. 14.22 Posture screening test.

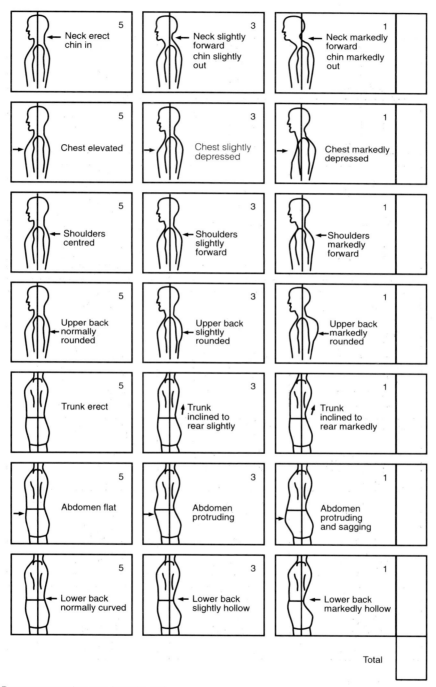

Fig. 14.22 Posture screening test (*continued*).

STRENGTH AND POWER

There is a variety of reasons why the coach or sport scientist would want to accurately assess the muscular strength and power of an athlete. These include:

- Establishing the relevance of strength and power to a particular sport
- Determining the strengths and weaknesses of an athlete by comparing test performances with group norms. By profiling the athlete in this manner, the test results can be used for the implementation of specific resistance training regimens
- Monitoring training progress or the progress of injury rehabilitation

GENERAL TESTING PRINCIPLES

Warm-up

As with any strenuous physical activity, it is important to warm the body prior to the performance of maximal strength or power testing. The warm-up should consist of several minutes of light aerobic exercise, such as riding a stationary bicycle, and be followed by light exercises for the muscle groups to be assessed. For example, light dumb-bell presses could be used to warm up the pectoral muscle group. Stretching exercises for the specific muscle groups should also be performed (see Chapter 10) and, prior to the performance of the test, several light practice trials should be permitted. The warm-up serves to facilitate performance by preparing the neuromuscular system for maximal exertion and also reduces the risk of musculoskeletal injuries.

Motivation, Rest Periods and Number of Trials

Prior to the administration of the test, subjects should be instructed to attempt to exert maximum effort. A subject's performance is often improved by vocal encouragement; however, since this is difficult to standardize, it is often more reliable not to encourage the subject during the performance of a test. The number of trials performed and the rest period used will be dependent upon the actual test undertaken. For example, a maximum isotonic test will typically be performed for only one trial, while four trials are recommended for high-speed isokinetic tests. Rest periods will also vary from test to test; however, a rest period of approximately 3 min is usually adopted between repeated trials.

There is a wide variety of methods that can be used to assess the qualities of muscular strength and power. These tests range from laboratory to field tests and include isometric, isotonic and isokinetic modalities.

ISOMETRIC TESTS

Strength Assessment

Isometric tests are a commonly used form of muscular strength assessment in the laboratory. Strength is generally defined as the force or torque (force multiplied by perpendicular distance to the axis of rotation) generated during a maximal isometric contraction (Atha 1981). Perhaps the main reason for the isometric mode having been the standard for strength assessment was due to the fact that the force developed in a concentric contraction decreases as a function of movement speed (see Force–Velocity Relationship in Chapter 9). Therefore the maximum force production would seem to occur during an isometric contraction, but more recently it has been observed that even greater forces can be recorded during eccentric contractions.

Isometric tests are performed against an immovable resistance, which is in series with a cable tensiometer (force shown as deflections of a dial), or load cell or strain gauge (whereby the transducer records the applied force as a change in voltage). For the latter devices, the voltage change is subsequently passed through an analogue to digital converter and recorded as an applied force by a computer or similar device. Subjects are required to give a maximal effort over a 3 or 4 s period. A series of isometric strength tests for the muscle groups most often assessed are presented in Figs 14.23 to 14.27.

The following guidelines for isometric strength assessment, which are adapted from those reported by Clarke and Clarke (1963), outline the specific requirements for limb and strap positioning and the precautions a tester should take to brace the subject for the tests in Figs 14.23 to 14.27.

HAND FLEXION

- Limb position — forearm in 90° of flexion and in mid-pronated position, hand in mid-position of its range of motion
- Strap position — proximal to the metacarpophalangeal joint
- Bracing — prevent elevation of the scapula and abduction of the arm; subject's free hand braces wrist being tested to prevent medial (internal) rotation of the arm

HAND EXTENSION

- Limb position — as for hand flexion
- Strap position — as for hand flexion
- Bracing — as above for the tester; subject's free hand braces wrist being tested to prevent lateral (external) rotation of the arm

FOREARM FLEXION

- Limb position — forearm in 115° of flexion and in a mid-pronated position

- Strap position — midway between wrist and elbow joints
- Bracing — prevent arm flexion and brace legs

FOREARM EXTENSION

- Limb position — forearm in 40° of flexion and in mid-pronated position
- Strap position — midway between wrist and elbow joints
- Bracing — prevent elevation of the scapula and trunk rotation

ARM FLEXION

- Limb position — forearm in 90° of flexion and in mid-pronated position
- Strap position — midway between elbow and shoulder joints
- Bracing — prevent trunk rotation

ARM EXTENSION

- Limb position — arm in 90° of flexion and medially (internally) rotated 90° (so forearm is across the body); forearm in 90° of flexion and fully pronated
- Strap position — midway between elbow and shoulder joints
- Bracing — prevent trunk rotation and arm adduction or abduction

ARM MEDIAL (INTERNAL) ROTATION

- Limb position — forearm in 90° of flexion and in mid-pronated position
- Strap position — midway between elbow and wrist joints
- Bracing — prevent arm flexion on test side and trunk rotation

ARM LATERAL (EXTERNAL) ROTATION

- Limb position — as for arm medial rotation

- Strap position — as for arm medial rotation
- Bracing — as for arm medial rotation

ARM ABDUCTION

- Limb position — forearm in 90° of flexion and in mid-pronated position; folded towels or pads supporting buttocks and shoulder to allow the passage of the strap underneath the trunk
- Strap position — at the distal end of the arm superior to the olecranon process
- Bracing — prevent arm flexion and lateral flexion of the trunk

ARM ADDUCTION

- Limb position — arm abducted to 90° and forearm flexed to 90°
- Strap position — midway between the shoulder and elbow joints
- Bracing — prevent rotation of the trunk

TRUNK FLEXION

- Limb position — arms folded across chest
- Strap position — around chest immediately beneath the axilla
- Bracing — prevent thigh flexion

TRUNK EXTENSION

- Limb position — arms adducted so that hands are clasped behind the trunk
- Strap position — as for trunk flexion
- Bracing — as for trunk flexion

THIGH FLEXION

- Limb position — test limb fully extended with other limb flexed at the hip and knee
- Strap position — midway between inguinal crease and superior border of patella. (Note: this position differs from that described by Clarke &

Clarke 1963 but improves the objectivity of the test)
- Bracing — prevent trunk flexion

THIGH EXTENSION

- Limb position — both limbs are fully extended in this prone lying position
- Strap position — as for thigh flexion
- Bracing — prevent trunk extension and raising of the hips

THIGH ABDUCTION

- Limb position — test limb fully extended with other limb flexed at the hip and knee
- Strap position — as for thigh flexion
- Bracing — prevent lateral flexion of the trunk

THIGH ADDUCTION

- Limb position — both limbs fully extended with upper limb held in slight abduction
- Strap position — as for thigh abduction
- Bracing — maintain support of the non-test limb

LEG FLEXION

- Limb position — leg in 165° of flexion
- Strap position — midway between knee and ankle joints
- Bracing — prevent extension of the trunk

LEG EXTENSION

- Limb position — leg in 115° of flexion, while arms may hold sides of bench
- Strap position — midway between knee and ankle joints
- Bracing thigh — prevent extension of the to raise buttocks

FOOT DORSI-FLEXION

- Limb position — foot in 125° of dorsi-flexion

	Isometric	Isokinetic	Isotonic
Hand flexion	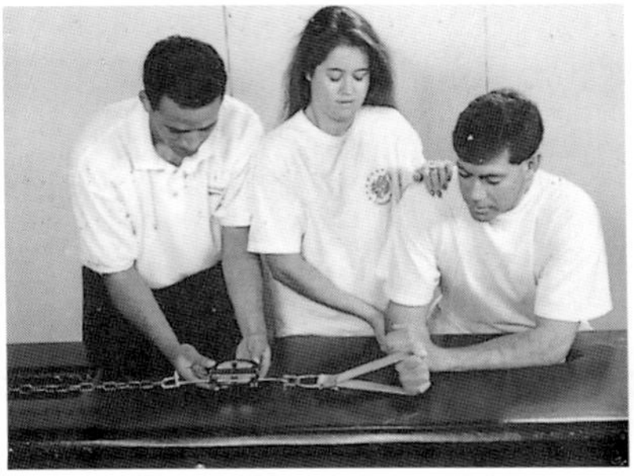	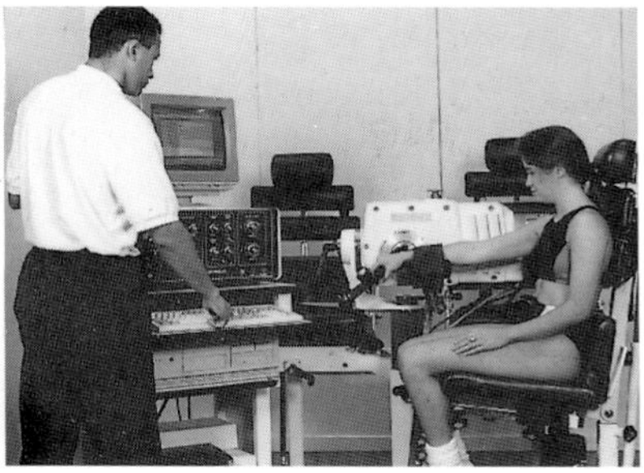 Biodex	Wrist curl (Fig. 9.72)
Hand extension	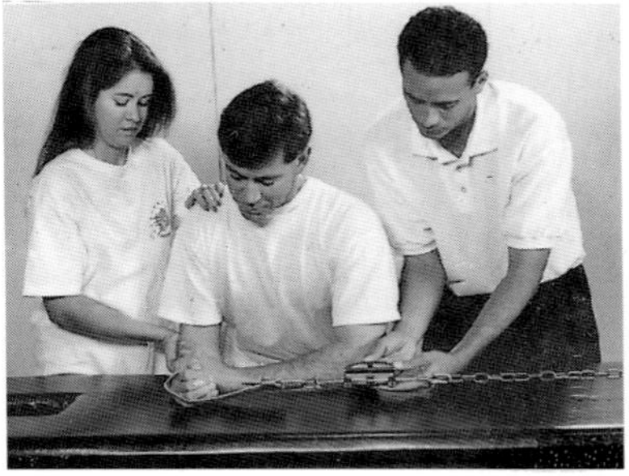	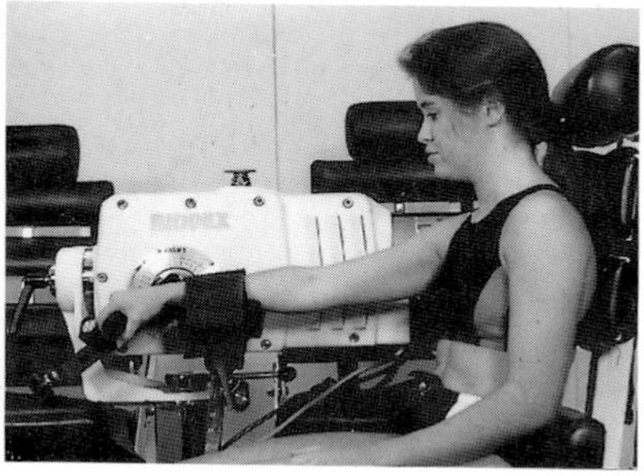	Reverse wrist curl
Forearm flexion	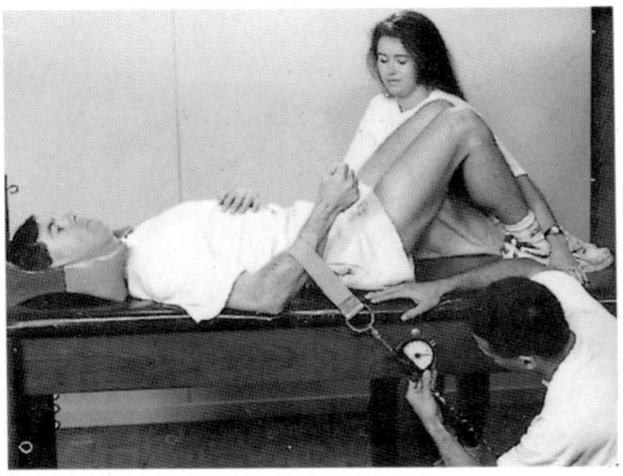	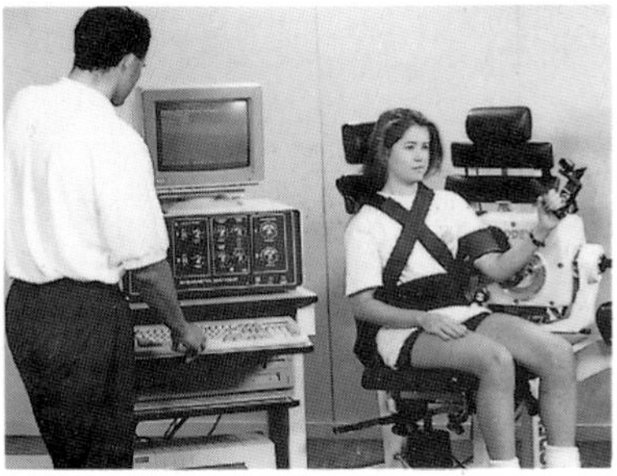 Biodex	Biceps curl (Fig. 9.11) Concentrated curls
Forearm extension	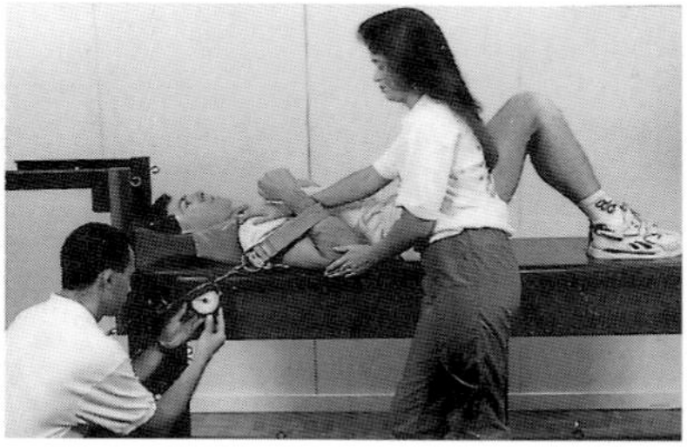	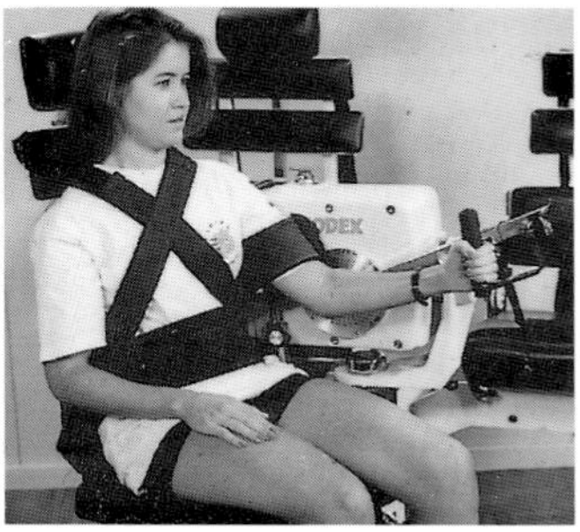	Triceps pushdown Lying triceps extension (Fig. 9.53) Military press

Fig. 14.23 Isometric, isokinetic and isotonic strength tests for hand flexion–extension and forearm flexion–extension. Note: Isokinetic exercise movements are performed reciprocally with the same equipment set-up.

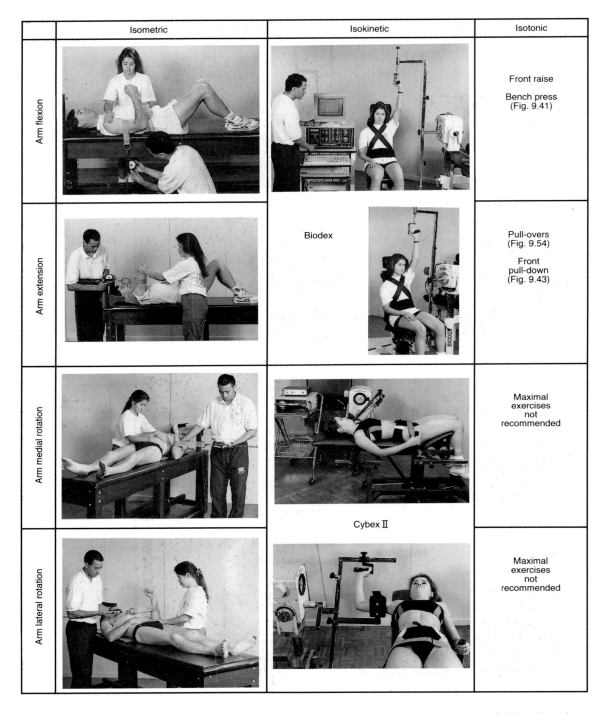

	Isometric	Isokinetic	Isotonic
Arm flexion			Front raise Bench press (Fig. 9.41)
Arm extension		Biodex	Pull-overs (Fig. 9.54) Front pull-down (Fig. 9.43)
Arm medial rotation			Maximal exercises not recommended
Arm lateral rotation		Cybex II	Maximal exercises not recommended

Fig. 14.24 Isometric, isokinetic and isotonic strength tests for arm flexion–extension and arm medial–lateral rotation. Note: Isokinetic exercise movements are performed reciprocally with the same equipment set-up.

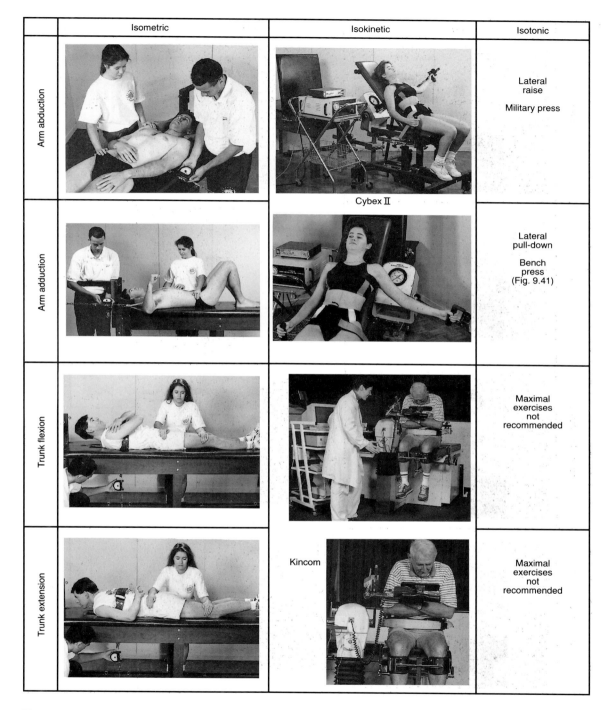

Fig. 14.25 Isometric, isokinetic and isotonic strength tests for arm abduction–adduction and trunk flexion–extension. Note: Isokinetic exercise movements are performed reciprocally with the same equipment set-up.

	Isometric	Isokinetic	Isotonic
Thigh flexion	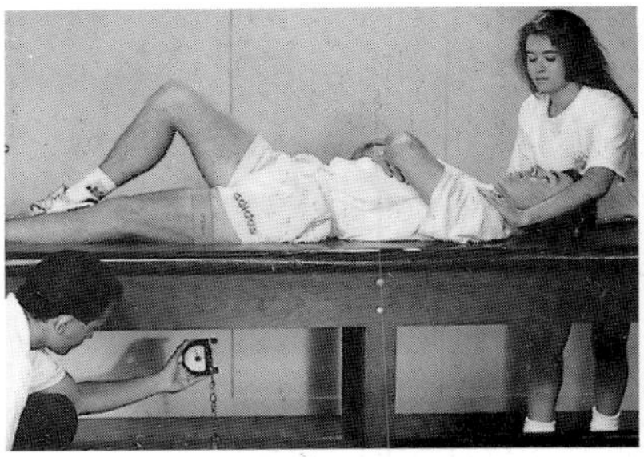	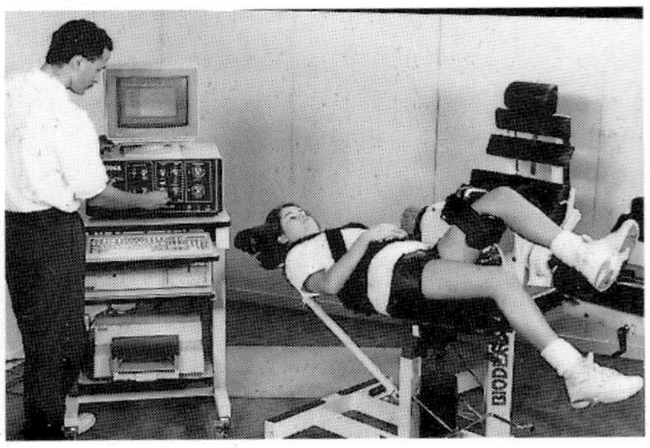 Biodex	Thigh flexion (Fig. 9.68)
Thigh extension	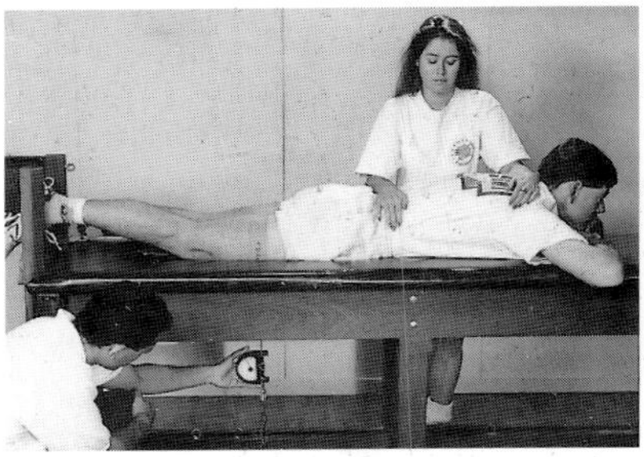	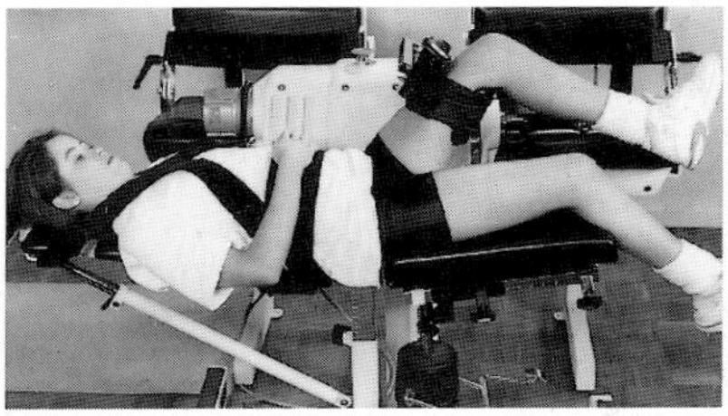	Thigh extension (Fig. 9.17) Squats (Fig. 9.61)
Thigh abduction	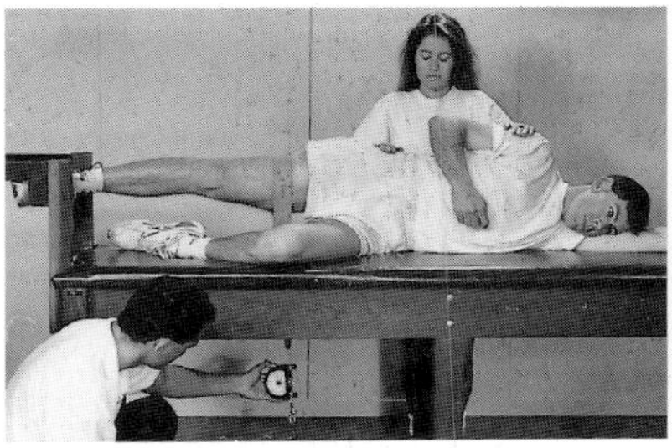	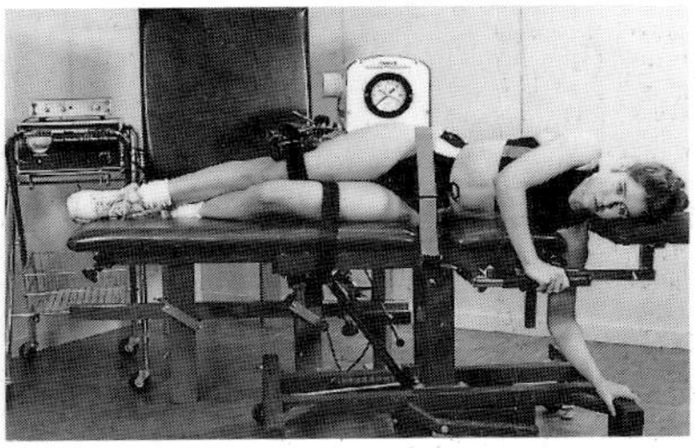 Cybex II	Thigh abduction (Fig. 9.66)
Thigh adduction	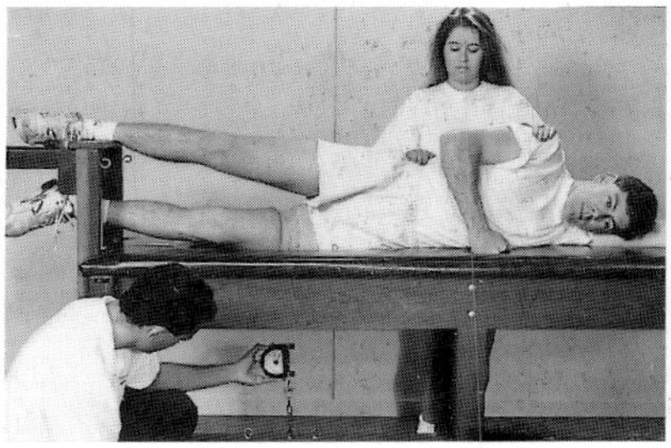	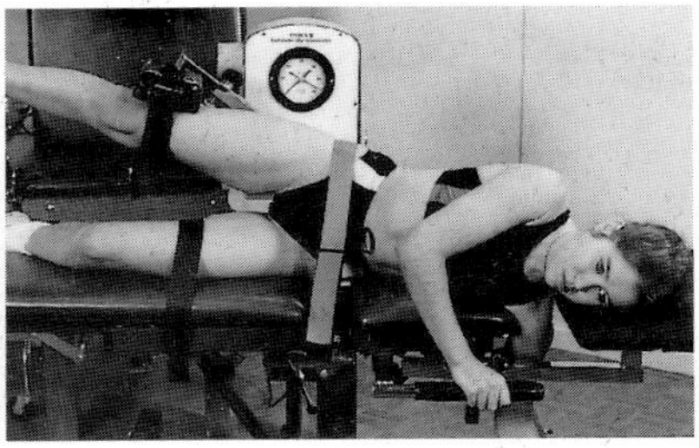	Thigh adduction (Fig. 9.67)

Fig. 14.26 Isometric, isokinetic and isotonic strength tests for thigh flexion–extension and thigh abduction–adduction. Note: Isokinetic exercise movements are performed reciprocally with the same equipment set-up.

	Isometric	Isokinetic	Isotonic
Leg flexion	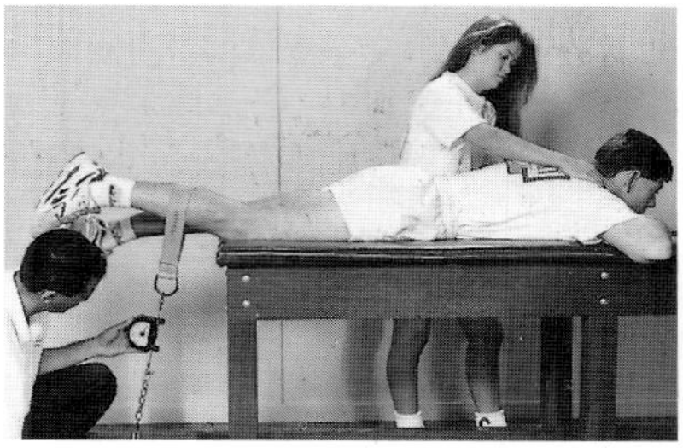	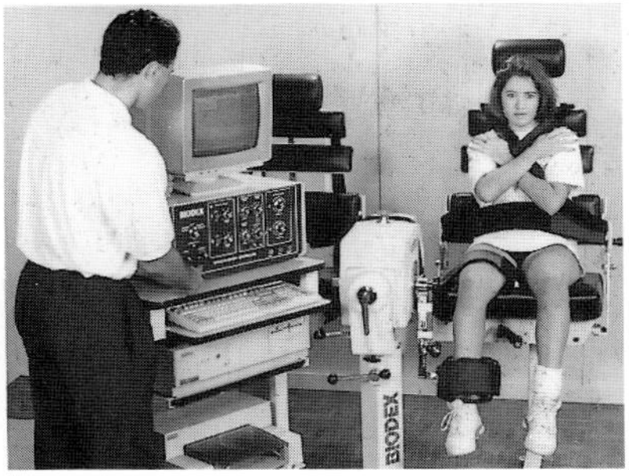	Leg curl (Fig. 9.16)
Leg extension	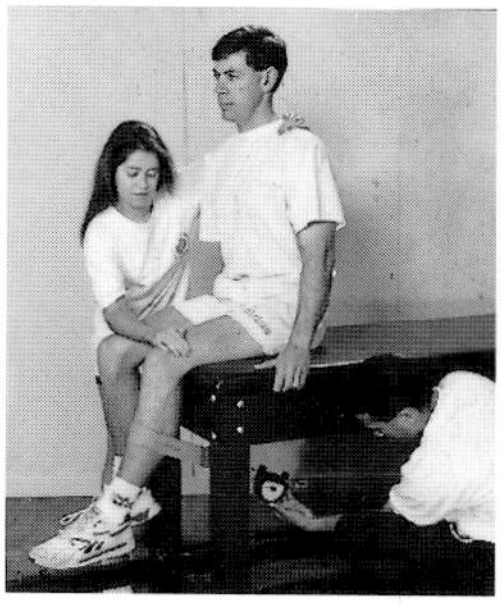	Biodex 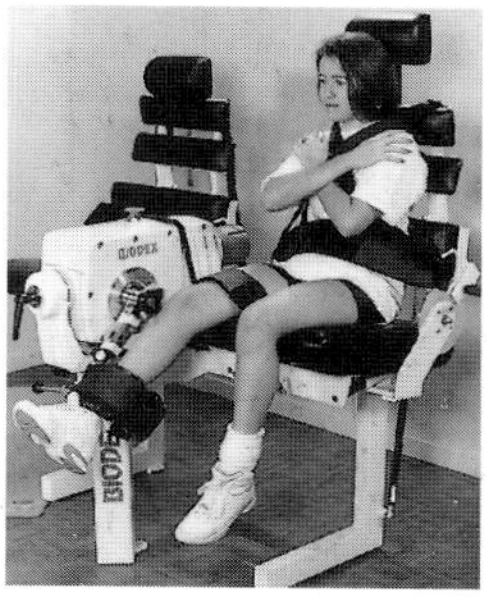	Leg extension (as shown in Fig. 9.74 without plyometric component)
Foot dorsi flexion	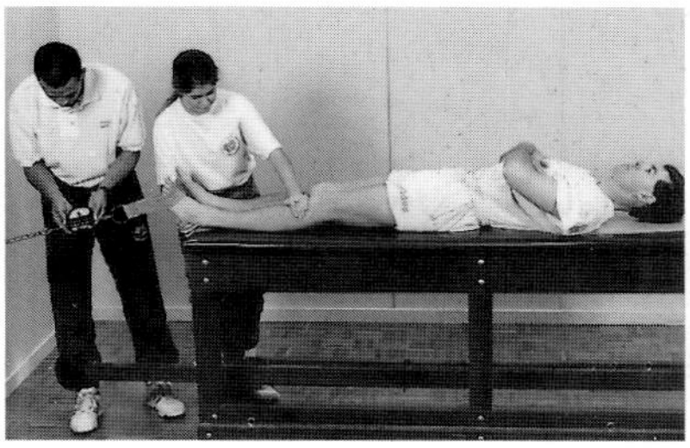	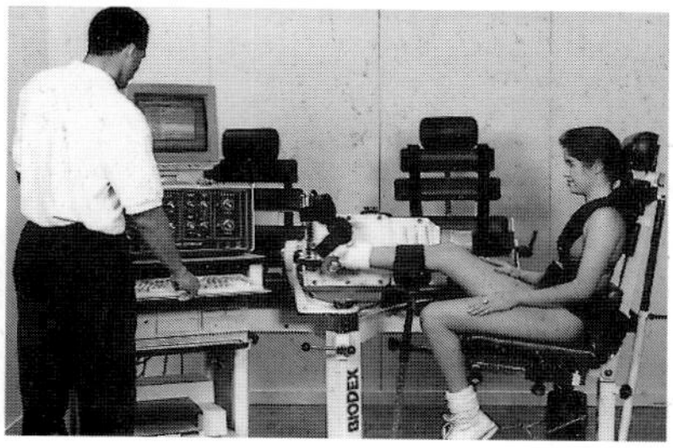	Ankle curls (Fig. 9.39)
Foot plantar flexion	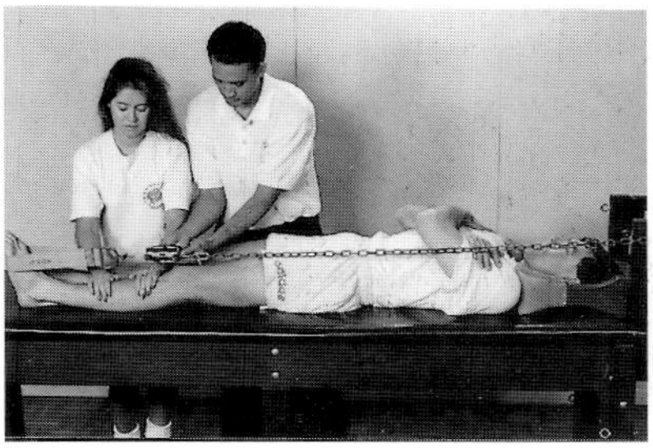	Biodex 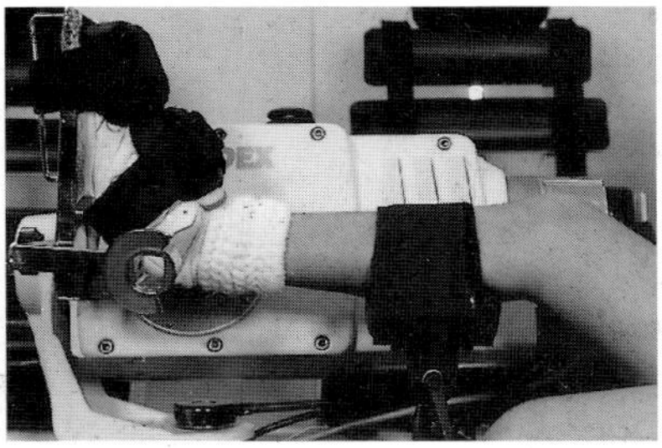	Calf raises

Fig. 14.27 Isometric, isokinetic and isotonic strength tests for leg flexion–extension and foot dorsi–plantar flexion. Note: Isokinetic exercise movements are performed reciprocally with the same equipment set-up.

- Strap position — distal to metatarso-phalangeal joint
- Bracing — prevent inversion/eversion of foot and flexion of thigh and leg

FOOT PLANTAR-FLEXION

- Limb position — foot in 90° of dorsi-flexion
- Strap position — as for foot dorsi-flexion
- Bracing — as for foot dorsi-flexion

RELIABILITY OF THE TEST

Maximal isometric strength tests have particularly high test–re-test reliability (Viitasalo *et al.* 1980; Bemben *et al.* 1992). Viitasalo *et al.* (1980) reported a high correlation between repeated maximal isometric trials which were conducted with a 5 min rest interval. Similar reliability values were obtained by Bemben *et al.* (1992) for subjects of differing ages. Greater reliability was achieved when several practice tests were provided prior to data collection and when the data were collected over a 2 day period and the values averaged.

LIMITATIONS OF THE TEST

One limitation of the isometric test is that it records the maximal force at only one joint angle and the results gained from this angle are not always representative of the strength of the muscle at other positions. Thus if information is required regarding force over a range of motion, the test will need to be repeated for a number of joint positions.

Due to the specificity of strength, which implies that individuals can be strong in some muscles but not in others, or even strong in particular ranges of motion but not others, it may be more valuable to perform strength tests in positions other than those for the standardized tests. Secher (1975) observed significant differences in isometric strength between rowers of varying ability, when tested in a position that simulated the initial pull phase in rowing. However, when standardized isometric tests were performed, these differences were not readily apparent between the rowers. Further, no significant relationship between isometric rowing strength and scores on the standard tests

for individual muscle groups, except grip strength, was observed.

Power Assessment

Mechanical power refers to the rate of change of performing work. It can also be defined as force multiplied by velocity. During an isometric muscular action no visible movement of a limb occurs, therefore no work is performed and hence, no power is achieved. However, the term 'power' is often used with respect to athletic performance relating to an explosive dynamic performance. While the calculation of a dynamic quality such as power through an isometric test does not appear empirically correct, such a test has been formulated and is becoming increasingly popular. Individuals are required to develop force quickly and with as much intensity as possible, against an immovable object, while an instantaneous recording of the force–time history is made throughout the contraction phase.

The rate of force development is seen to be a particularly important factor in many sports, as the time available for the exertion of force is very limited. For example, in sprinting the ground contact time is tyically 80–100 ms. Similarly, during the jumping events such as high and long jumps, the ground contact time is in the order of only 150 ms. Consequently the ability to rapidly generate force is of obvious importance.

QUANTIFICATION OF THE TEST

This physical capacity may be quantified in a variety of ways, with the most popular being the maximum rate of force development (Fig. 14.28). The time interval for calculation of this rate may vary from 5 ms (Viitasalo *et al.* 1980) through to 60 ms (Bemben *et al.* 1992). Other methods include determining the time taken to reach a criterion absolute level of force, or the time taken to reach a relative force level (such as 30% of the individual's maximum force). Alternatively, the level of force achieved in a specific period of time has also been used to quantify this parameter using an isometric test.

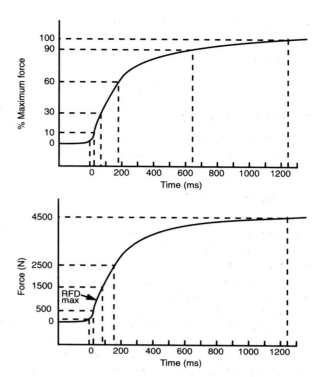

Fig. 14.28 Quantification of the isometric force–time curve. Note that several methods are used including calculation of the maximum rate of force development and the time taken to achieve an absolute or relative level of force (adapted from Sale 1991).

RELIABILITY AND VALIDITY OF THE TEST

The test for maximum rate of isometric force development has been shown to be reliable (Viitasalo et al. 1980; Bemben et al. 1992). For example, Bemben reported correlations between test scores administered on successive days for a variety of muscle groups of between 0.92 and 0.98.

The relationship between the rate of force development and athletic performance has received equivocal support from researchers. Mero et al. (1981) did not observe a relationship between maximal rate of force development and running speed. Similarly, Wilson et al. (1993) reported that this test was not a useful predictor of performance in running or cycling. However, Viitasalo and Aura (1984) reported a strong relationship between the average values of rate of force development for the quadriceps muscle group and high jumping performance, for eight nationally ranked high jumpers.

If one examines the force profiles and associated muscular activity of most competitive events

such as jumping or running, it is evident that force is developed during the eccentric phase of these activities and that during the concentric phase of the movement the force decreases in accordance with the force–velocity relationship of muscle (see Chapter 9). Consequently, the ability to rapidly develop force during an isometric or concentric contraction does not appear to be a relevant requirement of most sports that involve a dynamic eccentric contraction, as the majority of force is developed during the eccentric phase. In fact, during the concentric phase the dominant task would be to maintain the high force levels developed during the eccentric phase.

USES OF THE TEST

The shape of the isometric curve permits an assessment of relative abilities in strength and power development and has implications for the type of training that should be undertaken to enhance performance. For example, an individual who has a high level of force but a poor rate of force development, would be required to perform explosive resistance training to enhance performance. Traditional heavy weight training would be of little benefit for this individual, as the limitation to performance is not the level of strength, but the ability to apply it rapidly. Conversely, an individual with a rapid production of force, but a relatively poor level of maximum force, would appear to be limited by the low level of strength. In this instance, explosive power training would offer little benefit; however, traditional heavy weight training would serve to increase strength and enhance performance. One major limitation to the above use of the maximum rate of force development in strength diagnosis is the current lack of comparative normative data; however, test information is presently being compiled at the Australian Institute of Sport.

ISOTONIC TESTS

Strength Assessment

To assess strength isotonically a one repetition maximum (1 RM) test is performed. This test determines the maximum load one can lift for one complete repetition. The 1 RM test has been widely used for a variety of movements (see Figs 14.23 to 14.27), such as the bench press (Wilson *et al.* 1992), the squat, military press and power clean (Fry *et al.* 1991). Prior to the performance of the test subjects are warmed up and perform a series of submaximal lifts with progressively heavier loads. As the loads become relatively close to maximum, they are incremented by small amounts (2.5–10 kg, or 5–10% of maximum) until the lift cannot be completed. A 5 min recovery should be imposed between lifts. When using trained subjects who have a good knowledge of their maximum load, the process is relatively simple and generally requires no more than three or four lifts. Even when using the procedure with novice subjects the maximum is typically realized by the fourth trial. Anderson and Kearney (1982) reported that when performing a 1 RM with novice subjects, 60% of subjects required four trials, 30% required five trials and 10% required six trials.

When using novice subjects the process of determining the 1 RM using free weight movements is more difficult because of the skill component of the lifts. For this reason it is preferable that maximal isotonic tests be performed using weight machines whereby the skill component of the movement is greatly reduced. The effect of the skill component on isotonic strength was investigated by Rutherford *et al.* (1986). These researchers reported that following 12 weeks of resistance training, a 160–200% increase in weight was lifted during the isotonic exercises; however, maximum isometric force increased by only 3–20% over this same period. The large discrepancy between the two measures of strength was attributed to improvements in lifting technique.

The 1 RM test is seen by many to represent a superior measure of strength compared to an isometric test for experienced subjects, as it requires the production of force throughout a range of motion. However, the performance of maximal isotonic lifts is limited by the strength of the individual at the weakest point in the range of motion, often termed the sticking region (see Chapter 9). In fact during this part of the movement, the individual applies less force to the bar than the actual weight of the bar. The momentum developed earlier in the lift permits progress through this region, allowing the lift to be completed. Given the relatively small fluctuations in force applied during a maximal lift (see Chapter 9), the maximum load lifted can be considered a reasonable guide to the average strength of the individual over the range of motion prior to the deceleration phase.

SAFETY CONSIDERATIONS

During these tests where maximum loads are being lifted, it is imperative that they are performed with absolute safety. At all times at least one catcher or spotter for lifts such as the bench press, and at least two spotters for lifts such as squats, should be in attendance. It is also desirable to have the lifts performed in a rack, so that if the bar cannot be lifted it can be placed onto a rack or safety catches (Fig. 14.29). Further, it is important that the lifts are performed in a technically correct fash-

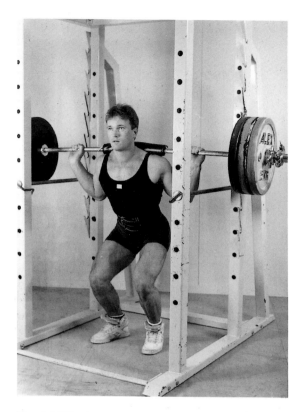

Fig. 14.29 Safety bars designed to limit the downward movement of the bar.

ion, particularly for exercises that involve the lower back, such as squats, power cleans or deadlifts. Small technique problems in such lifts can greatly alter the forces on the lower lumbar vertebrae and increase the risk of serious injury.

RELIABILITY OF THE TEST

Isotonic strength tests, when determined using experienced subjects, have high reliability. Sale (1991) for example, examined the reliability of a 1 RM bilateral forearm flexion movement in 11 young women and 12 young men. The maximal tests were conducted with 2 days of rest between repeated trials and highly significant test–re-test correlations were reported.

RELATIONSHIP TO PERFORMANCE

Maximal isotonic strength is a useful predictor of performance in athletic activities. Fry *et al.* (1991) reported that maximal isotonic strength differed significantly between volleyball players of varying ability, whereas no difference was reported for maximal isometric strength scores. Fry and Kraemer (1991) reported that there was a close relationship between the bench press and power clean exercises and the player's ability among American college football players.

Power Assessment

Power or dynamic performance has been estimated using an isotonic testing protocol by the performance of weighted squat jumps with various loads (Viitasalo 1985a,b; Hakkinen *et al.* 1987, 1988). The squat jumps were performed over a force plate which recorded the time of flight and from this the height of the jump was estimated using the equations of uniformly accelerated motion. A series of jumps was performed initially with body weight only and then with additional loads of 40, 80, 100 and 140 kg held to the back (Hakkinen *et al.* 1987, 1988). From this procedure a load–height curve was generated which is depicted in Fig. 14.30. This curve provides an approximation of the average force–velocity relationship of muscle (Viitasalo 1985b).

Such procedures should only be used on athletes who have had extensive experience in strength training, but even with this limitation it would appear that the risk of injury on landing would be reasonably high. This testing protocol is clearly not for the 'faint-hearted'!

RELIABILITY OF THE TEST

Viitasalo (1985b) examined the reliability of this testing protocol, both within a testing session and between test days, using loads from 0 to 80 kg. The author reported that the test had good reliability which, however, diminished for the heavier loads. To standardize the testing protocol, each load was performed in the following order: 0, 20, 40, 60, 80, 80, 60, 40, 20, 0 kg (Viitasalo 1985b).

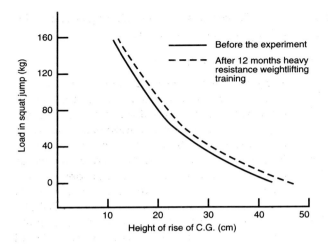

Fig. 14.30 Load–height curve derived by recording the height jumped at various loads. Note that the curve is similar to the average force–velocity curve (adapted from Hakkinen *et al.* 1987).

RELATIONSHIP TO PERFORMANCE

This procedure is a relatively recent development and has not yet been widely used. The test develops an estimate of the force–velocity relationship so that the performance of the muscle can be assessed throughout a wide range of conditions. Vertical jumps performed without additional load have been observed to be a valuable predictor of performance in many dynamic lower body domi-

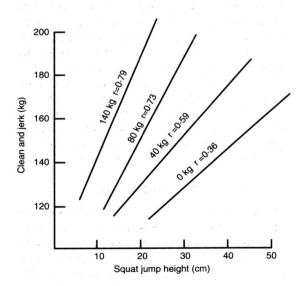

Fig. 14.31 Relationship between weightlifting performance in the clean and jerk lift and squat jump height (adapted from Sale 1991).

nated sports such as running and cycling. In activities where greater loads and forces are involved, such as in long and triple jumping or during the weightlifting events of the snatch and clean and jerk, the performance of heavily loaded vertical jumps are significantly better predictors of performance in comparison to unloaded jumps (Fig. 14.31).

Viitasalo (1985a) has used the loaded squat jump protocol to assess specific changes in muscular performance in response to training, using experienced volleyball players and high jumpers. These athletes performed explosive resistance training in the form of plyometrics over a 5 month period. Significant increases in jump height were recorded with no load and with an additional 20 kg load, although no significant changes were recorded for the jumps performed with the heavier load conditions.

NEW DEVELOPMENTS IN ISOTONIC TESTING

Future development of isotonic tests may include protocols based on a percentage of an individual's maximum strength as opposed to absolute loads, and the development of tests for other body movements. Furthermore, the results of the test may be more meaningful if expressed in terms of power rather than the vertical distance jumped.

Recently the Plyometric Power System (see Chapter 9) has been developed, which allows dynamically loaded activities such as squat jumps and bench press throws to be performed, with the option of engaging an electronically controlled brake to reduce potentially hazardous impact forces. The system permits the safe performance of these and many other standard resistance training movements. A rotary encoder, fixed to the shaft of the machine, records the direction and distance of bar movements and relays this information to a computer to enable the calculation of the distance moved, work done, average power output and peak velocity. The electronically controlled brake can be used to reduce the downward acceleration of the bar after it has reached maximum height. This serves to reduce the impact forces associated with landing from a heavily weighted squat jump or the impact force of catching a weighted bar in a bench press throw. The system is a relatively recent innovation but would appear to represent an exciting development in the isotonic assessment of muscular power.

ISOKINETIC TESTS

Strength Assessment

Isokinetic literally means 'same velocity' and refers to tests that are performed at a predetermined constant velocity. Isokinetic devices, commercially known as the Cybex II, Kin/Com, Biodex and so on, involve a dynamometer that is interfaced with a motor and which serves to provide equal and opposite resistance to the force provided by the musculature, once a predetermined velocity has been reached. These devices maintain a specific velocity and record the force, or more usually the torque applied by the athlete throughout the range of motion. A test of strength using these devices may be performed at the constant velocity of zero to produce an isometric contraction. Alternatively, these devices may be used to develop a force–velocity profile of the individual in a similar fashion to that described in the isotonic section of this chapter. However, rather than modifying the load and recording the performance parameters, these devices modify the velocity of motion. The subject set-up procedures for many of the standard measurement protocols are shown in Figs 14.23

to 14.27, where two images show global and detailed views of the equipment.

RELIABILITY OF THE TEST

Many scientists perceive isokinetic tests as the standard for assessment of the entire force–velocity curve. This is predominantly due to the large degree of control over the movement in terms of the velocity of motion. The movements required by the tests are easily standardized, involving for the most part, isolated muscular actions. For example, the popular leg extension test (Fig. 14.27) may be readily replicated with great reliability (Johnson & Siegel 1978) in comparison to multi-joint movement such as the vertical jump. It should be noted however, that isokinetic test results become less reliable as the velocity of movement increases. Therefore, while one or two repeat trials are usually sufficient at lower speeds (30–120°/s), four trials have been recommended at higher velocities (180–400°/s) to ensure reliable results (Osternig 1986).

ADVANTAGES OF ISOKINETIC TESTS

Isokinetic tests record the torque produced throughout the entire range of motion and allow for the identification of regions of strength or weakness within the range. In contrast, isotonic tests typically give a single, representative value for the entire movement, while isometric tests are specific to a single joint angle. Recent innovations, combined with the unilateral nature of many of the isokinetic machines, allow these systems to assess strength differences between alternate limbs, agonist and antagonist muscle groups and eccentric versus concentric movement phases.

LIMITATIONS OF ISOKINETIC TESTS

Isokinetic systems are not without their limitations and one of the most serious relates to the large proportion of movement that occurs prior to the achievement of a constant velocity. This is especially so when recording at high movement speeds. These dynamometers will only begin resisting the activity when the predetermined velocity has been achieved, and therefore at high velocities most of the movement is not isokinetic in nature. Osternig *et al.* (1982) reported that the movement phase was isokinetic for approximately 90% of the range when velocity was set at 50°/s. However, when the velocity was increased to 400°/s, the isokinetic phase represented only 15% of the total movement. For some activities such as kicking, however, where the swinging limb is rapidly accelerated prior to impact with a ball, this acceleration phase is specific to the skill and quite desirable.

A further limitation of isokinetic testing machines relates to the impact torque that is recorded at relatively high velocity settings. When the limb finally reaches the predetermined velocity, the dynamometer will engage to resist the limb and this has the effect of causing a collision between the lever arm and the rapidly accelerating limb (Fig. 14.32). This collision results in a large impact spike being recorded by the system (the magnitude of which is directly proportional to the velocity of the movement). Often this impact spike is the largest torque recorded during the movement and is often mistakenly perceived as the maximum ability of the contractile component to produce force at the predetermined velocity. This impact spike is an artefact and in most cases, efforts must be made to eliminate or ignore its presence in data analysis. Some dynamometers offer a ramp function which controls the acceleration of the limb prior to achieving the predetermined vel-

ocity, thereby reducing the extent of the impact torque.

RELATIONSHIP TO PERFORMANCE

Many strength practitioners perceive that the well controlled nature of isokinetic devices results in a lack of external validity. In controlling the movement velocity and performing isolated single joint movements that are not particularly representative of sporting actions, these devices are seen to lack application to competitive sports. Nevertheless, sport-specific isokinetic devices are available, such as the biokinetic swim bench, and these produce data that are often highly related to athletic performance. Sharp *et al.* (1982) trained four novice subjects on the biokinetic swim bench for a period of 4 weeks. The training resulted in a 19% increase in power output on the swim bench and a 4% improvement in swimming velocity. Further support for the value of isokinetic tests was supplied by Perrine and Edgerton (1975), who reported high relationships between isokinetic tests in a leg thrust exercise and performance in 40 yard sprint and vertical jump tests.

Power Assessment

Instantaneous power may be derived from the torque and angular velocity values when using an isokinetic dynamometer. The following equation describes the relationship between these variables.

$$W = \tau \cdot \omega$$

where W = instantaneous power (Watts)

            τ = instantaneous torque (Nm)

            ω = angular velocity (rad/s).

Power scores derived from this formula will only be valid for the period of time when the required velocity of movement has been achieved by the subject. A peak power score may also be computed by using the peak torque value in this formula.

Taylor *et al.* (1991) reported instantaneous leg extension power scores for elite power and endurance athletes at varying rotation velocities. All data were collected on a Biodex isokinetic

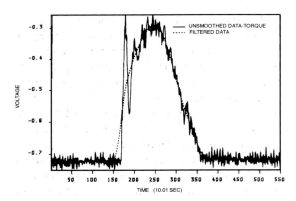

Fig. 14.32 A torque × time history recorded using an isokinetic dynamometer and showing a significant impact torque spike in the initial phase.

dynamometer. Regardless of the subject group, instantaneous peak power increased as a function of increasing movement velocity. However, the incremental gains in peak power were significantly greater for the power athletes compared to the endurance athletes, particularly when the movement velocity exceeded 180°/s.

COMPARISON BETWEEN TESTING MODALITIES

Although isometric, isotonic and isokinetic testing modalities can be used to test the same muscular functions, they often result in different scores. When comparing volleyball players of differing ability, Fry *et al.* (1991) reported significant differences between the groups for a range of isotonic strength measures. However, the same differentiation among subjects was not found using sport-specific isometric strength measures, nor for isokinetic strength assessed at 60, 180 and 300°/s. Hurley *et al.* (1988) compared peak torque for both the quadriceps and hamstring muscle groups between elite power-lifters and untrained control subjects who were matched for body mass. Despite recording significantly lower isotonic strength values than power-lifters, the control group recorded isokinetic peak torque values that were significantly greater for both muscle groups at 30°/s. The control group was subsequently trained for 4 months using a variety of isotonic exercises, resulting in a 40% increase in isotonic strength, whereas isokinetic strength remained unchanged. In addition, Wilson *et al.* (1993) have reported significant changes in athletic performance and isotonic tests of power as a consequence of resistance training; however, no change was apparent in the isometric rate of force development.

SPECIFICITY OF TESTING

The results from studies outlined above highlight one of the most important factors in testing, that is, the principle of specificity which suggests that the testing of muscular function should be specific to the method of training. When combined with the principle of specificity of training, it is clear that training and testing should both be specific to the competitive performance. Consequently, athletic performance and training in throwing events are probably best assessed by an isotonic power test that involves throwing or jumping with a load, whereas kicking skills may be best assessed using an isokinetic dynamometer set at relatively fast speeds.

FIELD TESTS OF POWER

Laboratory tests provide valuable information regarding an athlete's power generation; however, in many instances the necessary equipment is not readily available to the coach or athlete. In these instances field tests such as the vertical jump, standing broad jump, 40 m sprint, Margaria-Kalamen stair climb test and seated shot put can be used to assess this physical capacity.

Research has demonstrated that the field tests of lower body power are highly reliable (Gillespie & Keenum 1987; Mayhew et al. 1989), but that the tests were not closely related to each other. Therefore, good performance on one test item does not necessarily indicate a good performance on another. None of the field tests may be used to indicate general muscular power and consequently the test that is most specific to the competitive performance should be employed. That is, the vertical jump test may be effective in assessing leg power for basketball and volleyball players, but not for cyclists.

The relationship between various field tests and performance is dependent upon how closely the test and the activity are related. For example, the seated shot put test is a measure of upper body power and is significantly related to the power output recorded in a bench press lift (Gillespie & Keenum 1987). However, this test is not related to sprint swimming performance (Rohrs *et al.* 1990) even though swimming is strongly dependent upon upper body power. The reason for this disparity is that the bench press is a pushing movement involving a similar action to the seated shot put. Swimming is, however, a pulling activity involving movements that are quite different to the seated shot put.

Vertical Jump

The vertical jump test has been used as a test of leg power. Since the early part of this century when the test was first documented (Sargent 1921), many variations in protocol have been employed. This lack of standardization has limited the ability to pool data for comparative purposes. The resulting jump height is affected by many factors which need to be controlled in a standardized test. These factors include:

- The validity of the initial measure of standing reach height
- The starting position prior to the jump
- The use of the arms
- The existence of an unweighting phase in the preparation for the jump
- The method of scoring (i.e. chalk mark, time of flight, net ground reaction impulse)

ADMINISTRATION OF THE TEST

The following vertical jump protocol is designed to control many of the above factors.

- The athlete dips the fingers of the right hand in gym chalk and stands side on to the wall
- A mark is then made on the wall with the fingers after the athlete reaches as high as possible without lifting the heels from the ground
- The height of the standing reach is recorded
- The athlete then crouches and jumps as high as possible without taking a step, marking the wall at the peak of the jump (Fig. 14.33)
- This jump height is measured and the difference between standing reach height (to the nearest 0.5 cm) is noted
- The best score from three trials is subsequently recorded

DATA TREATMENT

Scores for the vertical jump test may be reported as the vertical distance between standing height and jumped height. Puhl *et al.* (1982) provide data for elite volleyball players, where the mean vertical distance for men (*n* = 8) was 67.0 cm and for women (*n* = 14) was 45.9 cm. Alternatively, a power score may be calculated using the Lewis nomogram

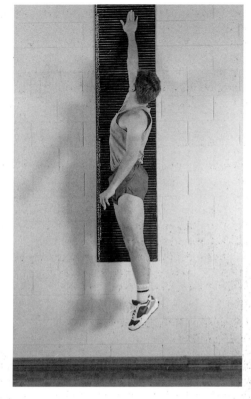

Fig. 14.33 An athlete marks the wall at the peak of the vertical jump test.

(Matthews & Fox 1976) based on equations of uniformly accelerated motion, summarized below:

$$P = \sqrt{4.9} \cdot W \cdot \sqrt{D}$$

where P = leg power (kg m/s)
W = weight of the athlete (kg)
D = vertical jump height (m).

Margaria-Kalamen Stair Climb Test

ADMINISTRATION OF THE TEST

The Margaria-Kalamen stair climb test requires the construction of suitable electronic timing equipment, shown in Fig. 14.34, and a suitable venue. Two switch mats, connected to an electronic timing device, are placed on the third and ninth steps of a staircase. The athlete begins from a standing

consider doing as 338 well.

start 6 m from the staircase, then runs as quickly as possible toward its base. Without losing momentum, the athlete leaps up to the third, sixth and ninth steps in quick succession. An elapsed time is recorded from foot contact with the third step until contact by the same foot with the ninth step. Three trials are permitted and the lowest time recorded.

DATA TREATMENT

Leg power is calculated using the following formula:

$$P = W \cdot D/T$$

where
- P = leg power (kg m/s)
- W = body weight (kg)
- D = the vertical distance between the third and ninth steps (m)
- T = the elapsed time (s).

STRENGTH–ENDURANCE ASSESSMENT

Strength–endurance can be assessed using a variety of methods. One popular method is to perform an exercise for a specific number of repetitions, often 20 or 30, and record the total work performed and the rate of fatigue. For example, an isokinetic leg extension movement can be per-

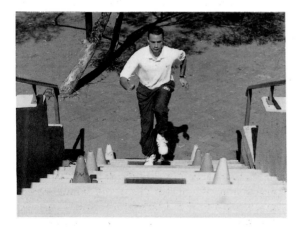

Fig. 14.34 The Margaria-Kalamen stair climb test of leg power.

formed for 30 maximal repetitions and total work and rate of fatigue recorded. Rate of fatigue is generally expressed as follows:

(maximum force – minimum force) / minimum force

A similar test can be performed isotonically using the Plyometric Power System (see Chapter 9) whereby 20–30 repetitions are performed on a jumping or throwing task and the total work and rate of fatigue recorded.

A slightly different approach was adopted by Fry *et al.* (1991), who required subjects to perform a series of jumps. The number of vertical jumps which exceeded 90% of maximum in a 30 s period was recorded. These and other researchers have also recorded the number of sit-ups, pull-ups and push-ups that could be performed in a set period of time.

Absolute and Relative Strength–Endurance

Gillespie and Gabbard (1984) and Anderson and Kearney (1982) quantified strength–endurance as the number of repetitions performed in an exercise at a specific submaximal load. Using this method, *absolute endurance* is assessed as the number of repetitions performed with a specified constant load, for example 50 kg. *Relative endurance* describes the number of repetitions performed with a load that is determined as a percentage of the athlete's maximum. Values for absolute endurance will be heavily dependent upon the maximum strength of an individual; however values of relative endurance will not. By determining an individual's absolute and relative endurance, valuable information can be obtained with implications for the formulation of specific resistance training routines.

IMPLICATIONS FOR TRAINING

If a strength–endurance athlete such as a 400 m runner possessed a high absolute endurance, but recorded a low relative endurance, it would suggest that the limitations to strength–endurance performance were the local muscle adaptations which promote local circulation, enhancing metabolism and waste removal. In this instance high repetition training should be more effective than pure strength training in facilitating the further development of strength–endurance. Conversely, if a strength athlete possessed a poor absolute endurance, but recorded a good relative endurance value, then the limitation to strength–endurance performance would be the athlete's strength. Consequently, strength training methods would be the most effective to further develop strength–endurance.

The number of repetitions that can be performed at various loads depends upon the exercises performed, the sex and the training status of the subject. Hoeger et al. (1990) have reported some normative data in relation to these loads, as outlined in Table 14.11. Furthermore, Anderson and Kearney

(1982) reported that approximately 40 repetitions were performed with a load of 40% of maximum, while Gillespie and Gabbard (1984) found that approximately 19 repetitions were performed with a load of 60% of maximum. Nevertheless, data can be collected on athletes at different times during the season and compared to previous values, in order to help formulate specific training routines.

RELIABILITY OF THE TEST

The reliability of the strength–endurance tests tends to be lower than for tests of strength or power. Particular care needs to be taken to ensure that all repetitions are performed with correct form. Furthermore, it is necessary to specify the rate of performance of the repetitions to improve the reliability of the test.

Table 14.11 Number of repetitions performed by trained subjects on various exercises at 40, 60 and 80% of maximum loads

Exercise	40%	60%	80%
Males (n = 25)			
LP	77.6±34.2	45.5±23.5	19.4±9.0
LD	42.9±16.0	23.5±5.5	12.2±3.7
BP	38.8±8.2	22.6±4.4	12.2±2.9
LE	32.9±8.8	18.3±5.6	11.6±4.5
SU	27.1±8.8	18.9±6.8	12.2±6.4
AC	35.3±11.6	21.3±6.2	11.4±4.1
LC	24.3±7.9	15.4±5.9	7.2±3.1
Females (n = 26)			
LP	146.1±66.9	57.3±27.9	22.4±10.7
LD	81.3±41.8	25.2±7.9	10.2±3.9
BP	—	27.9±7.9	14.3±4.4
LE	28.5±10.9	16.5±5.3	9.4±4.3
SU	34.5±16.8	20.3±8.1	12.0±6.5
AC	33.4±10.4	26.3±5.0	6.9±3.1
LC	23.2±7.7	12.4±5.1	5.3±2.6

Values are expressed as mean ± standard deviation.

LP = leg press (knees bent at 100° angle for the starting position); BP = bench press; LD = lateral pull-down (resistance pulled behind the head to the base of the neck); LE = leg extension; SU = sit-ups (horizontal board, feet held in place, knees at 100° angle and resistance held on chest); AC = arm curl (low pulley); LC = leg curl (to 90° of flexion).

FLEXIBILITY

Flexibility or joint mobility is influenced by a number of factors such as gender, age, body type, temperature and psychological stress. Their effects are explained more fully in Chapter 10 and provide the basis for the design of valid test protocols related to this capacity. A test of flexibility must have the following characteristics:

- The test must be specific to a single joint (with the exception of the vertebral column)
- The scoring system must be independent of the size or proportionality of the athlete
- Either a standardized warm-up or no warm-up must be permitted
- The posture adopted by the subject must not hinder nor enhance the attainment of maximum joint mobility
- The role of the tester in guiding the movement must be clearly defined

With these characteristics in mind, many of the 'field tests' of flexibility cannot be judged as valid. For example, the *sit and reach test* has been used by many as a 'general' test of hamstring and lower trunk mobility. However, the test is not valid due to the influence of proportionality in the scoring system and the fact that a single joint is not isolated. Individuals with varying upper and lower limb lengths, differences in hamstring extensibility, or who vary in the mobility of the lumbar vertebrae, may all obtain the same score on the sit and reach test.

In the procedures for a valid test, it must be clearly stated to what degree the tester may influence the movement. Since the amount of force provided by an assistant cannot be controlled, it is necessary that the body segments be moved only by the subject to reach the extreme points in the range of motion. Any assistance by the tester would invalidate the score and could cause soft tissue injury to the subject.

ASSESSMENT OF STATIC FLEXIBILITY

Scores on the following tests of static flexibility are independent of the dimensions of an athlete's body segments. They are designed to be performed *without* a warm-up and the positions must only be attained as a result of muscular contraction by the subject. That is, the tester must not force or assist the subject in any way except to keep the limb in the correct movement plane, or to prevent other movements of the body from affecting the test score.

Flexibility Screening

In this subjective screening test of flexibility the subject is asked to perform the following movements, whereupon a tester compares the position of maximum mobility with the diagrams in Fig. 14.35. The subject scores a rating of between 1.0 and 4.0 for each movement. Half scores (i.e. 1.5, 2.5 or 3.5) are also acceptable when the subject's position is perceived to be midway between the examples provided in Fig. 14.35.

ARM HORIZONTAL EXTENSION

The athlete adopts a prone lying position with the arms at right angles to the body and with the palms facing downwards. The arms are then lifted sideways.

ARM ABDUCTION

The athlete stands with one forearm flexed at the elbow joint behind the head and the fingers touching the upper back. The hand and forearm are then pushed down the back.

FOREARM FLEXION

The athlete stands with one arm held out horizontally in front of the body, then flexes the forearm towards the shoulder.

Flexibility Rating Form

Name: _____   Date: _____

Movement	1	2	3	4	Rating
Arm horizontal extension	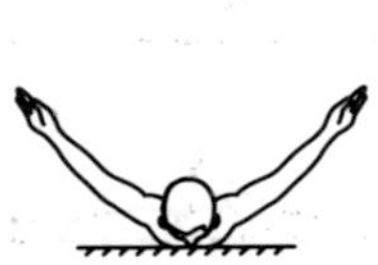	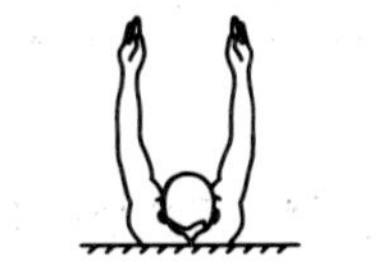	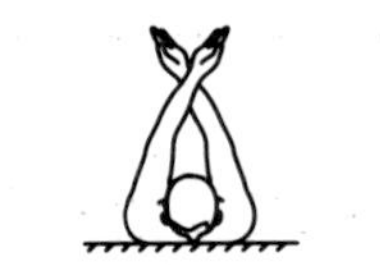	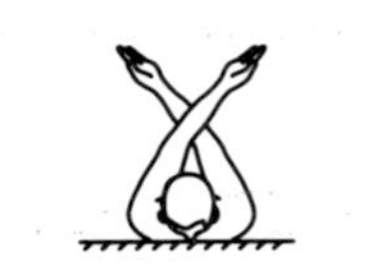	
Arm abduction	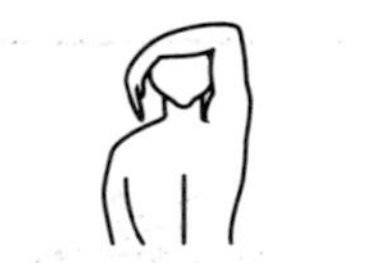	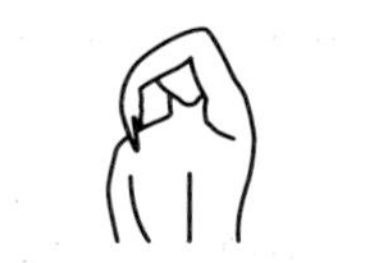	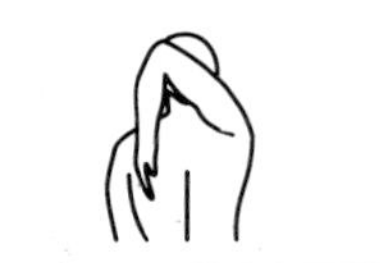	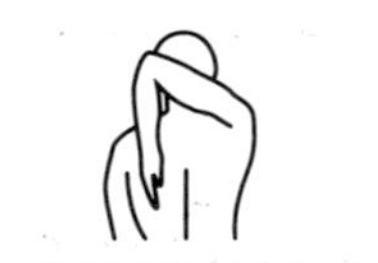	
Forearm flexion	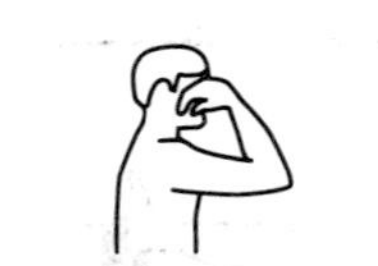	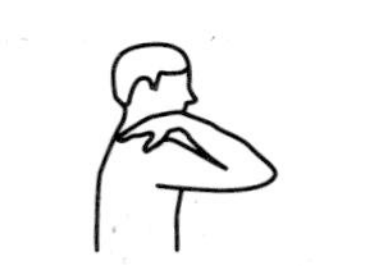	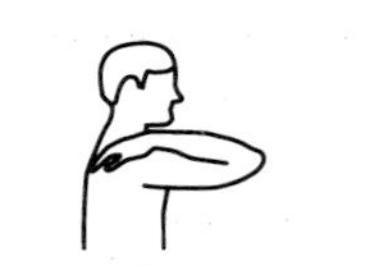	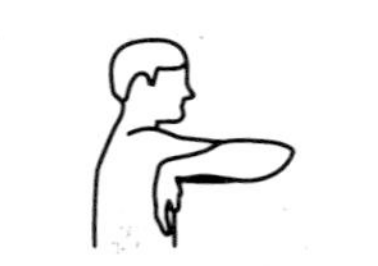	
Forearm hyper-extension	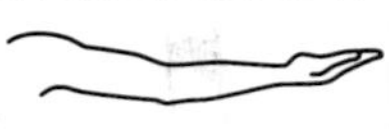	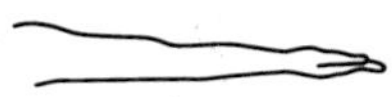	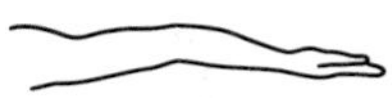	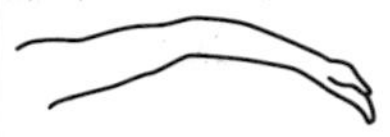	
Hand flexion	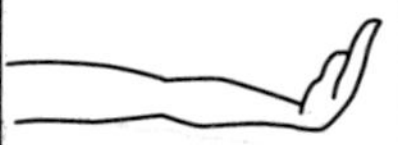	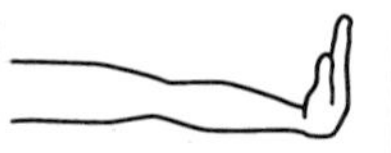	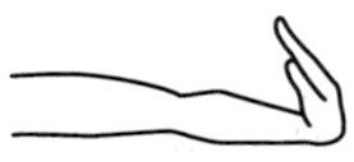	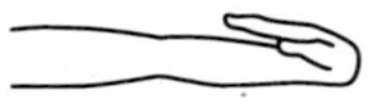	
Hand extension	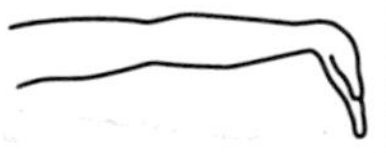	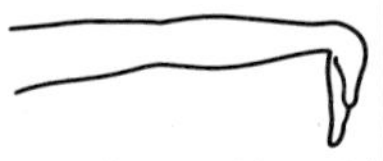	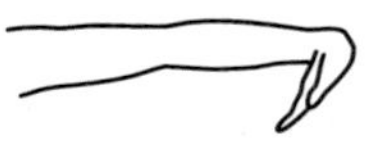	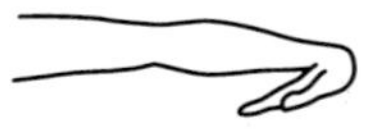	
Trunk flexion	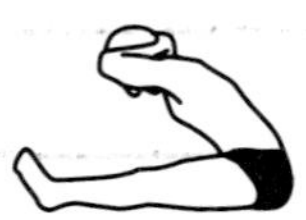	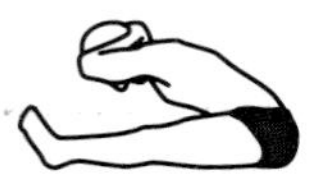	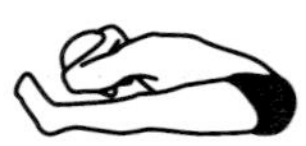	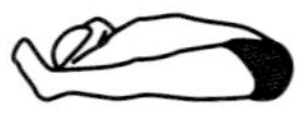	
Trunk hyper-extension	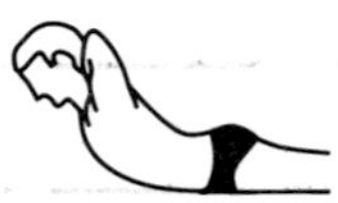	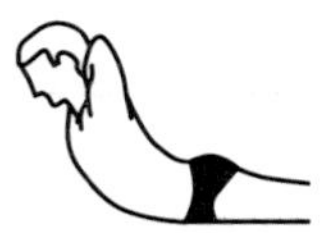	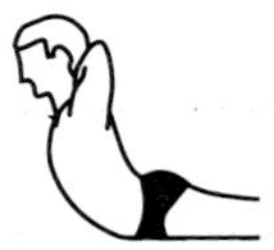	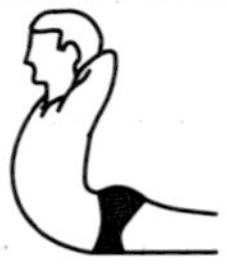	

Fig. 14.35 Flexibility screening test.

Movement	1	2	3	4	Rating
Trunk lateral flexion	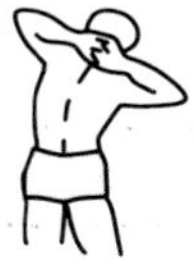	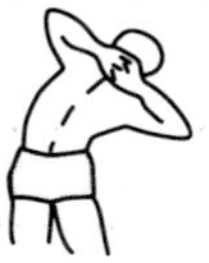	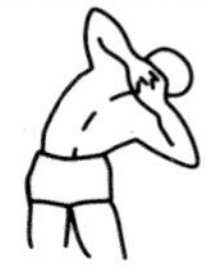	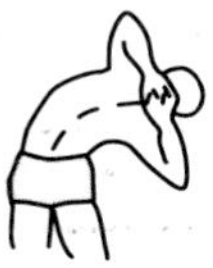	
Thigh flexion	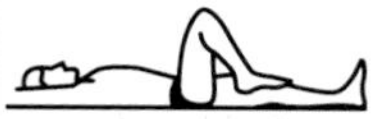	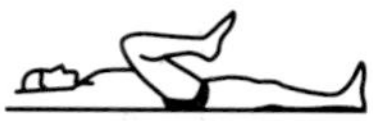	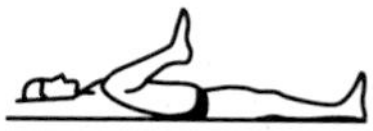	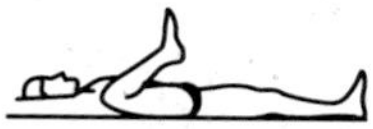	
Thigh extension	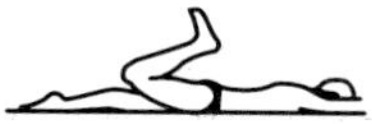	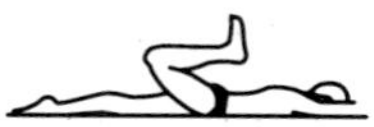	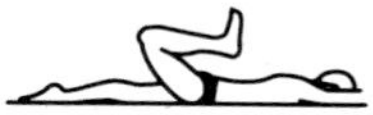	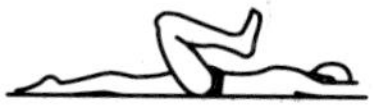	
Leg flexion	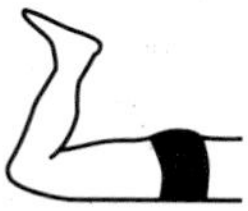	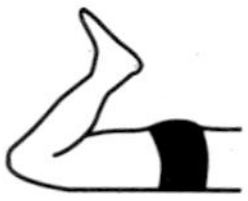	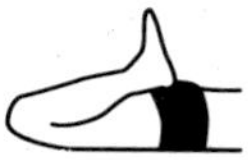	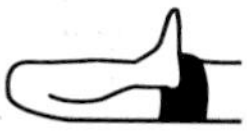	
Leg hyper-extension	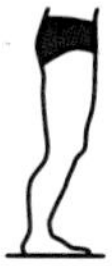	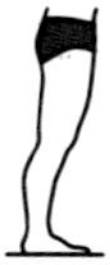	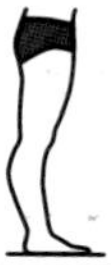	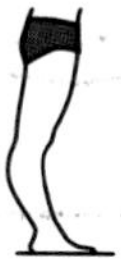	
Foot dorsi-flexion	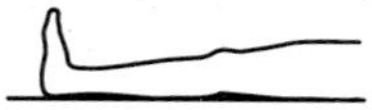	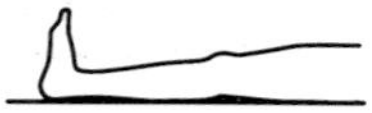	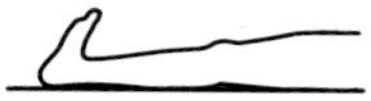	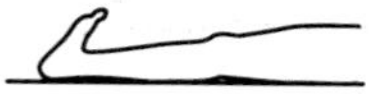	
Foot plantar-flexion	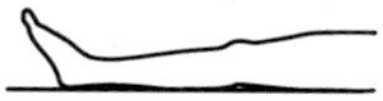	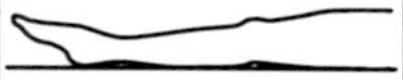	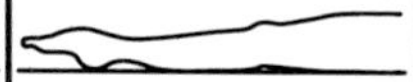	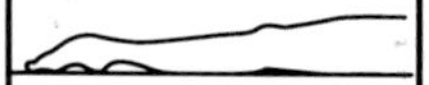	
Comments:					

Fig. 14.35 Flexibility screening test (*continued*).

FOREARM HYPEREXTENSION

The athlete stands with one arm held out straight and to the side of the body, then attempts to hyperextend the forearm at the elbow joint.

HAND FLEXION

The athlete stands with one arm held out straight and to the front, then flexes the hand at the wrist joint.

HAND HYPEREXTENSION

The athlete stands with one arm held out straight and to the front, then extends the hand at the wrist joint.

TRUNK FLEXION

The athlete adopts a long sitting position with the arms clasped behind the neck and the legs approximately 25 cm apart, then flexes the trunk forward towards the floor.

TRUNK HYPEREXTENSION

The athlete adopts a prone lying position with the hands clasped behind the neck and the partner holding the feet on the floor. The trunk is then slowly hyperextended.

TRUNK LATERAL FLEXION

The athlete stands with the hands clasped behind the neck, then laterally flexes the trunk to one side keeping the pelvis stationary.

THIGH FLEXION

The athlete adopts a supine lying position with one leg flexed at the knee and with the arms extended above the head and resting on the floor, then flexes the thigh at the hip joint.

THIGH EXTENSION

The athlete adopts a prone lying position with one leg flexed and with the arms extended in front of the shoulders, then extends the thigh at the hip joint.

LEG FLEXION

The athlete adopts a prone lying position with the arms extended in front of the shoulders and the non-assessed leg horizontal, then maximally flexes the leg at the knee joint.

LEG HYPEREXTENSION

The athlete stands in an upright position with the feet together, then pushes the knees backwards as far as possible.

FOOT DORSI-FLEXION

The athlete adopts a long sitting position with the hands on the ground close to the buttocks, then pulls the foot back toward the body.

FOOT PLANTAR-FLEXION

The athlete adopts a long sitting position with the hands on the ground close to the buttocks, then pushes the foot towards the ground without raising the knees.

The Leighton Flexometer

Developed by Leighton in 1942, the Leighton flexometer incorporates two weighted dials which may be locked in position at any point in the movement range. A strap connected to the back of the instrument is used to secure the flexometer to one of the subject's body segments.

In the list of movements described below, several pieces of equipment including benches and straps are employed to help to isolate the movement of the segment under scrutiny. The subject is instructed to move the segment to a position at one extreme of the range of motion, whereupon one of the weighted dials is locked. Then the segment is moved to the other end of the movement range and the second dial is locked. Since the inner dial is calibrated from 0 to 360° in both directions, extreme care must be taken to read the test score from the correct scale.

The following list of tests is not meant to be exhaustive, but includes those which are currently used by sport scientists to accurately assess athletes from many sports. Although the right limb is being tested in these examples, the dominant limb or both limbs may equally be chosen. For each test, two trials should be given and the greater score recorded to the nearest 1.0°.

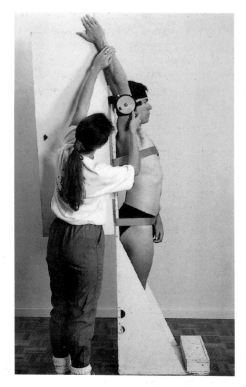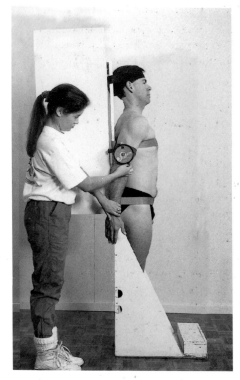

Fig. 14.36 Arm (a) flexion – (b) extension flexibility assessment.

ARM FLEXION AND EXTENSION

- The subject stands in the frame with arms inwardly rotated
- Ensure that the arm being tested hangs clear of the frame
- Place three straps around the body and frame at the forehead, chest and pelvic levels
- Strap the flexometer onto the lateral aspect of the arm, midway between the shoulder and the elbow
- Unlock both dials and, with a gentle guiding action, have the subject fully flex the arm so that it remains in the sagittal plane. Lock one of the dials at the end of this range (Fig. 14.36a)
- Guide the subject's arm down and back to a position of maximum extension in the sagittal plane. Lock the second dial (Fig. 14.36b)

ARM ABDUCTION

- The subject stands erect with the left shoulder touching a vertical wall and, to further prevent lateral trunk flexion, places the left hand (clenched) between the wall and the left thigh (Fig. 14.37)
- The flexometer is strapped to the posterior aspect of the right arm, midway between the shoulder and the elbow
- Unlock both dials
- Lock one dial and, with a gentle guiding action to keep the arm in the coronal plane, have the subject abduct the arm fully
- Lock the second dial

ARM LATERAL–MEDIAL ROTATION

- The subject stands in the frame so that the right arm hangs clearly to one side

345

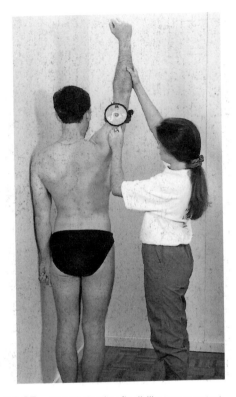

Fig. 14.37 Arm abduction flexibility assessment.

- Place three straps around the body and frame at the forehead, chest and pelvic levels
- Strap the flexometer to the posterior surface of the forearm, midway between the elbow and wrist
- Have the subject abduct the arm to 90° and flex the forearm to 90°
- Unlock both dials
- With gentle guidance, have the subject laterally (externally) rotate the arm (Fig. 14.38a). Lock one of the dials
- The subject then rotates the arm medially (internally). Lock the second dial (Fig. 14.38b)

FOREARM FLEXION AND EXTENSION

- The subject stands erect while the flexometer is strapped to the lateral aspect of the forearm, midway between the elbow and wrist
- Unlock both dials

- Instruct the subject to fully flex the forearm (Fig. 14.39a). Lock one of the dials
- The subject then fully extends the forearm and the second dial is locked (Fig. 14.39b)
- Ensure that the arm and trunk are vertically aligned at all times

THIGH FLEXION

- The subject lies in a supine position on a bench
- Place straps around the body and bench at the level of the chest and the knee of the limb not being tested (Fig. 14.40)
- Strap the flexometer to the lateral aspect of the thigh, midway between the hip and knee. Unlock both dials
- With the lower limb in a horizontal position, lock one of the dials
- Have the subject flex the thigh maximally, keeping the leg extended and then lock the second dial

THIGH EXTENSION

- The subject lies in a prone position on a bench
- Place straps around the body and bench at the level of the abdomen and the knee of the limb not being tested
- Strap the flexometer to the lateral aspect of the thigh, midway between the hip and knee. Unlock both dials
- With the lower limb in a horizontal position, lock one of the dials
- Keeping the leg extended, have the subject extend the thigh maximally (Fig. 14.41), then lock the second dial

THIGH ABDUCTION

- The subject stands erect with feet together and holds a rail located in front for stability
- Strap the flexometer to the posterior aspect of the thigh, midway between the hip and knee. Unlock both dials
- With the lower limb vertically aligned, lock one of the dials
- Have the subject abduct the thigh maximally in the coronal plane, keeping the leg extended (Fig. 14.42). Lock the second dial

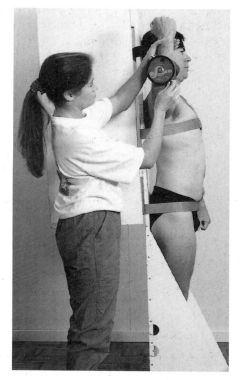
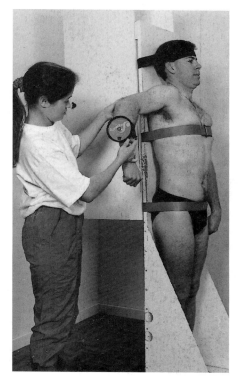

Fig. 14.38 Arm (a) lateral – (b) medial rotation flexibility assessment.

THIGH LATERAL–MEDIAL ROTATION

- The subject lies on a bench in a supine position with the feet vertically aligned and overhanging the end of the bench
- Place straps around the body and bench at the level of the chest, hips and knees
- Strap the flexometer to the plantar surface of the foot and unlock both dials
- Have the subject laterally (externally) rotate the thigh and lock one of the dials (Fig. 14.43a)
- Then the subject medially (internally) rotates the thigh and the second dial is locked (Fig. 14.43b)

LEG FLEXION

- The subject lies in a prone position on a bench
- Place straps around the body and bench at the mid-thigh level and the level of the abdomen

- Strap the flexometer to the lateral aspect of the leg, midway between the knee and ankle. Unlock both dials
- Lock one of the dials with the leg extended to a horizontal position
- The subject then maximally flexes the leg and the second dial is locked (Fig. 14.44)

FOOT DORSI–PLANTAR FLEXION

- The subject lies in a supine position on a bench with straps around the knees and hips. The ankle is suspended over the edge of the bench
- Strap the flexometer to the lateral border of the foot at the level of the metatarsals. Unlock both dials
- Instruct the subject to dorsi-flex the foot fully, then lock one dial (Fig. 14.45a)
- The subject then plantar-flexes the foot with-

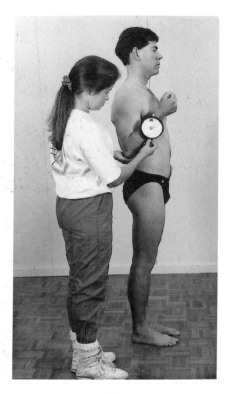
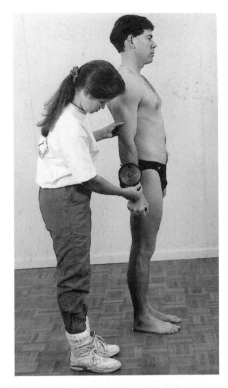

Fig. 14.39 Forearm (a) flexion – (b) extension flexibility assessment.

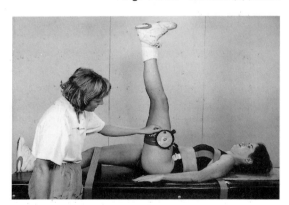

Fig. 14.40 Thigh flexion flexibility assessment.

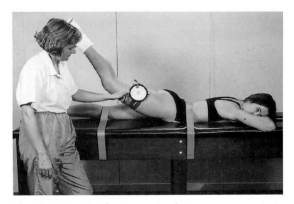

Fig. 14.41 Thigh extension flexibility assessment.

out raising the knee (Fig. 14.45b). Lock the second dial

TRUNK FLEXION

- The subject lies in a supine position on a bench with the lower limbs fully extended and fore-

arms crossed over the chest
- Place straps around the body and bench at the level of the knees and at mid-thigh
- Strap the flexometer to the side of the arm, with the strap also encircling the chest at the mesosternale level. Unlock both dials

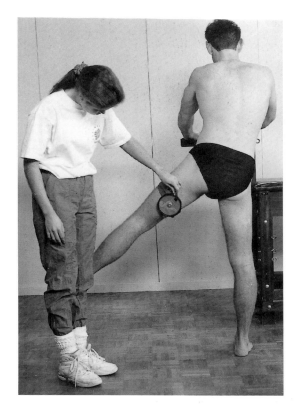

Fig. 14.42 Thigh abduction flexibility assessment.

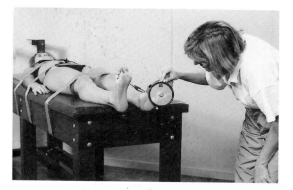

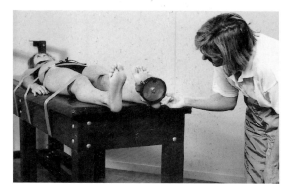

Fig. 14.43 Thigh (a) lateral – (b) medial rotation flexibility assessment.

- Lock one of the dials with the subject's trunk in a horizontal position (Fig. 14.46)
- Have the subject sit up to bring the chest as close to the knees as possible, then lock the second dial

NORMATIVE DATA

Flexibility values for athletes and non-athletes measured using a Leighton flexometer are presented in Table 14.12. A total score for combined actions is presented for some of these movements, with the data shown adjacent to the brackets in this table.

Other Devices

A number of other devices have been employed to determine the range of motion of a body segment. These include the goniometer and arthrodial protractor. Both instruments perform essentially the same function as the Leighton flexometer and, while they are not as adaptable to the variety of movements that may be assessed using the flexometer, they do represent a less expensive alternative.

ASSESSMENT OF FUNCTIONAL FLEXIBILITY

Assessment of the range of motion exhibited by an athlete during performance requires that some device be used to record the action. As the signal is subsequently replayed, measures of segmental ranges of motion can then be derived. Such devices have typically included high-speed photography or video, or a single axis electrogoniometer attached to a pen recorder. However, the time lag between performance and the provision of feed-

Table 14.12 Mean range of motion values (degrees) for male athletes and non-athletes

Movement	Non-athletes[1,2] (<19 years)	(>19 years)	Swimmers[3]	Gymnasts[4]	Field athletes[3]
Arm flexion–extension	236	222	223	224	208
Arm abduction	185	183	199	190	172
Arm lateral–medial rotation	178	167	200	192	201
Forearm flexion–extension	146	141	163	152	151
Thigh flexion	—	78	} 107	} 126	} 110
Thigh extension	7	12			
Thigh abduction	52	40	55	58	53
Thigh lateral–medial rotation	101	89	108	72	86
Leg flexion	144	141	149	145	138
Foot dorsi–plantar flexion	71	67	70	54	56
Trunk flexion	—	—	73	68	65

[1]Boone & Azen (1979). [2]Ekstrand *et al.* (1982). [3]Leighton (1957a). [4]Leighton (1957b).
[5]Ekstrand & Gillquist (1982). [6]Sigerseth & Haleski (1950). [7]Sharratt *et al.* (1986).

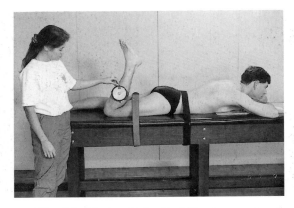

Fig. 14.44 Leg flexion flexibility assessment.

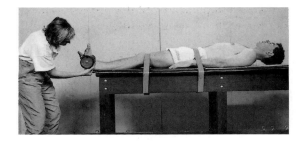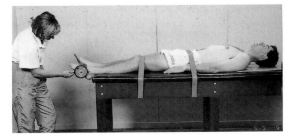

Fig. 14.45 Foot (a) dorsi – (b) plantar flexion flexibility assessment.

Table 14.12 Mean range of motion values (degrees) for male athletes and non-athletes (*cont'd*)

Movement	Soccer players[5]	American footballers[6]	Baseball players[3]	Basketball players[3]	Wrestlers[4,7]
Arm flexion–extension	—	246	221	198	207
Arm abduction	—	—	188	160	176
Arm lateral–medial rotation	—	—	195	187	183
Forearm flexion–extension	—	148	157	151	148
Thigh flexion	81	93	} 101	} 105	} 122
Thigh extension	—	—			
Thigh abduction	34	56	56	55	53
Thigh lateral–medial rotation	—	—	113	88	63
Leg flexion	137	115	143	138	149
Foot dorsi–plantar flexion	—	55	75	58	52
Trunk flexion	—	—	78	68	76

[1]Boone & Azen (1979). [2]Ekstrand *et al.* (1982). [3]Leighton (1957a). [4]Leighton (1957b). [5]Ekstrand & Gillquist (1982). [6]Sigerseth & Haleski (1950). [7]Sharratt *et al.* (1986).

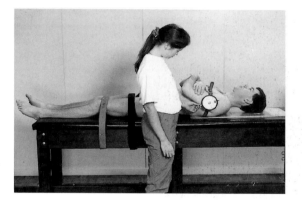

Fig. 14.46 Trunk flexion flexibility assessment.

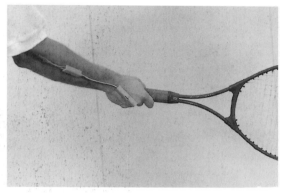

Fig. 14.47 Assessing functional flexibility of the hand with an electrogoniometer.

back using these devices is often too great for effective technique modification to be made.

Recently a series of two- and three-dimensional electrogoniometers have been developed, with the advantage that they do not severely encumber the movement pattern. Furthermore, the signal may be recorded by a data logger, or transmitted directly to a recording device. The latter option would permit a real time analysis and instantaneous feedback of the data to the coach and athlete.

The Penny and Giles electrogoniometer shown in Fig. 14.47 is set up to record flexion–extension and abduction–adduction movements of the hand during the performance of a backhand ground stroke in tennis.

SPEED, AGILITY AND BALANCE

Tests for speed, agility and balance require that the subject be dressed appropriately for maximal performance. That is, lightweight clothing and training shoes should be worn for all general tests of speed and agility, whereas the normal playing attire should be worn for the specific sport tests.

Ideally, the tests should be administered prior to any vigorous training sessions so that they are not limited by fatigue or soreness. In addition, it is preferable that the subjects do not ingest food within a 2 hour period preceding the tests. A thorough warm-up involving aerobic activity and muscle stretching exercises plus other activities related to the specific tests must be completed prior to their administration to prevent injury and permit the recording of a maximal effort.

GENERAL TESTS OF SPEED

40 Metre Dash

ADMINISTRATION

A 40 m track is marked with cones on a suitable, level surface (Fig. 14.48). The track should be set up cross-wind to negate any environmental influence on the obtained scores. The subject stands behind the starting line and on the signal to start (a verbal command — 'go', as well as a visual action such as a sudden drop of the hand), sprints past the 40 m mark. Two recorders with stopwatches are positioned at the 40 m mark and begin timing on the starter's signal. The watches are stopped as the runner's trunk passes the 40 m mark and an average time for the two recorders is noted. Two trials are permitted and the lower mean score is recorded to the nearest 0.1 s. For greater accuracy and measurement precision, photoelectric cell timing gates can be employed in the administration of this test and this obviates the need for stopwatches.

40 Yard Dash (36.6 m Dash)

ADMINISTRATION

The 40 yard dash is set up and administered in a similar fashion to the 40 m dash. Extensive normative data have been collected, particularly for American football players, although rarely published in scientific literature. Subjects may either begin from a standing start or with a 'flying start', although the former is normally used. Under the latter protocol, the subject begins to sprint from a position 15 yards behind the starting line and the time is recorded from the starting to finishing lines (40 yards). The use of timing gates is almost essential in the scoring of this test, but stopwatches may be used if resources are limited.

SPECIFIC TESTS OF SPEED

A number of specific speed tests have been developed for certain sports which better reflect the

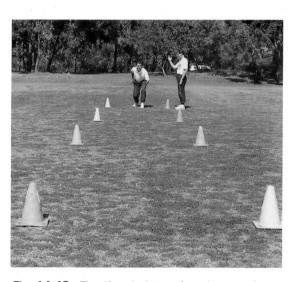

Fig. 14.48   The 40 m dash test of running speed.

particular requirements of those sports compared to the previously mentioned tests. The following examples of specific speed tests provide both administrative details and normative data.

Baseball Speed Test

ADMINISTRATION

This is a three-stage test of speed performed on a regulation baseball diamond. Each player attempts three sprints and the combined score is recorded to the nearest 0.1 s (Fig. 14.49).

- Each player begins at the batting box with a bat and in batting stance
- A ball is pitched and the player bunts
- When contact is made a timekeeper begins the watch and the player sprints through first base. The elapsed time is recorded from bunt to the touch at first base (T1)
- The player then jogs back to first base and takes up a 'sidestep' position with the left foot in contact with the base
- On the command 'go' the player runs from first base, touches second base and runs through third base. The elapsed time from first to third base is recorded (T2)
- The player jogs to home plate and prepares for the final sprint
- On the command 'go' the player runs from home plate around all bases (touching each) and this time is also recorded (T3)
- Sum T1, T2 and T3 to obtain a composite score

Normative Data

Comparative data for junior and senior players were reported by Draper et al. (1991) and are presented in Table 14.13.

20 Metre Dash for Tennis Players

The purpose of the 20 m dash for tennis players is to determine a player's ability to accelerate from a stationary position and move quickly over 20 m. The administration of this test is identical to that

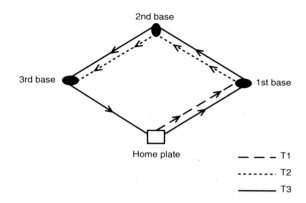

Fig. 14.49 Sport-specific speed test — baseball.

Table 14.13 Normative data for Australian junior (<18 years) and senior baseball players on the baseball speed test

	Junior		Senior	
Component	$\overline{x}$	Range (s)	$\overline{x}$	Range (s)
Home to first (T1)	4.50	3.87–4.92	4.37	3.72–4.75
First to third (T2)	8.46	7.69–8.84	8.23	7.37–9.46
Home to home (T3)	18.85	17.09–20.05	17.63	16.47–19.75
Total	31.81	28.65–33.81	30.23	27.56–33.96

for the 40 m dash with the obvious exception of the length of the course. According to Groppel et al. (1989), average scores for male and female professional players are 3.16 and 3.58 s, respectively.

All Direction Line Sprint

The all direction line sprint is specifically for tennis players but may be easily modified for other court sports. As the time for completion is 50–60 s, this test relies heavily on anaerobic glycolysis, rather than the creatine phosphate energy system which is used almost exclusively for the 40 m, 40 yard and 20 m tests.

ADMINISTRATION

The subject begins at the intersection of the centre and base lines (S) and on the command 'go' performs the following tasks, always in the same order:

- Sprint to the intersection of the centre and service lines (Fig. 14.50), sidestep to the right singles sideline, sidestep to the left singles sideline, sidestep back to the centre line, then back-pedal to S
- Sprint to the intersection of the service line and the right singles sideline, back-pedal to S, then sidestep across the baseline to the right singles sideline and back to S
- Repeat the previous series of runs, but to the left side of the court
- Sprint to the intersection of the net and the right doubles sideline, back-pedal to S, then sidestep across the baseline to the right doubles sideline and back to S
- Repeat the previous series of runs, but to the left side of the court
- Finish with a sprint from S to the net along the centre line

NORMATIVE DATA

According to Groppel *et al.* (1989) the average scores obtained from 30 touring professional players were 53.37 s for men and 60.90 s for women.

GENERAL TESTS OF AGILITY

As described in Chapter 12, the term agility refers to an ability to move and rapidly change direction or body position. Several general agility tests have been evaluated and reported in the literature (Draper & Lancaster 1985), but almost all lack standardization of protocols, established validity, or published normative data for various populations. However the Illinois agility run described below, has been used extensively in the physical education field and normative data are available.

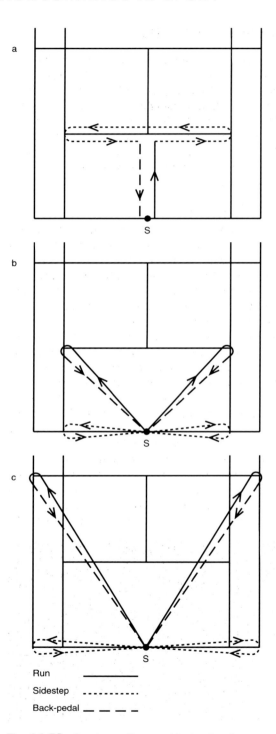

Run _____
Sidestep ....
Back-pedal _ _ _ _ _

Fig. 14.50 Sport-specific speed test — tennis.

The Illinois Agility Run

This test is a modified version of that described by Getchell (1985). A non-slip ground or floor surface at least 15 m long and 6.5 m wide is required for this test. A rectangle measuring 9.14 m by 3.65 m must be clearly marked and divided in half along its length by four cones positioned at equidistant intervals. The centres of the first and fourth cones must be positioned directly over the mid-point of the 3.65 m sides (Fig. 14.51).

ADMINISTRATION

The subject starts in a front lying position with the vertex of the head on the starting line, forearms flexed at the elbows and hands just outside the shoulders. Two recorders with stopwatches are positioned at the start–finish line. On the command 'go' they start their watches and the subject rises from the lying position, runs as quickly as possible to the end line, stops as one foot touches or crosses it, then turns and sprints back to the starting mark. After turning again, the subject then weaves in and out around the centre cones toward the end line and back to the starting line. At this point the subject again sprints to the end line, turns as one foot touches or crosses it and sprints back through the finishing line.

The watches are stopped as the subject's trunk crosses the finishing line, both times are averaged and the resulting score, to the nearest 0.1 s, is noted. Each subject should be permitted one practice run at a slow pace, then two trials, with the

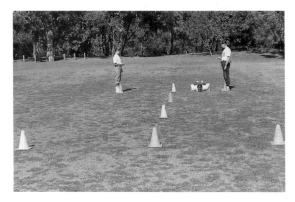

Fig. 14.51 The Illinois agility run.

lower elapsed time of these trials eventually recorded. It should be noted that grounds for disqualification of a trial score are:

- Straying outside the side boundaries of the rectangle
- Any failure to touch or cross a line at either end of the rectangle
- Touching a cone, even if accidentally
- Failure to follow the prescribed course

NORMATIVE DATA

The comparative data for men and women displayed in Table 14.14 are adapted from that reported by Getchell (1985).

Table 14.14 Comparative norms for the Illinois agility run with respect to ratings of excellent (1) to poor (7)

Category	Men (s)	Women (s)
1	<16.1	<17.1
2	16.7	19.0
3	17.3	20.4
4	17.9	21.7
5	18.5	23.1
6	19.1	24.4
7	>19.3	>24.9

SPECIFIC TESTS OF AGILITY

Basketball Zigzag Agility Drill

ADMINISTRATION

- Marking cones (30 cm high) are placed at the four corners of the basketball key as shown in Fig. 14.52
- Two recorders with stopwatches are required to measure the elapsed time
- The player begins at cone 1 with the hand in contact with the cone and feet behind the baseline
- On a whistle or 'go' command the player sprints to cones 2, 3 and 4, then back to cone 1
- Each cone must be touched during the circuit
- The average elapsed time from 'go' until the subject returns to touch cone 1 is noted and the better of two trials recorded

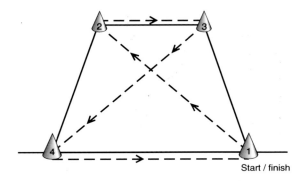

Start / finish

Fig. 14.52 Sport-specific agility test — basketball (zigzag drill).

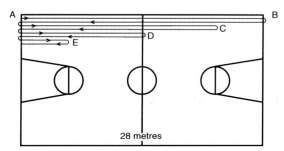

28 metres

Fig. 14.53 Sport-specific agility test — basketball (ladder drill).

NORMATIVE DATA

Comparative data for Australian age-group and senior players were reported by Draper *et al.* (1991) and are presented in Table 14.15.

Ladder Drill/Suicides

ADMINISTRATION

- Check that the length of the court from base-line to baseline is 28 m (Fig. 14.53)
- Two recorders with stopwatches are required
- The player begins at position A using a stand-ing start posture with the leading foot behind the baseline

- On the command 'go' the player runs to, and touches the opposite baseline B with one foot, turns and runs back to the starting line
- Immediately, the player turns and runs to C and back to A, then D and back to A, then E and back to A
- As the player's foot crosses baseline A for the last time, the elapsed time is read to the nearest 0.1 s
- The average time is noted
- After exactly 2 min rest the player is permitted a second attempt and the better score recorded
- It should be noted that this is also a test of anaerobic capacity, resistance to fatigue and running speed, rather than merely one of agil-ity

Table 14.15 Normative data for Australian age-group and senior basketball players on the zigzag agility run

Team	Mean (s)	Range (s)
Female		
National senior team	6.6	5.9–7.5
National junior team	6.8	6.2–7.8
17 years	6.9	6.1–7.7
16 years	7.1	6.3–7.9
15 years	7.1	6.7–7.7
14 years	7.3	6.4–7.8
Male		
17 years	6.4	5.8–7.0
16 years	6.4	5.9–7.2
15 years	6.5	6.0–7.3
14 years	6.7	6.1–7.4

Table 14.16 Normative data for Australian age-group and senior basketball players on the ladder drill

Team	Mean (s)	Range (s)
Female		
National senior team	30.1	28.6–33.1
National junior team	30.8	29.3–34.5
17 years	32.0	29.2–36.4
16 years	31.7	28.7–35.7
15 years	31.6	29.3–33.5
14 years	32.6	30.6–34.1
Male		
17 years	28.1	26.7–29.5
16 years	28.2	26.7–30.1
15 years	28.5	27.5–29.5
14 years	29.0	28.5–29.4

NORMATIVE DATA

Comparative data for Australian age-group and senior players were reported by Draper *et al.* (1991) and are presented in Table 14.16.

Baseball and Softball Agility Test

ADMINISTRATION

- A course is prepared on a level grass field as shown in Fig. 14.54, with a catcher located within a circle of 1.5 m diameter, and a baseball or softball placed on the ground at the indicated position
- Two recorders with stopwatches are required
- On the command 'go' the player sprints around cones A and B to the ball
- On reaching the ball, the player picks it up and throws to the catcher
- A score is only recorded if the ball reaches the mitt without the catcher having to leave the circle
- The average elapsed time from 'go' until the ball reaches the catcher's mitt is noted
- The lower score of two trials is recorded
- It should be noted that test scores are also influenced by throwing ability

NORMATIVE DATA

Normative data were reported by Draper *et al.* (1991) for Australian junior (under 18 years) and senior baseball players. The mean and range of scores for the junior players were 6.53 and 5.50–7.23 s, respectively, while for senior players they were 6.13 and 5.75–6.55 s, respectively.

Modified SEMO Agility Test

The modified SEMO agility test was designed for tennis players to determine their agility on court. A smooth surface with a 20 × 20 foot area (6.1 × 6.1 m) is required for this test, as well as space to run around the perimeter of this square. Four cones, A, B, C and D, are placed in each corner of the area.

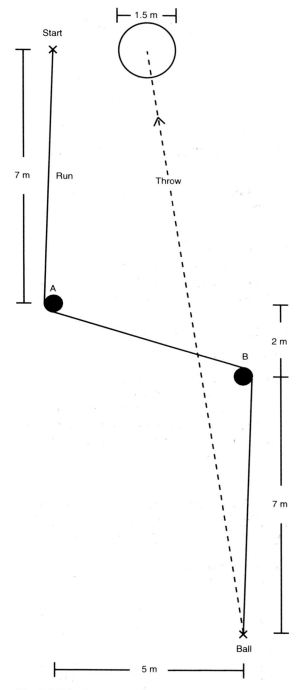

Fig. 14.54 Sport-specific agility test — softball and baseball.

ADMINISTRATION

- The subject begins facing cone A with his or her back to the course (Fig. 14.55)
- On the command 'go', the subject sidesteps from A to B, passing outside B
- From there the subject back-pedals to and around D, then sprints forward to and around A
- The subject back-pedals from A to C, then sprints forward to B
- From B, the subject sidesteps to the finish line at A
- One practice circuit should be permitted and

the better score from two trials recorded. A recovery time of 2 min should be enforced between trials

NORMATIVE DATA

Average scores for male and female players are 12.8 and 14.2 s respectively, according to Groppel *et al.* (1989).

The Quinn Test

The Quinn test is designed to measure dynamic balance and response time of tennis players, as

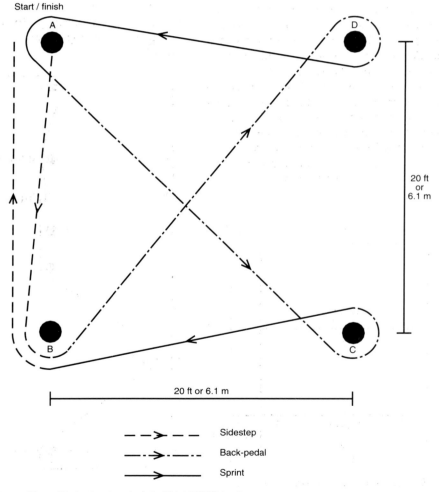

Fig. 14.55 Sport-specific agility test — tennis (modified SEMO test).

well as their agility. It should be administered on half a tennis court as shown in Fig. 14.56.

ADMINISTRATION

The subject begins standing at the intersection of the service line and centre line without a racquet. While holding a tennis ball, the tester takes up a position on the centre line, approximately 2 m behind the net. On the command 'go', the tester will point to one of the eight positions on court using the ball and begin the stopwatch. The subject then sprints to that position, touches the spot with one foot, then sprints back to the start position.

Immediately, the tester points to another position selected at random, whereupon the subject must run to touch the spot and return to the start position. This continues until all eight positions have been visited and the subject returns to the start position for the final time. The elapsed times for two trials are noted and the better score recorded. It is important to stress that the subject must watch the tennis ball which is held by the tester at all times. This requirement is designed to help simulate the game situation. A 3 min recovery time should be interposed between trials.

NORMATIVE DATA

Average scores for male and female players on the Quinn test are 29.4 and 34.5, respectively, according to Groppel et al. (1989).

The Rugby Agility Run

The rugby agility run is designed to measure the ability of a player to accelerate and change direction (A. R. Morton, pers. comm. 1993).

ADMINISTRATION

The course is set out in Fig. 14.57. Cones are used to mark positions A to G and the finishing line. Tall markers, which are constructed of plastic tubing and are approximately 1500 × 30 × 30 mm in size to simulate opponents, are located at positions H to L.

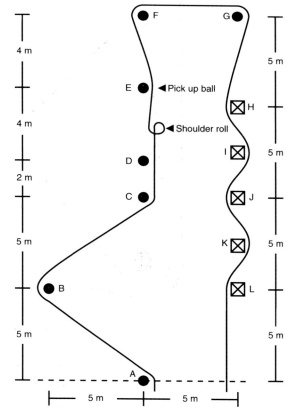

Fig. 14.57 Sport-specific agility test — rugby.

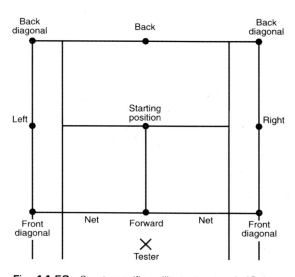

Fig. 14.56 Sport-specific agility test — tennis (Quinn test).

The tester should stand at the finishing line to ensure the most accurate timing. Subjects begin by lying on their backs with the head on the starting line at cone A. On the command to 'go', the subject gets up and sprints around cone B, cuts back to cone C and performs a shoulder roll at cone D. Quickly accelerating from the roll to cone E, the subject then picks up a ball, passes around cones F and G and accelerates toward the tall markers. The subject weaves around the tall markers H to L and then sprints to the finishing line to score a try. Two trials are permitted and the lower time recorded to the nearest 0.1 s.

NORMATIVE DATA

The data in Table 14.17 were collected by A. Morton, G. Treble and B. Hopley and are unpublished (University of Western Australia), but represent a compilation of scores from Western Australian rugby union state representatives as well as selected players from the Sydney (New South Wales) first grade clubs. These results are reported for players in various positions and the differences in mean scores reflect their respective roles. The *tight five* group (group A) includes the props, hooker and second rowers, while Group B contains the lock and breakaways. Group C is composed of scrum half and fly half, whereas those in Group D include the centres, the wingers and the fullback.

TESTS OF STATIC BALANCE

A number of static balance tests have been used in the field of human movement development to assess the maturity of the neuromuscular system of children. These tests cannot be applied with any great effect to adolescent or adult athletes because they do not tax the mature neuromuscular system.

More sophisticated tests and test apparatus are required to assess the athlete's ability to maintain balance in a static situation. This ability is vitally important for many performers in sports such as archery, pistol and rifle shooting, golf and diving. Static balance may be analysed using a combination of high-speed video or film to detect postural adjustments, and centre of pressure movements recorded on a force platform. Movements of the body are detected as a change in the centre of pressure within the base of support (Fig. 2.12). Postural adjustments made by the subject to counter these movements of the centre of pressure may be gross or subtle, hence the need for a visual record of the test.

TEST OF DYNAMIC BALANCE

Dynamic balance refers to the ability to execute movements and maintain balance while in motion. A successful test of this capacity needs to assess the ability of the neuromuscular system to assimilate information from visual, auditory, vestibular and kinaesthetic receptors and to coordinate a series of motor responses. At a subjective level of analysis, this may be done by recording movement and analysing the performance of athletes under competitive conditions.

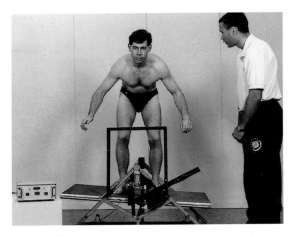

Fig. 14.58 Assessing dynamic balance using the stabilometer.

Table 14.17 Normative data for rugby players on the rugby agility run

Group	Mean agility run time (s)
A	15.78
B	14.41
C	14.50
D	14.68

A more objective assessment of this capacity requires the use of a less specific task, such as with the dynamic balance platform or stabilometer shown in Fig. 14.58. A potentiometer, located at the axis of rotation of the platform, records deviations from the horizontal position. These deviations may be recorded on a pen recorder or input into a computer for post-analysis.

The test is usually conducted over a period of 15–30 s with subjects adopting either a 'jockey' position with the feet parallel, shoulder width apart and in a single transverse plane, or a 'surfing position' with one foot forward with respect to the other. The total area under the displacement time curve, together with the proportional deviations to the left and right, are generally used to score this test.

CONCLUSION

The tests outlined in this section provide a valid and reliable means of assessing human physical capacity. Consequently the results may then be used to construct a profile for an individual athlete or normative data for an athletic population as discussed in Section 2. When employing these tests it is imperative that particular care be exercised to follow the exact protocols. This will ensure that results are derived with precision and accuracy and that meaningful athlete comparisons can be made.

REFERENCES

Adams R., Daniel A. & Rullman L. (1975) *Games, Sports and Exercises for the Physically Handicapped*, pp. 101–116. Lea & Febiger, Philadelphia.

Ackland T. & Bloomfield J. (1992) Functional anatomy. In Bloomfield J., Fricker P. & Fitch K. (eds) *Textbook of Science and Medicine in Sport*, pp. 2–28. Blackwell Scientific Publications, Melbourne.

Anderson T. & Kearney J. (1982) Effects of three resistance training programs on muscular strength and absolute and relative endurance. *The Research Quarterly for Exercise and Sport* **53**, 1–7.

Atha J. (1981) Strengthening muscle. In Miller D. (ed.) *Exercise and Sport Science Reviews*, Vol. 9, pp. 1–73. Franklin Institute Press, Philadelphia.

Bailey D., Martin A., Houston C. & Howie J. (1986) Physical activity, nutrition, bone density and osteoporosis. *Australian Journal of Science and Medicine in Sport* **18**, 3–8.

Behnke A., Feen B. & Welham W. (1942) The specific gravity of healthy men. *Journal of the American Medical Association* **118**, 495–498.

Behnke A., Guttentag O. & Brodsky C. (1959) Quantification of body weight and configuration from anthropometric measurements. *Human Biology* **31**, 213–234.

Behnke A. & Wilmore J. (1974) *Evaluation and Regulation of Body Build and Composition*, pp. 75–81. Prentice-Hall, Englewood Cliffs, NJ, USA.

Bemben M., Massey B., Boileau R. & Misner J. (1992) Reliability of isometric force–time curve parameters for men aged 20 to 79 years. *Journal of Applied Sport Science Research* **6**, 158–164.

Bloomfield J., Fricker P. & Fitch K. (eds) (1992) *Textbook of Science and Medicine in Sport*, p. 5. Blackwell Scientific Publications, Melbourne.

Boone D. & Azen S. (1979) Normal range of motion of joints in male subjects. *Journal of Bone and Joint Surgery* **61**, 756–759.

Bray G., Greenway F., Molitch M., Dahms W., Atkinson R. & Hamilton K. (1978) Use of anthropometric measures to assess weight loss. *American Journal of Clinical Nutrition* **31** 769–773.

Burkinshaw L., Jones P. & Krupowicz D. (1973) Observer error in skinfold thickness measurement. *Human Biology* **45**, 273–279.

Buskirk E. (1961) Underwater weighing and body density: a review of procedures. In Brozek J. & Henschel A. (eds) *Techniques for Measuring Body Composition*. National Academy of Sciences National Research Council, Washington.

Carter J. & Heath B. (1990) *Somatotyping — Development and Applications*, pp. 352–397. Cambridge University Press, Cambridge.

Carter J. & Ackland T. (1994) *Kinanthropometry in Aquatic Sports*. Human Kinetics Publishers, Champaign, IL, USA.

Carter J. & Marfell-Jones M. (1994) Somatotypes. In Carter J. & Ackland T. (eds) *Kinanthropometry in Aquatic Sports*: Human Kinetics Publishers, Champaign, IL, USA.

Chaffin D. & Andersson G. (1984) *Occupational Biomechanics*, pp. 147–232. John Wiley and Sons, New York.

Clarke H. & Clarke D. (1963) *Developmental and Adapted Physical Education*, pp. 79–96. Prentice-Hall, Englewood Cliffs, NJ, USA.

Clarys J., Martin A. & Drinkwater D. (1984) Gross tissue weights in the human body by cadaver dissection. *Human Biology* **56**, 459–473.

Dietz W. (1987) Childhood obesity. *Annals of the New York Academy of Sciences*. **499**, 47–54.

Donnelly J. & Sintek S. (1986) Hydrostatic weighing without head submersion. In Day J. (ed.) *Perspectives in Kinanthropometry*, pp. 251–256. Human Kinetics Publishers, Champaign, IL, USA.

Draper J. & Lancaster M. (1985) The 505 test: A test for agility in the horizontal plane. *The Australian Journal of Science and Medicine in Sport* **17**, 15–18.

Draper J., Minikin B. & Telford R. (1991) *Test Methods Manual*. Section 3. Australian Sports Commission, Canberra, Australia.

Drinkwater D. (1984) An anatomically derived method for the anthropometric estimation of body composition. PhD thesis. Simon Fraser University, Burnaby, BC, Canada.

Drinkwater D. & Ross W. (1980) The anthropometric fractionation of body mass. In Ostyn M., Beunen G. & Simons J. (eds) *Kinanthropometry II*. University Park Press, Baltimore.

Drinkwater D., Bach T., Ackland T. & Kerr D. (1994) Data management and reports. In Carter J. & Ackland T. (eds) *Kinanthropometry in Aquatic Sports*. Human Kinetics Publishers, Champaign, IL, USA.

Ekstrand J. & Gillquist J. (1982) The frequency of muscle tightness and injuries in soccer players. *American Journal of Sports Medicine* **10**, 75–78.

Ekstrand J., Wiktorsson M., Oberg B. & Gillquist J. (1982) Lower extremity goniometric measurements: A study to determine their reliability. *Archives of Physical Medicine and Rehabilitation* **63**, 171–175.

Fry A. & Kraemer W. (1991) Physical performance characteristics of American football players. *Journal of Applied Sport Science Research* **5**, 126–138.

Fry A., Kraemer W., Weseman C. *et al.* (1991) Effects of an off-season strength and conditioning program on starters and non-starters in women's collegiate volleyball. *Journal of Applied Sport Science Research* **5**, 174–181.

Garrett J. & Kennedy W. (1971) *A Collation of Anthropometry*, Vols 1–2. National Technical Information Services, Springfield, VA, USA.

Getchell B. (1985) *Physical Fitness: A Way of Life*, 3rd edn. Macmillan Publishing Co., New York.

Gillespie J. & Gabbard C. (1984) A test of three theories of strength and muscular endurance development. *Journal of Human Movement Studies* **10**, 213–223.

Gillespie J. & Keenum S. (1987) A validity and reliability analysis of the seated shot put as a test of power. *Journal of Human Movement Studies* **13**, 97–105.

Gordon C., Chumlea W. & Roche A. (1988) Stature, recumbent length and weight. In Lohman T., Roche A. & Martorell R. (eds) *Anthropometric Standardization Reference Manual*, pp. 3–8. Human Kinetics Publishers, Champaign, IL, USA.

Groppel J., Loehr J., Melville D. & Quinn A. (1989) *Science of Coaching Tennis*, pp. 10–75. Leisure Press, Champaign, IL, USA.

Guo S., Roche A., Chumlea W., Miles D. & Pohlman R. (1987) Body composition predictions from bioelectrical impedance. *Human Biology* **59**, 221–233.

Hakkinen K., Komi P., Alen M. & Kauhanan H. (1987) EMG, muscle fibre and force production characteristics during a one year training period in elite weightlifters. *European Journal of Applied Physiology* **56**, 419–427.

Hakkinen K., Pakarinen H., Alen M., Kauhanen H. & Komi P. (1988) Neuromuscular and hormonal adaptations in athletes to strength training in two years. *Journal of Applied Physiology* **65**, 2406–2412.

Harrison G. (1987) The measurement of total body electrical conductivity. *Human Biology* **59**, 311–317.

Hoeger W., Hopkins D., Barette S. & Hale D. (1990) Relationship between repetitions and selected percentages of one repetition maximum: A comparison between untrained and trained males and females. *Journal of Applied Sport Science Research* **4**, 47–54.

Houtkooper L. (1986) Validity of whole body impedance analysis for body composition assessment in non obese and obese children and youth. PhD thesis. The University of Arizona, Tucson (unpubl.).

Houtkooper L., Lohman T., Going S. & Hall M. (1989) Validity of bioelectrical impedance for body composition assessment in children. *Journal of Applied Physiology* **66**, 814–821.

Hurley J., Hagberg J. & Holloszy B. (1988) Muscle weakness among elite powerlifters. *Medicine and Science in Sport and Exercise* Suppl. **20**, S81.

Hutcheson L., Latin R., Berg K. & Prentice E. (1988) Body impedance analysis and body water loss. *The Research Quarterly for Exercise and Sport* **59**, 359–362.

Jensen D. (1976) *The Principles of Physiology*, pp. 83–88. Prentice-Hall, Englewood Cliffs, NJ, USA.

Johnson J. & Siegel D. (1978) Reliability of an isokinetic movement of the knee extensors. *Research Quarterly* **49**, 88–90.

Katch F. & Katch V. (1983) Computer technology to evaluate body composition, nutrition and exercise. *Preventative Medicine* **12**, 619–631.

Kerr D. (1988) An anthropometric method for fractionation of skin, adipose, bone, muscle and residual tissue masses in males and females age 6 to 77 years. MSc thesis. Simon Fraser University, Burnaby, BC, Canada (unpubl.).

Leighton J. (1942) A simple, objective and reliable measure of flexibility. *Research Quarterly* **13**, 204–216.

Leighton J. (1957a) Flexibility characteristics of three specialized skill groups of champion athletes. *Archives of Physical Medicine and Rehabilitation* **38**, 24–28.

Leighton J. (1957b) Flexibility characteristics of three specialized skill groups of champion athletes. *Archives of Physical Medicine and Rehabilitation* **38**, 580–583.

Lukasaki H. (1988) Methods for the assessment of human body composition: Traditional and new. *American Journal of Clinical Nutrition* **47**, 7–11.

Malina R. (1987) Bioelectrical methods for estimating body composition: An overview and discussion. *Human Biology* **59**, 329–335.

Martin A. (1984) An anatomical basis for assessing human body composition: Evidence from 25 cadavers. PhD thesis. Simon Fraser University, Burnaby, BC, Canada (unpubl.).

Martin A., Ross W., Drinkwater D. & Clarys J. (1984) Prediction of body fat by skinfold callipers: assumptions and cadaver evidence. *International Journal of Obesity* **7**, 17–25.

Martin A., Drinkwater D., Clarys J. & Ross W. (1986) The inconsistency of the fat free mass: A reappraisal with implications for densitometry. In Reilly T., Watson J. & Barnes J. (eds) *Kinanthropometry III*, pp. 92–97. Spon, London.

Matiegka J. (1921) The testing of physical efficiency. *American Journal of Physical Anthropology* **4**, 223–330.

Matthews D. & Fox E. (1976) *The Physiological Basis of Physical Education and Athletics*, p. 500. W. B.

Saunders Co., Philadelphia.

Mayhew J., Piper F., Schwegler T. & Ball T. (1989) Contributions of speed, agility and body composition to anaerobic power measurement in college football players. *Journal of Applied Sport Science Research* **3**, 101–106.

Mero A., Luhtanen P., Viitasalo J. & Komi P. (1981) Relationship between the maximal running velocity, muscle fiber characteristics, force production and force relaxation of sprinters. *Scandinavian Journal of Sport Science* **3**, 16–22.

Osternig L. (1986) Isokinetic dynamometry: Implications for muscle testing and rehabilitation. *Exercise and Sport Sciences Reviews* **14**, 45–80.

Osternig L., Sawhill J., Bates B. & Hamill J. (1982) A method for rapid collection and processing of isokinetic data. *The Research Quarterly for Exercise and Sport* **53**, 252–256.

Perrine J. & Edgerton V. (1975) Isokinetic anaerobic ergometry. *Medicine and Science in Sports* **7**, 78.

Puhl J., Case S., Fleck S. & van Handel P. (1982) Physical and physiological characteristics of elite volleyball players. *Research Quarterly for Exercise and Sport* **53**, 257–262.

Rohrs D., Mayhew J., Arabas C. & Shelton M. (1990) The relationship between seven anaerobic tests and swim performance. *Journal of Swimming Research* **6**, 15–19.

Ross W. & Wilson N. (1974) A stratagem for proportional growth assessment. *Acta Paediatrica Belgica* Suppl. **28**, 169–182.

Ross W., Eiben O., Ward R., Martin A., Drinkwater D. & Clarys J. (1986) Alternatives for the conventional methods of human body composition and physique assessment. In Day, J. (ed.) *Perspectives in Kinanthropometry.* pp. 203–219. Human Kinetics Publishers, Champaign, IL, USA.

Ross W., Leahy R., Mazza J. & Drinkwater D. (1994) Relative body size. In Carter J. & Ackland T. (eds) *Kinanthropometry in Aquatic Sports.* Human Kinetics Publishers, Champaign, IL, USA.

Ross W. & Marfell-Jones M. (1991) Kinanthropometry. In MacDougal J., Wenger H. & Green H. (eds) *Physiological Testing of the High Performance Athlete,* 2nd edn, pp. 255–258. Human Kinetics Publishers, Champaign, IL, USA.

Rutherford O., Greig C., Sargent A. & Jones D. (1986) Strength training and power output: Transference effects in the human quadriceps muscle. *Journal of Sport Sciences* **4**, 101–107.

Sale D. (1991) Testing strength and power. In MacDougall J., Wenger H. & Green H. (eds) *Physiological Testing of the High Performance Athlete,* 2nd edn, pp. 21–106. Human Kinetics Publishers, Champaign, IL, USA.

Sargent D. (1921) The physical test of a man. *American Physical Education Review* **26**, 188–194.

Secher N. (1975) Isometric rowing strength of experienced and inexperienced oarsmen. *Medicine and Science in Sports* **7**, 280–283.

Segal K., Gutin B., Presta E., Wang J. & Van Itallie T. (1985) Estimation of human body composition by electrical impedance methods: A comparative study. *Journal of Applied Physiology* **58**, 1565–1571.

Segal K., Van Loan M. & Fitzgerald P. (1988) Lean body mass estimation by bioelectrical impedance analysis: A four-site cross-validation study. *American Journal of Clinical Nutrition* **47**, 7–11.

Sharratt M., Taylor A. & Song T. (1986) A physiological profile of elite Canadian freestyle wrestlers. *Canadian Journal of Applied Sport Sciences* **11**, 100–105.

Sharp R., Troup J. & Costill D. (1982) Relationship between power and sprint freestyle swimming. *Medicine and Science in Sports and Exercise* **14**, 53–56.

Sigerseth P. & Haleski C. (1950) The flexibility of football players. *Research Quarterly* **21**, 394–398.

Taylor N., Cotter J., Stanley S. & Marshall R. (1991) Functional torque-velocity and power-velocity characteristics of elite athletes. *European Journal of Applied Physiology* **62**, 116–121.

Viitasalo J. (1985a) Effects of training on force–velocity characteristics. In Winter D., Norman R., Wells R., Hayes K. & Palta A. (eds) *Biomechanics IX-A,* pp. 91–95. Human Kinetics Publishers, Champaign, IL, USA.

Viitasalo J. (1985b) Measurement of force–velocity characteristics for sportsmen in field conditions. In Winter D., Norman R., Wells R., Hayes K. & Palta A. (eds) *Biomechanics IX-A,* pp. 96–101. Human Kinetics Publishers, Champaign, IL, USA.

Viitasalo J., Saukkonen S. & Komi P. (1980) Reproducibility of measurements of selected neuromuscular performance variables in man. *Electromyography and Clinical Neurophysiology* **20**, 487–501.

Viitasalo J. & Aura O. (1984) Seasonal fluctuation of force production in high jumpers. *Canadian Journal of Applied Sport Science* **9**, 209–213.

Ward R., Ross W., Leyland A. & Selbie S. (1989) *The Advanced O-Scale Physique Assessment System,* pp. 6–26. Kinemetrix Ltd, Burnaby, BC, Canada.

Weltman A. & Katch V. (1981) Comparison of hydrostatic weighing at residual volume and total lung capacity. *Medicine and Science in Sports* **13**, 210–213.

Wilmore J. (1969) A simplified method for determination of residual lung volumes. *Journal of Applied Physiology* **27**, 96–100.

Wilson G., Elliott B. & Wood G. (1992) Stretch shorten cycle performance enhancement through flexibility training. *Medicine and Science in Sports and Exercise* **24**, 116–123.

Wilson G., Newton R., Murphy A. & Humphries B. (1993) The optimal training load for the development of dynamic athletic performance. *Medicine and Science in Sports and Exercise* **25**, 1279–1286.

INDEX